W0050009

Editor-in-Chief: F. Cavalli (Bellinzona)
Associate Editor: H. M. Pinedo (Amsterdam)

Editorial Office: *Annals of Oncology*, Via Soldino 22, CH-6903 Lugano, Switzerland

Editorial Board

G. Bonadonna, Milan, Italy
J. C. Cerottini, Epalinges, Switzerland
H. Cortes-Funes, Madrid, Spain
D. Crowther, Manchester, UK
H. H. Hansen, Copenhagen, Denmark
C. Jasmin, Villejuif, France

G. Klein, Stockholm, Sweden
B. Leyland-Jones, Montreal, Canada
J. G. McVie, London, UK
R. Mertelsmann, Freiburg, Germany
S. Monfardini, Aviano, Italy
F. M. Muggia, Los Angeles, USA
M. Ogawa, Tokyo, Japan

M. F. Rajewsky, Essen, Germany
S. Seeber, Essen, Germany
K. Sikora, London, UK
J. F. Smyth, Edinburgh, UK
S. Tanneberger, Bologna, Italy
E. van der Schueren, Leuven, Belgium
R. Zittoun, Paris, France

Editorial Staff and Consultants
(Editorial Committee)
A. Goldhirsch, Lugano, Switzerland
  (Coordinator)
J. Bernier, Bellinzona, Switzerland
M. D'Incalci, Milan, Italy

R. Gelber, Boston, USA
C. Hürny, Bern, Switzerland
R. Joss, Luzern, Switzerland
S. Leyvraz, Lausanne, Switzerland
R. Malinverni, Bern, Switzerland
A. Mantovani, Milan, Italy

U. Metzger, Zürich, Switzerland
A. Pedrazzini, Bellinzona, Switzerland
A. Santoro, Milan, Italy
C. Sessa, Bellinzona, Switzerland
P. Valagussa, Milan, Italy

Annals of Oncology is covered in *Current Contents/Clinical Medicine®, Science Citation Index®, Index Medicus/MEDLINE/MEDLARS, Excerpta Medica (Embase*

Fourth International Conference on Malignant Lymphoma ___

June 6–9, 1990 – Lugano, Switzerland

Selected Papers _____

Guest editors:

John E. Ultmann & Brian L. Samuels
Section of Hematology/Oncology, Department of Medicine,
The University of Chicago Cancer Research Center, Chicago, Illinois, USA

Organizing Committee:
F. Cavalli, *Bellinzona*
G. Bonadonna, *Milan*
T.A. Lister, *London*
M. Rozencweig, *Wallingford*
J.E. Ultmann, *Chicago*
R. Zittoun, *Paris*

Advisory Board:
C.W. Berard, *Memphis*
S.B. Murphy, *Chicago*
H. Rappaport, *Duarte*
S.A. Rosenberg, *Stanford*
R.C. Young, *Philadelphia*

Technical Editor:
Joan A. David

This Supplement was published with the financial contribution of
the Organizing Committee, Mr E. Camponovo (Chiasso, Switzerland) and
an educational grant provided by the Government of Canton Ticino (Switzerland).

ISBN 978-1-4899-7294-1   ISBN 978-1-4899-7305-4 (eBook)

DOI 10.1007/978-1-4899-7305-4

Editor-in-Chief: F. Cavalli (Bellinzona)

Associate Editor: H.M. Pinedo (Amsterdam)

Editorial Office: *Annals of Oncology*, Via Soldino 22, CH 6903 Lugano, Switzerland

Editorial Board

G. Bonadonna, Milan, Italy

J.C. Cerottini, Epalinges, Switzerland

H. Cortes-Funes, Madrid, Spain

D. Crowther, Manchester, UK

H.H. Hansen, Copenhagen, Denmark

C. Jasmin, Villejuif, France

G. Klein, Stockholm, Sweden

B. Leyland-Jones, Montreal, Canada

J.G. McVie, London, UK

R. Mertelsmann, Freiburg, Germany

S. Monfardini, Aviano, Italy

F.M. Muggia, Los Angeles, USA

M. Ogawa, Tokyo, Japan

M.F. Rajewsky, Essen, Germany

S. Seeber, Leverkusen, Germany

K. Sikora, London, UK

J.F. Smyth, Edinburgh, UK

S. Tanneberger, Bologna, Italy

E. Van der Schueren, Leuven, Belgiu

R. Zittoun, Paris, France   m

Editorial Staff and Consultants
  (Editorial Committee)

A. Goldhirsch, Lugano, Switzerland
  (Coordinator)

J. Bernier, Bellinzona, Switzerland

M. D'Incalci, Milan, Italy

R. Gelber, Boston, USA

C. Hürny, Bern, Switzerland

R. Joss, Luzern, Switzerland

S. Leyvraz, Lausanne, Switzerland

R. Malinverni, Bern, Switzerland

A. Mantovani, Milan, Italy

U. Metzger, Zürich, Switzerland

A. Pedrazzini, Bellinzona, Switzerland

A. Santoro, Milan, Italy

C. Sessa, Bellinzona, Switzerland

P. Valagussa, Milan, Italy

All right reserved   ISSN 0923–7534

© 1991 Springer Science+Business Media Dordrecht

Originally published by Kluwer Academic Publishers in 1991

No part of the material protected by this copyright notice may be reproduced or utilised in any form or by any means, electronic or mechanical, including photocopying, recording or by any information storage and retrieval system, without written permission from the copyright owner

Printed on acid-free paper

Publication programme 1991: Volume 2 (10 issues).

Subscription prices: Dfl. 476.–/US$270.– including postage and handling. ASCO members may subscribe at the reduced rate of Dfl. 308.–/US$ 163.– including postage and handling. Application to mail at second-class postage rate is pending at Rahway, NJ, ISSN 0923–7534. U.S. mailing agent: Expediters of the Printed Word Ltd., 2323 Randolph Ave., Avenel, NJ 07001, U.S.A.. Subscriptions should be sent to *Kluwer Academic Publishers Group, P.O. Box 322, 3300 AH Dordrecht, The Netherlands*, or at *P.O. Box 358 Accord Station, Hingham, MA 02018-0358, U.S.A.*, or to any subscription agent. Changes of mailing address should be notified together with our latest label. For advertisement rates, prices of back volumes, and other information, please apply to Kluwer Academic Publishers, P.O. Box 17, 3300 AA Dordrecht, The Netherlands.

Photocopying.

In the U.S.A.: This journal is registered at the Copyright Clearance Center, Inc., 27 Congress Street, Salem, MA 01970. Authorisation to photocopy items for internal or personal use, or the internal or personal use of specific clients, is granted by Kluwer Academic Publishers for users registered with the Copyright Clearance Center (CCC) Transactional Reporting Service, provided that the base fee of $ 1.00 per copy plus $ 0.15 per page per copy is paid directly to CCC. For those organisations that have been granted a photocopy licence by CCC, a separate system of payment has been arranged. The fee code for users of the Transactional Reporting Service is 91/0923–7534/$ 1.00 + 0.15. Authorisation does not extend to other kinds of copying, such as that for general distribution, for advertising or promotional purposes, for creating new collective works, or for resale.

In the rest of the world: Permission to photocopy must be obtained from the copyright owner. Please apply to Kluwer Academic Publishers, P.O. Box 17, 3300 AA Dordrecht, The Netherlands.

Annals of Oncology is covered in *Current Contents/Clinical Medicine®, Science Citation Index®, Index Medicus/MEDLINE/MEDLARS* and *Excerpta Medica (Embase)*.

Contents

Continued overleaf

Annals of Oncology, Supplement 2 to Volume 2: 1–7, 1991.
© 1991 *Kluwer Academic Publishers*.

An overview ———————————————

The fourth international conference on malignant lymphoma

Brian L. Samuels & John E. Ultmann

Department of Medicine and Cancer Research Center, University of Chicago, Chicago, Illinois, USA

Introduction

The Fourth International Conference on Malignant Lymphoma was held in Lugano, Switzerland, from June 6th to June 9th, 1990. It was attended by over 1100 delegates from around the world. As at previous Conferences, a large number of invited papers, brief presentations, and posters were presented on a wide variety of topics in the field of lymphoma research. A great deal of excitement was generated by the advances presented in the basic science sessions. Although steady progress is being made in the therapy of lymphomas, few major advances were reported in the clinical arena. In contrast, the application of the techniques of immunology and molecular genetics has resulted in fascinating discoveries that are increasing our understanding of the fundamental nature of lymphoproliferative disorders. These discoveries may lead to innovative therapeutic strategies unlike any currently in use.

This introductory overview clearly cannot include all of the work presented at the Conference. This volume is a collection of selected clinical papers with summaries of some of the workshops held during the Conference. A few basic science papers have been included with the relevant clinical material, rather than in a separate basic science section. We will therefore attempt to give an idea of the breadth of presentations, with emphasis on the basic science papers that have not been included.

At the Third International Conference in 1987, it was evident from the work presented that the field of lymphoma research was beginning to be caught up in the biological revolution. It became clear during the Fourth Conference that major strides have now been made in understanding the biology of lymphoma. Much of this work has been possible as a result of the advances in technology that are an integral part of that intellectual revolution.

New information regarding the biology of lymphoma was presented, mainly in the areas of etiology and pathobiology. In addition, it was evident that more insight has been gained into the prognostic factors that are of true importance in lymphomas.

The nature of the Reed-Sternberg cell

The etiology of Hodgkin's disease and the nature of the Reed-Sternberg cell continue to fascinate investigators. Hodgkin's disease was virtually the first neoplasm to be curable with combination chemotherapy, even in advanced cases. Paradoxically, a quarter century later, we understand far less about the biology of Hodgkin's disease than about many solid tumors, for which no effective therapy yet exists.

Most evidence favors a lymphoid origin for Hodgkin's disease. Previously, immunologic and molecular evidence for both T and B cell lineage has been published, as well as data suggesting a macrophage origin and an association with interdigitating reticulum cells.

Data were presented at the Conference to indicate that the Epstein-Barr virus may be causally involved in Hodgkin's disease. Although the association of Epstein-Barr virus and Hodgkin's disease has long been established, many have felt that Epstein-Barr virus infection was a consequence of the immune defect seen in patients with Hodgkin's disease. Stein presented data to demonstrate that Epstein-Barr virus genome is incorporated into host DNA in 57% of Hodgkin's disease patients. In cases in which the location was determined, the Epstein-Barr virus DNA was in the Reed-Sternberg cells, rather than the reactive lymphocytes. Moreover, the Epstein-Barr virus genome was clonal, suggesting that incorporation occurred before rather than after malignant transformation.

Evidence was presented by Uccini to show that Epstein-Barr virus genome was present in 20% of the malignant cells in AIDS-associated Hodgkin's disease. It is possible that an immune defect, leading to Epstein-Barr virus infection, might be involved in the initial stages of neoplastic transformation in this situation.

Relationship of Hodgkin's disease and non-Hodgkin's lymphoma

A striking finding was recently reported by Cossman and colleagues and was discussed by Rosenberg at the tact (the so-called 'juxtacrine' effect). Dexter also discussed the intriguing possibility of using growth inhibitors at the time of chemotherapy to protect marrow stem cells by taking them temporarily out of cycle. There might even be a protective effect for other rapidly cycling tissues, such as the oral and intestinal mucosa.

Sporn discussed the role of negative regulation of growth by factors such as transforming growth factor-β (TGF-β). TGF-β controls the growth and differentiation of immune effector cells and the growth and proliferation of target cells. It functions as a suppressor of proliferation, particularly in lymphocytes and epithelial cells. Almost all normal cells have TGF-β receptors. Transformed lymphocytes have been shown to have lost their TGF-β receptors and thus are released from the negative control of this factor. This may lead to uncontrolled proliferation of these cells. Use of differentiating agents such as retinoids or phorbol esters which up-regulate expression of TGF-β receptors, may have a role in treating a large variety of neoplasms, including lymphoproliferative disorders. High concentrations of such agents may even stimulate transformed cells to secrete TGF-β itself, thus restoring an autocrine feedback.

The characterization of the hematopoietic growth factors and the cloning of their genes represent a major theoretical and clinical advance. A number of clinical studies using various growth factors in an attempt to ameliorate myelosuppression from chemotherapy were presented at the Conference. Molecular genetic analyses show that many growth factor genes and growth factor receptor genes are found at loci that are significant for translocations and deletions.

The pace of discovery is accelerating. New factors continue to be described almost monthly. The increasing number of available factors and their myriad interactions on each other, on hematopoiesis, and on many nonhematopoietic organs and physiologic functions are a potential morass. There is a danger of squandering time and resources in trying every permutation of growth factor and chemotherapeutic agent. Intensive research is now under way to try to determine the most effective way to take advantage of the promise offered by these proteins.

It will be important that thoughtful and well designed studies are carried out in order to do this. For example, the use of specific factors in the appropriate sequence may greatly enhance the resulting effect on hematopoiesis. If this careful design phase is carried out, it is likely that growth factor therapy will revolutionize the way chemotherapy will be administered in the 1990s.

Relevance of prognostic factors

Whereas for Hodgkin's disease, four clinical stages (each with two substages) and four histologic subtypes, have been sufficient for practical prognostication; for non-Hodgkin's lymphoma there has been a plethora of prognostic factors described over the years, possibly because none are adequate. Most have been derived from retrospective analysis of patients treated with a specific regimen. In this sense, they are statistical phenomena only, and possibly of relevance only to that particular patient group. A truly relevant prognostic factor should be relatively independent of the exact regimen used, otherwise it will be of little use to the practicing clinician. With increasingly detailed knowledge of the biology of lymphoma, it is to be expected that more fundamental and important prognostic indicators will thereby be identified.

A workshop on prognostic factors in large cell lymphoma was held prior to the Conference and was reported by Canellos. It was agreed that a new staging system is required, since the Ann Arbor system is unsatisfactory for non-Hodgkin's lymphoma. In essence, stage, measured tumor bulk, lactate dehydrogenase level, and possibly β-2 microglobulin, were the critical determinants identified. All are clearly indirect evaluations of total tumor burden. It is clear that a single, accurate marker of tumor burden is required. A start has been made towards determining the utility of prognostic factors generated by analysis of one lymphoma database in predicting outcome of patients in a different database. It was agreed that this should be continued and that in particular, the databases of the French GELA group Study Group for Aggressive Lymphomas, the Dana Farber Cancer Institute, and the M.D. Anderson Hospital should be evaluated in this fashion. Data presented by Crowther and by Felman suggested that measurement of the proliferative activity of the tumor did not offer additional prognostic information. However, during the Conference, Armitage reported a study in which proliferative activity was highly correlated with survival. The relevance of proliferative activity clearly will require further study. It was felt that the prognostic importance of patient age may currently be underestimated because many aggressive chemotherapy protocols have routinely excluded elderly patients. The importance of adequate statistical analysis, including multivariate analysis was stressed. It was agreed that there are not yet sufficient data to allow formulation of a new staging system. However, with intergroup and interinstitutional cooperation, it is hoped that such data will become available in the future.

Prognostic factors in Hodgkin's disease

Patients with Hodgkin's disease have higher serum levels of circulating interleukin-2 receptor (CD25) than normal subjects. From data presented by Pfreundschuh, the degree of elevation appears to correlate with clinical stage, outcome of initial therapy, and prognosis for relapse. In addition, soluble CD30 antigen in the serum of Hodgkin's patients appears to indicate a lower complete response rate and a higher relapse rate. It is not yet clear whether such immunologic prognostic parameters are regimen independent and whether they provide independent prognostic information.

Prognostic factors in non-Hodgkin's lymphoma

Markers that may be of biological significance for prognosis in non-Hodgkin's lymphoma were discussed by several investigators. They included immunological markers, molecular genetic markers, and cytogenetic markers.

The list of nonrandom cytogenetic abnormalities associated with non-Hodgkin's lymphoma continues to grow. This list is considerably longer than the one that was available at the time of the Third Conference in 1987. Schouten discussed the relevance of specific, recurrent cytogenetic abnormalities as indicators of prognosis. In addition, the concept of cytogenetic progression (or its equivalent molecular genetic change) as a predictor of later histologic progression was discussed.

Clonal excess as a prognostic factor

Some reputed prognostic factors may not stand the test of time. The clonal excess technique attempting to predict relapse was reported at the last conference. At least one report at the meeting suggested that there may be no prospective predictive ability for this test. Future studies may resolve the question, using increasingly sensitive detection techniques.

Biology of lymphomas — Summary

Progress has been exciting in basic science research in the lymphoma field. This bodes well for the future of clinical as well as basic science. At present, there are not many significant clinical advances being reported in either Hodgkin's disease or non-Hodgkin's lymphoma, but this situation is likely to change as new understanding of biology suggests new and possibly radically different approaches to therapy.

Influence of drug resistance on protocol design

DeVita delivered a thoughtful discussion of the ways in which protocol design should be manipulated to take account of knowledge of drug resistance mechanisms. In the Henry Kaplan Memorial Lecture, he explored what is known about drug resistance and the kinetics of resistance development. In particular, the Goldie-Coldman hypothesis predicts a relationship between tumor size and likelihood of resistance developing by somatic mutation. The prediction from this would be that all effective drugs should be used in the initial

therapeutic regimen. As DeVita discussed, this aspect of the theory has not been proven in an adequate, prospective fashion. Unfortunately, such tests may be very hard to carry out. DeVita also discussed the concept of dose intensity as contrasted with total dose administered. In curable malignancies such as lymphoma, outcome analysis suggests that total dose may influence median survival, but the cure rate is more dependent on dose intensity. There are many potential mechanisms for clinical resistance to chemotherapy. Strategies to overcome this resistance must be developed. Several were discussed by DeVita, including attention to dose intensity and scheduling and pharmacologic modulation of multidrug resistance. Future chemotherapy regimens must be designed with these mechanisms and kinetics in mind.

Clinical aspects of Hodgkin's disease

Rosenberg gave his perspective as to where staging and therapy for Hodgkin's disease are heading. He stressed the importance of patient age as a prognostic variable as well as the continuing role of lymphangiography and the evolving role of MRI in staging. In a disorder in which 83% of all patients survive 16 years or more, toxicity of therapy is becoming an increasingly important parameter. Short-term toxicity may be addressed by modifying treatment programs commensurately with risk level. In this regard, Ann Arbor stage and histologic subtype seem to be less important than patient age and tumor bulk. The reduction of therapy for good-risk cases and the early application of intensive therapy for poor-risk patients would be the goals of such an approach. The concept of tailoring treatment to the patient's status would be enhanced by a better understanding of the biology and genetics of Hodgkin's disease. If this could be achieved, distinct subsets defined by immunologic or molecular genetic techniques could be singled out for specific therapeutic approaches.

One of the problems that continue to plague clinicians dealing with a curable neoplasm in largely young patients is that of the long-term toxicities of therapy. These are now well known, as confirmed by Cosset in reporting the overall EORTC (European Organization for Treatment and Research of Cancer) experience in over 1650 patients. Late gastrointestinal, pulmonary, and cardiac complications and secondary malignancies are among the prominent toxicities described. One response to this problem is to attempt to minimize therapy in good prognostic subgroups. This may be achieved by using reduced amounts of both chemotherapy and radiation. For example, regimens were described by Anderson and by Brice that utilized short courses of chemotherapy in addition to radiation for early stage Hodgkin's disease. A cautionary note was sounded in the Pediatric Lymphoma session however. The omission of procarbazine from a regimen resulted in a major decrease in efficacy in a German Cooperative study.

The question of the optimal initial therapy continues to cause debate. The CALGB (Cancer and Leukemia Group B) data from a large randomized trial reported the superiority of ABVD over MOPP in a North American population, but failed to show an additional advantage to alternating MOPP with ABVD. However, both the alternating regimen and the combination MOPP-ABV 'hybrid' regimen gave more striking results in Milan, approaching a 90% complete response rate in advanced disease.

Relapsed/refractory Hodgkin's disease

The problem of relapsed disease continues to be a vexing one, given the generally poor prognosis when this occurs. One approach is to improve the results of initial therapy so as to reduce the number of relapses. In the EORTC experience reported here, as well as the experience of many other groups, many relapses occur at the site of original disease. It was suggested that adding involved field radiation to chemotherapy might reduce the relapse rate. The role of salvage radiation in relapsed disease of limited extent was also discussed. The duration of remission before relapse continues to have prognostic importance. Canellos reported that the EVA (etoposide, vinblastine, Adriamycin) regimen was equivalent to the ABVD regimen in salvaging patients who had failed MOPP therapy. Several reports were also given relating to developments in the field of high-dose chemotherapy with autologous bone marrow rescue for relapsed Hodgkin's disease. This approach is becoming safer and more appropriately utilized among specific subgroups of patients most likely to benefit.

Hodgkin's disease — Challenges for the 1990s

We have seen that the biology of Hodgkin's disease remains mysterious. If enough effort is directed towards elucidating the pathologic processes which cause Hodgkin's disease, further improvements in therapy will follow almost automatically. This should also allow more definitive description of biologically significant prognostic factors. With this, allocation to therapy groups should be more precise, enabling many young people to escape the potential complications of chemotherapy.

Therapy of aggressive lymphomas

Armitage defined four subgroups of patients with aggressive lymphomas which should be the subjects of particular research interest in the near future. These are patients with localized disease, elderly patients, patients with HIV-related lymphoma, and patients with high grade lymphomas. The controversy over whether more is better rages on. The data reviewed by Armitage suggest that dose intensity and schedule are important, rather than number of drugs in a regimen. This implies that CHOP administered in full dose, on time, may be as good as a third generation regimen.

The matter is far from settled, however. The EORTC data presented here suggested that, all other factors being equal, a more aggressive regimen gives better results. The SWOG (South West Oncology Group) data suggest that there may be no difference in outcome between the various third generation regimens. Analysis of dose intensity will be essential in any future attempts to compare the efficacy of treatment regimens.

Autologous bone marrow reinfusion

Philip discussed the therapy of relapsed lymphoma, stressing that aggressive therapy may be necessary. However, he noted that at this time the interim data from the PARMA randomized trial show no difference in outcome between aggressive conventional chemotherapy and high dose therapy with autologous bone marrow rescue.

For patients with relapsed lymphoma, the situation is relatively straightforward, in that action is immediately required. Should high risk patients have aggressive consolidation therapy in first remission, without waiting for relapse to occur? An example would be the use of high dose chemotherapy for patients with lymphoblastic lymphoma in remission, as reported by Santini.

High-risk B-cell malignancies may also benefit from the approach of transplantation in the first remission, as was discussed by Freedman.

The place of autologous bone marrow rescue in the therapy of follicular lymphomas continues to be controversial, as was discussed by Lister and by Rohatiner. Evidence is now emerging to suggest that patients with follicular lymphoma who relapse after therapy have a relatively poor prognosis. In this situation, the role of high-dose chemotherapy with or without bone marrow rescue, is probably to consolidate gains made with more conventional therapy and attempt to secure more durable subsequent remissions. Again, it was suggested that transplantation in first remission may be advantageous, if a reliable way to determine risk of second relapse could be determined, so that unnecessary treatment could be avoided.

Growth factors

The preclinical promise of growth factor therapy as a means of reducing myelosuppression is starting to become reality. Phase I and II trials with four growth factors: granulocyte colony stimulating factor (G-CSF), granulocyte-macrophage colony stimulating factor (GM-CSF), multi-colony stimulating factor (M-CSF), and interleukin-3, have been carried out. Three other agents – interleukin-1, interleukin-4, and interleukin-6 – are still in initial trials. Good randomized studies have not as yet been done. The conclusion reached from these early trials is that there appears to be some benefit in terms of the rate of recovery from neutropenia and depth of the nadir count when growth factors are used after conventional chemotherapy drugs. In some series, the time to first appearance of myeloid cells was not changed, suggesting that the agent was not acting on the very earliest precursors, but on later, more committed progenitor cells.

Non-Hodgkin's lymphoma — Challenges for the 1990s

Identification of biologically significant prognostic subgroups is a major challenge, as was recognized at this conference. With new understanding of the biology of follicular lymphoma, new approaches to therapy are now possible. The matter of CHOP versus the newcomers may take years to resolve, as the data from randomized studies mature. In the interim, a logical approach, based on the available data, may be indicated. Similarly, a great deal of thought and planning now will save many blind alleys and false negative results when clinical results of trials involving chemotherapy and growth factors are analyzed.

Speculations

What topics will be discussed at the Fifth International Conference in 1993? There are several possibilities for translating the recent basic science advances into clinical strategies:

As knowledge of lymphoma biology increases, it should become possible to tailor therapy more to specific prognostic groups. Thus excessive toxicity may be avoided in patients likely to be cured anyway and high risk patients may be given more intensive therapy from the start.

With increasing evidence of viral involvement in the etiology of some lymphomas, the use of antiviral therapy and of molecular strategies to reverse the viral lesion may become feasible. Reversing the malignant phenotype in such a fashion is now within sight, using, for example, antisense oligonucleotides to turn off overexpressed oncogenes.

Alternatively, where tumor suppressor genes are deleted, it may become possible to replace the missing gene product, much as insulin is replaced today. If such suppressor genes are demonstrated to be implicated in the pathogenesis of lymphoma, the therapy of lymphoma may change radically within a very few years.

Correspondence to:
Brian L. Samuels
Department of Medicine and Cancer Research Center
University of Chicago
Chicago, Illinois, USA

Annals of Oncology, Supplement 2 to Volume 2: 9–21, 1991.
© 1991 Kluwer Academic Publishers.

Original article ———————————————————————

Molecular biology of lymphoid malignancies*

Jacob Kagan & Carlo M. Croce

Fels Institute for Cancer Research and Molecular Biology, Temple University School of Medicine, Philadelphia, Pennsylvania, USA

Over the last decade advances in our understanding of the pathogenesis of human cancer have largely been established upon the recognition that frequent and consistent chromosomal abnormalities, occurring in a variety of human cancers, are the cytogenetic markers for molecular genetic changes which underlie oncogenesis [1].

In 1960, Nowell and Hungerford discovered a marker chromosome, the Philadelphia chromosome Ph' which is consistently associated with chronic myelogenous leukemia (CML) [2]. The Ph' chromosome is a shortened chromosome 22 that arises from the t(9;22)(q34;q11) reciprocal translocation [3]. This translocation occurs in the majority (~95%) of patients with CML and in a smaller proportion (~10%) of patients with acute lymphoblastic leukemia (ALL) or acute myelogenous leukemia (2%) (AML) [4]. The Ph' translocation results in transposition of the cellular abl (c-abl) gene from its location on chromosome 9 to chromosome 22 [2, 4, 5].

A second striking observation was reported in 1972 by Manolov and Manolova, who detected a marker chromosome 14 (14q⁺) associated with a majority (75–80%) of Burkitt's lymphomas [6]. Zech et al. [7] subsequently showed that the 14q⁺ chromosome results from the reciprocal translocation t(8;14)(q24;q32). Interestingly, in both cases the translocation breakpoints are at the sites of the human homologue of a viral oncogene. In CML, as a result of the t(9;22)(q34;q11) translocation, c-abl, the human homologue of the v-abl oncogene of the Abelson leukemia virus, is translocated from its normal position on chromosome 9 band q34 to chromosome 22 band q11 [8]; and in the t(8;14)(q24;q32) translocation of Burkitt's lymphoma, c-myc, the human homologue of the v-myc oncogene present in avian myelocytomatosis virus, normally located on chromosome 8 band q24 is translocated to the immunoglobulin heavy chain locus on chromosome 14 band q32 [9, 10].

There are two main categories of oncogenic activation by chromosomal translocation. The first mechanism is exemplified by 95% of CML cases in which the c-abl oncogene is recombined with the bcr gene, re-

sulting in the expression of a hybrid c-abl-bcr protein product with acquired tyrosine kinase activity [12]. The second mechanism is observed in Burkitt's lymphomas and involves the juxtaposition of the c-myc gene to the immunoglobulin heavy chain (IgH) locus by the t(8;14) translocation [11]; the deregulation of c-myc is a consequence of its proximity to cis-activating elements within the IgH locus. This mechanism was observed in other malignancies although either the activated oncogene (e.g., bcl-2) or the cis-activating element (e.g., T-cell receptor [TCR] loci) may vary. These findings strongly suggest that chromosomal translocations alter the regulation or the structure of the cellular proto-oncogene, leading to malignancy.

I. Molecular analysis of chromosomal translocations in Burkitt's lymphomas

Burkitt's lymphoma is an extremely aggressive B-cell malignancy primarily affecting children and young adults. In equatorial Africa, more than 70% of the endemic Burkitt's lymphoma (eBL) cells carry Epstein-Barr virus (EBV) [11]. The majority of these tumors express cell surface IgM, and a smaller proportion exhibit surface IgG; in rare cases there is no expression of cell surface immunoglobulin [13]. In the sporadic form of Burkitt's lymphoma (sBL), found in North America and Europe, only 15–20% of the cases occur in association with EBV, and the cells express more cell surface immunoglobulin [13] and secrete more IgM [11].

Chromosomal translocations observed in Burkitt's lymphoma are characterized by reciprocal chromosome translocations involving chromosome 8 at band q24 [6, 7], the location of the c-myc gene [9]. The other chromosomal regions involved in the translocation are either chromosome 14 band q32 (in 80% of the cases) or chromosome 22 band q11 (in 15% of the cases) and chromosome 2 band p11 (in 5% of the cases). These regions carry the human immunoglobulin heavy chain (IgH), lambda light chain (Igλ), and kappa light chain (Igκ), respectively [14, 15]. Somatic cell genetic analysis of the t(8;14) translocation revealed that the human

* This work was supported by a grant from the National Cancer Institute CA39860 (CMC).

IgH locus was interrupted by the chromosomal translocation; the c-*myc* gene may be truncated or translocated in its entirety to chromosome 14. In the variant t(2;8) and t(8;22) chromosome translocations, the c-*myc* gene remains on chromosome 8 while the locus for either the Igλ or Igκ constant region translocates 3' to the c-*myc* gene [17, 18]. At the molecular level the chromosomal breakpoints on chromosome 8 and 14 are scattered. Breakpoints in the IgH locus have been localized within D_H segments [19], J_H segments [20], upstream of the switch Sµ [22], Sγ [23] and Sα regions [24].

The variant translocations may occur within the Vκ [25] or Jκ segments on chromosome 2 or 5' to the Cλ region on chromosome 22 [17, 27]. On chromosome 8 the translocations are similarly dispersed. Chromosomal breakpoints were found 75 kb 5' of c-*myc* [19, 20, 27, 28], immediately upstream of the first exon of *myc* [23, 29, 30] or within the first intron of *myc* in the t(8;14) translocations [29, 30]. However, in both types of the variant translocations, the breakpoints occur at a minimum distance of 47 kb 3' of *myc* [32]. In several cases the breakpoints were reported to fall within 140 kb [33] and 300 kb [34] distal from c-*myc*, in a region homologous to the rodent pvt1/mis1 locus [35]. The function of the human pvt1-like locus 3' to c-*myc* is unknown, although it is speculated that the pvt1 gene could, upon rearrangement, either deregulate c-*myc* expression in trans or contribute independently to tumor formation [33–35].

The chromosomal breakpoints and structural rearrangements of the *myc* locus in (8;14) translocations differ for endemic and sporadic forms of Burkitt's lymphoma. The first type, found in most eBL and EBV-positive AIDS-associated lymphoma, involves sequences on chromosome 8 upstream from *myc* and sequences within or near the J_H or D_H regions on chromosome 14 [19, 20, 30]. The second type, found in most sBL, involves sequences within or immediately 5' to *myc* on chromosome 8 and sequences within or near the IgH switch (S) regions on chromosome 14 [19, 20, 30, 36, 37]. In addition, eBL expresses only cytoplasmic or membrane-bound immunoglobulin, indicative of early B-cells, whereas the sporadic type secretes immunoglobulin, indicating a more advanced stage of B-cell differentiation. As we have previously suggested [19, 20], chromosomal translocations involving J_H and D_H segments may occur at the time of $V_H D_H J_H$ joining in the immature eBL B-cells, whereas translocations involving S sequences may occur during isotype class switching in more differentiated B-cells, as observed in sBL. However, at least in one case, the translocation may have occurred after $V_H D_H J_H$ rearrangement, or during $V_H D_H J_H$ joining; but additional genetic changes were necessary for the full expression of the aggressive phenotype [36].

A consistent finding in almost all Burkitt's lymphomas indicates that the *myc* protein is unaffected, suggesting that the physiological function of the *myc* protein is not altered in the malignant cells. However, as a consequence of the chromosomal translocation, the *myc* gene is transcribed constitutively at elevated levels [38–42]. To explain the mechanism that alters *myc*'s expression, several hypotheses were proposed: (1) deregulation as a result of loss of physiological promoters, due to translocation occurring within the first exon or first intron of *myc* [21]; (2) loss of transacting control regions 5' of *myc* [43]; and (3) mutations in the noncoding or coding regions of *myc* [44, 45]. None of these hypotheses could explain cases where the translocations occurred far 5' or 3' from *myc*, leaving the gene and its proposed 5' control region intact, and thus allowing *myc* to utilize its own physiological promoters.

The hypothesis that gives the best explanation for *myc*'s deregulation in Burkitt's lymphoma relies on the cis activation of *myc* transcription from the translocated allele, due to *myc*'s proximity to enhancer elements or enhancer-like elements of the immunoglobulin loci [21, 46]. Several observations support this proposition. First, DNA transfection experiments with constructs containing *myc* and immunoglobulin enhancer resulted in high levels of *myc* transcripts [21, 47]. Constructs that lacked *myc*'s 5' exon were not transcribed [47]. Thus, it appears that 5' truncation of *myc* in itself is not sufficient for deregulation. The transcription deregulation of the translocated allele is influenced by the transformed B-cell context, since stable transfection of eBL's translocated allele into fibroblasts resulted in the expression of this translocated allele at levels indistinguishable from the normal *myc* allele. Therefore, the expression of translocated *myc* requires a particular environment [48].

Second, somatic cell hybrid studies have shown that in almost all cases the translocated allele is constitutively expressed in Burkitt's lymphoma, whereas the nontranslocated allele is silent [39]. However, expression of the translocated *myc* allele is dependent on the stage of differentiation of the involved Burkitt's lymphoma cell. This was demonstrated in experiments where the translocated *myc* gene was expressed in cell hybrids between Burkitt's lymphoma and murine plasmacytoma cells, but not in hybrids with lymphoblastoid cells. Furthermore, the expression of the translocated *myc* allele is specific for B-cells; hybrids with fibroblast do not transcribe. Thus, it appears that the translocated *myc* activation depends on enhancer-like elements present in all of the immunoglobulin loci that are activated by transacting factors expressed in Burkitt's lymphoma and plasma cells, but not in less-differentiated B-cells (lymphoblastoid cells) [46].

The third observation in support of the cis-acting transcriptional control model of *myc* deregulation comes from studies on transgenic mice into which activated *myc* genes were introduced [49, 52]. Introduction of the *myc* gene coupled to an immunoglobulin enhancer element (µ or κ) results in aggressive B lineage tumors which occur at high frequency [49]. Constructs utilizing intact or truncated *myc* genes were virtually ineffective in inducing tumors [49]. These findings strongly suggest that the tissue-specific activation of c-*myc* observed in Burkitt's lymphomas occurs through a similar mechanism of transcriptional deregulation in cis.

One criticism of this hypothesis is that in some cases the IgH chain locus enhancer is translocated to the $8q^-$ chromosome rather remaining on the $14q^+$ chromosome, or alternatively the juxtaposed enhancer to *myc* is placed too far away to effect activation. However, the IgH chain enhancer can activate tandem V_H promoters separated by nearly 20 kb [53]. In addition, in early B-cell ontogeny, most V_H segments are in a configuration accessible to activation [53]. Since the V_H segments span hundreds of kilobases of DNA, it is obvious that the transcriptional mechanism is able to transcribe over a huge distance.

II. Activation of other oncogenes by the IgH locus

Over 60% of human non-Burkitt's B-cell lymphomas carry translocations involving chromosome 14 band q32, the chromosomal location of the human IgH locus; however, these translocations usually do not involve chromosome 8 band q24, the location of the human c-*myc* gene [1, 38, 46].

1. Translocations at the bcl-2 locus on chromosome 18q21

About 90% of follicular B-cell lymphomas and ~20% of large diffuse B-cell lymphomas carry the t(14;18)(q32;q21) translocation [54], which directly involves the IgH locus on chromosome 14. Like the *myc* translocations in Burkitt's lymphomas, the t(14;18)(q32;q21) translocation occurs 5' or 3' to the *bcl*-2 gene, but not within the protein coding portion of the gene [51–52]. The association of the *bcl*-2 gene with the heavy chain locus results in high levels of *bcl*-2 expression [56]. The follicular lymphoma translocations are structurally much more uniform than those of Burkitt's lymphoma. In about 70% of human follicular lymphomas the breakpoints are clustered with the 3' untranslated region of the gene (designated major breakpoint region [mbr] [56]; in another 10–20% of the cases the breakpoints are clustered in a region more than 20 kb downstream from *bcl*-2's second exon (designated minor cluster region [mcr] [57]. In some cases, the translocations were detected near the 5' exon [58]. A variant translocation in which the IgL chain loci are translocated into the *bcl*-2 locus was detected in ~10% of the cases of chronic lymphocytic leukemia [59, 60]. In these cases the translocations were clustered 5' to *bcl*-2's first exon on chromosome 18. The breakpoints in the IgL chain's loci were mapped within V_λ of rearranged $V_\lambda J_\lambda$ segments and, in another case, within the 5' flanking region of $J_\kappa 4$. The breakpoint of the reciprocal translocation at the κ locus on chromosome $2q^-$ was in the $V_\kappa J_\kappa 3$ rearranged segment [60]. These findings suggest that the translocation occurred after $V_\kappa J_\kappa$ joining, or alternatively, during $V_\kappa J_\kappa$ joining. In the latter case, additional rearrangement of V_κ to J_κ occurred [60]. Interestingly, different cluster regions of translocation breakpoints at the *bcl*-2 locus are associated with different types of disease. In CLL, the breakpoints are clustered within 1 kb 5' of *bcl*-2's first exon [59, 60]; while in follicular lymphoma, 80% of the translocation breakpoints were clustered in two regions located 3' of *bcl*-2 [56, 57] and ~20% were clustered 5' of the first exon [58]. Furthermore, it appears that in follicular lymphoma, the translocations took place in pre-B-cells during the rearrangement of the IgH chain locus [56, 61], while in CLL the translocation occurred in more mature B-cells during or after IgL chain loci rearrangement [59, 60].

The *bcl*-2 gene codes for two overlapping protein products with molecular masses of 26 kd (*bcl*-2 alpha) and 22 kd (*bcl*-2 beta) [61, 62]; *bcl*-2 was shown to be an insoluble membrane-bound protein predominately localized in the rough endoplasmic reticulum and nuclear envelope [63, 64, 65]. In contrast to the initial reports [63, 64], it is expressed in normal T and B lymphoid cells and in a variety of lymphomas with and without chromosomal rearrangements at the *bcl*-2 locus, although the highest expression was detected in follicular lymphomas carrying the t(14;18) translocation [66]. The biochemical role of *bcl*-2 is unclear [67], although some data suggest that it may have GTP-binding activity [65]. Although the physiological activity of *bcl*-2 is unknown, the elevated levels found in cells with *bcl*-2 rearrangements are thought to contribute to the pathogenesis of these B-cell neoplasms. Some gene transfer experiments have suggested that *bcl*-2 can regulate the growth of human and murine B-cells in vivo and in vitro [59–65]. The consistent finding of *bcl*-2 involvement in follicular lymphoma and in a fraction of CLLs strongly suggests that the *bcl*-2 product plays a role in lymphoid differentiation and proliferation.

2. Translocations at the bcl-1 locus on chromosome 11q13

The t(11;14)(q13;q32) chromosomal translocation is associated with B lymphocytic malignancy. This abnormality has been reported in chronic lymphocytic leukemia, multiple myeloma, and diffuse B-cell lymphoma [1, 75]. At the molecular level, the IgH chain locus is split 5' to the J_H segment or within the V_H segment [76–81]. On chromosome 11q13, four of the reported translocations are clustered within 1 kb of DNA in a region termed *major translocation cluster* (*mtc*) [76, 77, 81]. Additional translocations have been reported to occur 27 kb telomeric to *mtc* in prolymphocytic leukemia [79]; 36 kb telomeric to *mtc* in multiple myeloma [80]; and 67 kb telomeric to *mtc* in a case of chronic lymphocytic leukemia [81]. Although, more than 100 kb of DNA at the *bcl*-1 locus was cloned, a transcription unit has not been identified. By analogy to *myc* and *bcl*-2 translocations, the proto-oncogene *bcl*-1 should be telomeric to the translocation region on chromosome 11. Thus, we assume that the *bcl*-1 gene lies more than 63 kb telomeric to *mtc*.

3. Translocations occurring at the bcl-3 locus on chromosome 19q13.1

The $(14;19)(q32.3;q13.1)$ is a recurrent translocation found in the neoplastic cells of some patients with CLL [82–84]. In two cases analyzed so far, the translocations involve the switch $C\alpha_1$ region of the IgH chain $C\alpha$ locus on chromosome 14q32. On chromosome 19q13.1 the translocation breakpoints are separated by 19 kb. The involvement of the α switch region in the translocations of both patients suggests that this translocation resembles sporadic cases of the $t(8;14)$ translocation in Burkitt's lymphoma [30], in which breaks usually occur in a switch region. This indicates that the translocation occurred in a mature B-cell probably during an attempt at isotype switch. A transcription unit was identified adjacent to one of the translocation breakpoints on chromosome 19 [84]. The gene sequence, termed *bcl*-3, predicts a protein containing seven tandem copies of the SW16/cdc10 motif, previously identified in yeast [85]. The cdc10 is one of two genes in the yeast *Schizosaccharomyces pombe* known to be required for commitment to the start of the cell cycle [86]. In invertebrates, cdc10 relates to a transmembrane protein involved in cell differentiation pathways. As expected, leukemic cells with the $t(14;19)(q32;q13.1)$ translocation show elevated expression of this gene as compared to other CLL samples [85]. Thus, it seems that the *bcl*-3 proto-oncogene may contribute to malignant transformation when abnormally expressed.

4. The t(9;14)(p11;q32) translocation

Chromosome 9 band p11 has been found to be involved in several nonrandom abnormalities: a $t(9;12)(p11;p12)$ translocation is found in 2% of childhood B-cell precursor ALLs [87], and other alterations in T-cell lymphomas [88].

(a) The $t(9;14)(p11;q32)$ chromosomal translocation breakpoint was cloned from a case of malignant lymphoma occurring in human alpha heavy chain disease (αHCD) [89], a lymphoproliferative disorder characterized by the production of immunoglobulin molecules consisting of an incomplete heavy chain and devoid of the light chain [89, 90]. Molecular analysis revealed that the breakpoint occurred 3' to the IgH J_H6 segment and 5' to the Sα region on chromosome 14. On chromosome 9, the breakpoint region was flanked by two nearly identical inverted repeats. It was suggested that these repeats may have been involved in local pairing between chromosomes 9 and 14 leading to the chromosomal translocation [89]. The proposed proto-oncogene in the vicinity of the translocation breakpoint has not yet been identified [89].

(b) A $t(9;14)(p13;q32)$ chromosome translocation was reported in the diffuse large-cell lymphoma cell line Kish [91]. In this case, the breakpoint on chromosome 14 was 265 bp downstream from the 3' border of the J_H6 joining segment. Class switch recombination deleted most of the constant gene of IgH and juxtaposed the $C\alpha_2$ to a transcriptionally active region on chromosome 9. The 11-kb RNA transcript was detected in several other human B-cell lines. The sequence and function of this gene are as yet unknown [91].

Although both of the translocations occurred at the short arm of chromosome 9, the breakpoint regions were different.

5. The t(5;14)(q31;q32) chromosome translocation

The $t(5;14)(q31;q32)$ chromosomal translocation is a distinct subtype of ALL with B-lineage phenotype [92, 93]. Molecular cloning of the translocation breakpoint revealed that the IgH chain J_H segment is juxtaposed to the promoter region of the interleukin-3 gene in opposite transcriptional orientation [94]. It is suggested that, as for the *myc* and *bcl*-2 translocations, the IgH enhancer element may activate the IL-3 gene, resulting in the neoplastic transformation and the associated eosinophilia [94].

III. Activation of oncogenes by T-cell receptor genes

Chromosomal abnormalities nonrandomly associated with T-cell leukemia and lymphoma frequently involve chromosome 14 band q11, the location of the T-cell receptor α locus (TCRα) [95]. Less frequently the translocations involve chromosome 7 band q35 and chromosome 7 band p13, the locations of TCRβ and TCRγ respectively [96, 97]. The analogy between the involvement of the immunoglobulin genes in B-cell malignancies and the implication of the TCR loci in T-cell neoplasia is quite evident. The TCR genes are organized similarly, rearrange during cellular differentiation, and are expressed in a tissue-specific manner [98].

1. Translocations at the TCL-1 locus on chromosome 14q32.1

T-cell leukemias frequently carry the inv(14;14)(q11;q32) and/or the $t(14;14)(q11;q32)$ chromosomal translocation [99, 100].

Molecular analysis of the inv(14)(q11;q32) revealed that the inversion occurred between the TCRα locus at band q11 and the IgH locus at band q32, resulting in a chimeric gene composed of V_H-J_α-C_α [101]. Similar inversion was described in an acute B-cell leukemia cell line [102]. Inversions between the IgH and TCRα loci on chromosome 14 or inversions between the TCRβ

locus at band 7q35 and the TCRγ locus at band 7p13, were observed in ataxia telangiectasia (AT) and in healthy donors [103]. Furthermore, translocations which result in chimeric γ/δ genes were described in DNA from healthy donors [104]. Thus, although the inversions and translocations which produce chimeric receptors between immunoglobulin and TCR genes are results of errors in the recombination process [104, 105], their pathogenic significance is doubtful. A second class of inversions and translocation breakpoints, found in T-cell tumors from AT and non-AT patients, involves chromosome 14 band q32.1, which is 10–20 Mbp centromeric to the IgH locus [106, 107]. Molecular analysis of chromosomal breakpoints involving this locus revealed that in the t(14;14)(q11; q32.1) translocations and the inv(14;14)(q11;q32.1) inversions, the breakpoints occurred in the TCRJα segments; in the t(7;14)(q35;1432.1) translocation the breakpoint occurred in TCRJβ segment [106–112]. On chromosome 14q32.1, at the TCL-1 locus, the breakpoints are spread over a large distance which was not connected by chromosomal walking techniques [106–112]. At present, the proposed oncogene tcl-1 has not been identified.

2. Translocations at the TCL-2 locus on chromosome 11 band p13

The t(11;14)(p13;q11) translocation was originally described in a pediatric patient with CD2+ T-ALL and is observed in about 10–15% of T-ALL cases [113]. Somatic cell hybrid analysis showed that the translocation splits the TCRα locus between V_α and C_α [114]. Molecular cloning revealed that the translocations occurred at the TCRδ locus probably during an attempt to rearrange a V segment next to J_δ, $D_\delta D_\delta$ or $D_\delta D_\delta J_\delta$ segments [115]. Most of the breakpoints studied so far (5 of 10) are clustered within a stretch of 2 kb on 11p13, while the rest fall within a region of 25 kb on chromosome 11p13 [116]. At present no transcript has been identified within ~100 kb of the cloned TCL-2 locus [116].

3. Translocations at the TCL-3 locus on chromosome 10 band q24

Chromosome 10 band q24 is another locus nonrandomly associated with T-cell leukemias and high-grade T-cell lymphomas [99, 117, 118].

Somatic cell genetic analysis of leukemic cells carrying the t(10;14)(q24;q11) translocations clearly demonstrated that the TCRα locus has been split between V_α and C_α [119]. On chromosome 10 the breakpoint occurred distal to the human terminal deoxynucleotidyltransferase gene [119]. Molecular cloning of the breakpoint junctions in three acute T-lymphoblastic leukemias carrying the t(10;14)(q24;q11) chromosome translocation revealed that the involved TCRδ sequences are made from the $D_\delta 2$ segment. The chromosome breakpoints are clustered within a region of 263 bp of chromosome 10 [120]. Recently, another two translocation breakpoints were reported to fall in a region 1.5 kb telomeric to the breakpoints reported by us [121]. Interestingly, a 2.9-kb RNA transcript was detected with a probe derived from a region of chromosome 10 expected to translocate to the der [14] chromosome [121]. In this case, it is important to note that the probe which detects the transcriptionally active region on chromosome 10 is translocated downstream of the V_α locus on chromosome 14 at band q11, and not to the TCRδ enhancer region [122]. However, in Burkitt's lymphoma and follicular lymphoma translocations, the myc and bcl-2 oncogenes are translocated and juxtaposed to immunoglobulin enhancer regions [46–52, 55–60]. The sequence of this gene, its deregulation due to the chromosomal translocation, and its potential oncogenic activity are as yet unknown [121]. Recently, a variant t(7;10)(q35;q24) translocation was cloned and shown to fall within band q24, the location of the breakpoint region with reference to the TCL-3 cluster region was not determined [123].

4. Translocations at the TCL-5/SCL/TAL locus on chromosome 1 band p32

Human chromosome 1 band p32 aberrations have been detected in acute T-cell leukemia [124], human cutaneous malignant melanoma [125] and human neuroblastomas [126].

We and Begley reported the cloning of the t(1;14)(p32;q11) translocation breakpoint in human leukemic stem cell line DU528, derived from a patient with acute T-lymphoblastic leukemia [127, 128]. The translocation breakpoint on the 1p+ chromosome occurred at the TCRδ diversity ($D\delta_2$) segment and the reciprocal chromosomal joining on the 14q⁻ chromosome occurred at the TCRδ diversity segment, $D\delta_1$ [127]. The involvement of Dδ segment at the translocation junctions suggests that the translocation occurred during an attempt at $D\delta_1 D\delta_2$ joining in a stem cell. The segment of chromosome 1 at band p32 adjacent to the chromosomal breakpoint encodes a transcriptional unit designated TCL-5/SCL/TAL (T-cell leukemia/ lymphoma 5/stem cell leukemia/T cell acute leukemia) [127, 128, 130]. Another three translocation breakpoints ~10 kb centromeric to the one reported by us were cloned recently [129, 130], indicating the existence of a breakpoint cluster region on chromosome 1p32. The TCL-5/SCL/TAL gene sequence predicts a protein with primary amino acid sequence homology to the previously described amphipathic helix-loop-helix (HLH) DNA binding and dimerization motif of the lyl-1 [132], myc, myo D, and the immunoglobulin enhancer-binding family of genes [131]. From the cDNA clones obtained it appears that the gene may be expressed in several different forms due to alternate usage of 5' exons [130, 131]. The predicted proteins would have conserved HLH domains, but distinct amino terminal ends. Antisera against specific peptides immunoprecipitated two distinct proteins with molecular masses of 37 and 41 kd. Since the gene is preferentially expressed in immature hematopoietic cell lines and has 84% homology within the HLH domain of other genes like *lyl*-1 (which is also expressed in primitive hematopoietic tissue), it is possible that the TCL-5/SCL/TAL protein is a transcription factor with a possible role in hematopoietic differentiation [130, 131].

5. The t(11;14)(p15;q11) chromosomal translocation at the Ttg-1 locus on chromosome 11p15

The t(11;14)(p15;q11) chromosomal translocation was initially described in a T-cell line, RPMI 8402, established from the malignant cells of a patient with T-cell acute lymphoblastic leukemia [133]. The translocation breakpoint joins chromosome 11p15 sequences with the TCRδ $D\delta_1 D\delta_2 J\delta_1$ rearranged segment. The reciprocal translocation on the der (14q⁻) chromosome joins a chromosome 11p15 heptamer-like sequence to the recombination signal 5′ of the TCRδ $D\delta_1$ segment [134, 135]. A gene located near the breakpoint on the der (14q⁻) chromosome was identified [134] and cloned [135, 136]. The *ttg*-1 gene (T-cell translocation gene-1) [135] is transcribed from two distinct promoters with unrelated sequences. The gene has two alternative first exons which code for two species of proteins differing in a single amino acid [136]. The 1.4-kb cDNA encodes a potential zinc finger protein, which may bind DNA [135]. As yet it is unclear whether this gene is an oncogene, especially since our previous studies of Burkitt's lymphoma and follicular lymphoma translocations indicate that *myc* and *bcl*-2 deregulation occurs as a result of the juxtaposition of the oncogenes to immunoglobulin or TCR constant regions [46–52, 55–60, 137]. Nevertheless, additional studies on the oncogenic potential of this gene will answer this question.

6. Translocation at the lyl-1 locus on chromosome 19 band p13

In this locus a single case with t(7;19)(q35;p13) chromosomal translocation in acute T cell leukemia was repeated [138]. The translocation breakpoint involved the TCRβ Jβ.11 segment and a transcriptionally active region on chromosome 19p13 termed *lyl*-1 (lymphoid leukemia gene-1) [138]. The t(7;19) translocation breakpoint occurred in intron 1 of the *lyl*-1 gene, resulting in the loss of exon 1 and juxtaposition of the truncated *lyl*-1 gene with the TCRβ gene in opposite transcriptional orientation. The predicted *lyl*-1 product contains an HLH DNA binding domain also found in several proteins involved in the control of cell differentiation and proliferation [132].

7. The (7;9)(q34;q34) chromosomal translocation

The translocation breakpoint cloned from the T cell line SUpT1 occurred 5′ to the Dβ2.1–Jβ2.2 TCRβ rearranged segment on chromosome 7 band q34 and in a transcriptionally active sequence on chromosome 9 band q34 [139]. The nature of this gene and its pathogenic role was not reported.

8. Translocations involving the TCR gene and the c-myc oncogene

In this category the reported translocations juxtaposed TCRα/δ gene enhancer regions 3′ of the *myc* oncogene [137, 140–143]. These translocations are analogues to those found in Burkitt's lymphoma variant t(2;8) and (8;22) translocations, where one of the IgL chain genes (κ on chromosome 2 or λ on chromosome 22) is translocated to the 3′ end of *myc*. The reported translocations were detected in T cells [137, 140–142] and in a B cell line [143]. The translocations were probably mediated by recombinase, since heptamer-like sequences were detected in most of the cases [137, 140–143].

IV. Chromosomal translocations resulting in generation of chimeric proteins

In this category there are two known examples, the t(9;22) and the t(1;19) translocations which result in production of BCR-ABL and E2A-PRL chimeric proteins, respectively [144–152].

1. The Philadelphia chromosome

The Ph′ chromosome is a shortened chromosome 22 that arises from a reciprocal translocation t(9;22)(q34;q11) [13]. This cytogenetic aberration is detected in the majority (90–95%) of patients with CML and in much smaller proportions in patients with ALL (10–15%) or AML (~2%) [4]. A small subset of CML (<5%) usually exhibits variant Ph′ translocations, most of which seem to involve chromosome 9q34 [153, 154]. In some cases, where no cytogenetic evidence was available, detection of molecular rearrangements of the characteristic regions on chromosome 9 and 22 indicated the type of the disease [155]. The c-*abl* proto-oncogene, the cellular homologue of the Abelson murine leukemia virus transforming gene v-*abl* is located on the long arm of chromosome 9 band q34 in a region involved in the t(9;22) translocation [5, 156]. The c-*abl* locus spans at least 230 kb of genomic DNA, contains at least 11 exons and is oriented with its 5′ end towards the centromere [144, 145, 157]. The gene has two alternative first exons, 1a and 1b. Exon 1b is more than 200 kb proximal to the second exon; and exon 1a is 19 kb proximal to the second exon [145]. The consequence of this genomic organization is the production of two messages of 6 kb and 7 kb. The 6 kb consists of exons

1a through 11, while the 7 kb begins with exon 1b, omits exons 1a, and joins to exons 2 through 11. An analogous genomic organization was reported in mice, which have four types of c-abl transcripts with distinct first exons [158]. Thus, all c-abl transcripts share a set of 3' exons starting from exon 2. The splice-acceptor site associated with exon 2 is remarkable, since it can accept multiple exon donor sites and can ignore nearby exons in favor of those further away. These features are pivotal to the tumorigenicity of this gene, since they also permit c-abl to be fused with chromosome 22 sequences and thus become activated. Cloning of the t(9;22) translocation breakpoint regions revealed that the breakpoints on chromosome 9 occurred 5' to c-abl [156]. On chromosome 22, in most CML cases, the translocation breakpoints were clustered within a 5.8-kb region, termed the breakpoint cluster region (bcr) [159]. The bcr locus is transcriptionally active and spans at least 90 kb [146, 160, 161]. The bcr gene is transcribed as 4.5-kb and 6.7-kb mRNAs [144] which are expressed almost in all tissues examined [161]. The gene codes for a 160-kd protein (p160bcr) [162] with unknown physiological activity [161].

In most of the CML patients the breakpoint in the t(9;22) translocations occurred between bcr exons 2 and 3 or 3 and 4. As a result of the reciprocal translocation, the 3' bcr gene exons distal to the breakpoint within bcr are relocated to chromosome 9. Proximal 5' bcr exons (including exons 1 and 2 with or without exon 3) remain on chromosome 22. Simultaneously, the c-abl is translocated to chromosome 22q11. The breakpoints on chromosome 9 can be scattered over an extended region of ≥200 kb at the 5' end of the c-abl gene [157]. However, exons 2–11 are always included in the chromosome 9 region which is juxtaposed to chromosome 22; exons 1b and 1a can be included as well [144]. The end result of the translocation is that the proximal BCR gene sequences are juxtaposed to abl sequences in a head-to-tail fashion and form a chimeric bcr-abl gene on chromosome 22 [144]. Thus, during the process of mRNA formation, the splice-acceptor site associated with c-abl exon 2 can skip splice donor sites in c-abl exons 1b and 1a to fuse with the splice donor sites of the bcr-juxtaposed exons [145]. The chimeric bcr-abl is expressed as an 8.5-kb mRNA that codes for the p210 fusion protein [12, 163]. Another breakpoint region, associated frequently with the t(9;22) translocation in ALL, occurs within the first intron of the bcr gene. In these cases, only the first exon of the bcr gene is fused with c-abl [147] resulting in expression of a 7-kb bcr-abl chimeric transcript that codes for the p185 fusion protein [148–150, 164]. Variations in the bcr-abl p210 protein arise because of differences in transcripts which may or may not include bcr's exon 3 [165]. The c-abl protein, a 145-kd (p145cabl) is a tyrosin kinase protein; v-abl is formed by substitution of a gag (core) viral moiety for the N terminal part of c-abl. Hence, the v-abl 160-kd protein is a fusion gag-abl product. The gag-abl fusion protein

confers on the abl-MULV the capacity to transform a variety of hematopoietic cells in vitro [166, 167]. In vivo, v-abl causes primarily B-cell leukemias in susceptible murine hosts infected with abl-MULV [166, 167]. The p210 and p185 fusion proteins have tyrosine kinase activity, like the p160 v-abl fusion protein of the acutely transforming abl-MULV [164]. Since the tyrosine kinase activity of p160 is essential for cell transformation by abl-MULV [166, 167], the bcr-abl kinase activity of p210 and p185 is expected to be important in conferring a growth advantage to Ph'-positive cells.

2. The t(1;19)(q23;p13) chromosomal translocation

The t(1;19)(q23;p13) chromosomal translocation is a characteristic feature of approximately 30% of pre-B-cell leukemias and 6% of pediatric acute leukemias [168–170]. As a result of the translocation, a fusion protein is formed from joined regions of the E2A gene (a chromosome 19 gene which codes for the immunoglobulin-enhancer factors E12/E47 [171–172] and the PRL homeogene (a chromosome 1 pre-B-cell leukemia gene) [151, 152, 173]. The fusion protein has features of a chimeric transcription factor in which the DNA binding domain of E2A has been replaced by the putative DNA binding domain of the PRL gene [151, 152]. Two alternative splicing forms of the fusion protein exist, resulting in predicted products of 85 and 80 kd [151, 152]. RNase protection experiments and polymerase chain reaction analysis of RNA from cells carrying the t(1;19) translocation showed that, in all cases examined so far, the same E2A and PRL sequences are joined together [151]. This suggests that the specific fusion of these proteins is pathogenically important in leukemic cells carrying the t(1;19) translocation [151, 152]. The PRL gene codes for predicted 46- and 41-kd proteins which result from alternative 3' splicing [174]. All PRL-expressing cells contain both forms of the protein. Identical alternative splicing of the PRL portion in the E2A-PRL fusion transcript was also detected; its significance is unknown [151]. The PRL proteins have a homeodomain with 36% homology to the yeast MATal and 30% homology to any of the higher eukaryotic homeodomains [151].

Conclusion

The molecular analysis of cytogenetic abnormalities has proved to be useful in studying and understanding the malignant processes that arise due to perturbations in the functions of cellular proto-oncogenes [175]. The development of a large number of molecular probes has further improved our understanding and our ability to detect genetic changes unique to cancerous cells, such as deletions [176–178] and masked chromosomal translocations [179–181].

Tumor-specific probes that detect specific DNA rearrangement due to chromosomal translocations or deletions are unique diagnostic markers in monitoring the clonal expansion of tumor cells. The degree of detection is crucial in monitoring early relapse and minimal residual disease during clinical remission. Application of polymerase chain reaction technology further improves that diagnostic value of molecular probes [182, 183]. Finally, it is reasonable to predict that the knowledge acquired in studying the molecular genetic mechanisms that deregulate oncogenes will soon be applied in designing new therapies.

Acknowledgements

The authors are grateful to George F. Christopher and Pamela J. Bennett for help in preparation of this manuscript.

References

1. Yunis JJ. The chromosomal basis of human neoplasia. Science 1983; 221: 227–236.
2. Nowell PC, Hungerford DA. A minute chromosome in chronic granulocytic leukemia. Science 1960; 132: 1497.
3. Rowley JD. Identification of the constant chromosome regions involved in human hematologic malignant disease. Science 1973; 216: 749–751.
4. Fourth International Workshop on chromosomes in Leukemia. Abnormalities of chromosome 22. Cancer Genet Cytogenet 1982; 11: 316–18.
5. Bartram CR, de Klein A, Hagemeijer A, van Agthoven T, van Kessel AG, Bootsma D, Grosveld G, Ferguson-Smith MA, Davies T, Stone M, Heisterkamp N, Stephenson JR, Groffen J. Translocation of c-abl oncogene correlates with the presence of a Ph' chromosome in chronic myelocytic leukemia. Nature 1983; 306: 277–80.
6. Manolov G, Manolova Y. Marker band in one chromosome 14 from Burkitt's Lymphoma. Nature 1972; 237: 33–34.
7. Zech L, Haglund V, Nilson N, Klein G. Characteristic chromosomal abnormalities in biopsies and lymphoid cell lines from patients with Burkitt and non Burkitt lymphomas. Int J Cancer 1976; 17: 47–56.
8. Groffen J, Stephenson JR, Heisterkamp N, de Klein A, Bartram CR, Grosreld G. Philadelphia chromosomal breakpoints are clustered within limited region, bcr, on chromosome 22. Cell 1984; 36: 93–99.
9. Dalla-Favera R, Bregni M, Erikson J, Patterson D, Gallo RC, Croce CM. Assignment of the human c-myc oncogene to the region of chromosome which is translocated in Burkitts Lymphoma cells. Proc Natl Acad Sci USA 1982; 79: 7824–7827.
10. Dalla Favera R, Martinotti S, Gallo RC, Erikson J, Croce CM. Translocation and rearrangement of the c-myc oncogene in human differentiated B cell Lymphoma. Science 1983; 219: 963–967.
11. Klein G, Klein E. Evolution of tumors and impact of molecular oncology. Nature 1985; 315: 190–95.
12. Konopka JB, Watanabe SM, Witte ON. An alteration of the human c-abl protein in K562 leukemia cells unmasks associated tyrosine kinase activity cell 1984; 37: 1035–42.
13. Benjamin D, Magrath IT, Maguire R, Janus C, Todd HD, Parsons RG. Immunoglobulin secretion by cell lines derived from African and American undifferentiated lymphomas of Burkitt's and non Burkitt's type. J Immunol 1982; 129: 1336–42.
14. Croce CM, Shander M, Martinis J, Cicurel L, D'Ancona GG, Dolby TW, Koprovkski H. Chromosomal location of the human immunoglobulin heavy chain genes. Proc Natl Acad Sci USA 1979; 76: 3416–17.
15. Erikson J, Martinis J, Croce CM. Assignment of the human genes for lambda immunoglobulin chain to chromosome 22. Nature 1981; 294: 173–75.
16. McBride DW, Heiter PA, Hollis GF, Swan D, Otey MC, Leder P. Chromosomal location of human kappa and lambda immunoglobulin light chain constant region gene. J Exp Med 1982; 155: 1480–90.
17. Croce CM, Theirfelder W, Erikson J, Nishikura K, Finan J, Lenoir G, Nowell PC. Transcriptional activation of an unrearranged and untranslocated c-myc oncogene by translocation of a Cλ locus in Burkitt lymphoma cells. Proc Natl Acad Sci USA 1983; 80: 6922–26.
18. Erikson J, Nishikura K, ar-Rushdi A, Finan J, Emanuel BS, Lenoir G, Nowell PC, Croce CM. Translocation ofm an immunoglobulin k locus to a region 3' of an unrearranged c-myc oncogene enhances c-myc transcription. Proc Natl Acad Sci USA 1983; 80: 7581–85.
19. Haluska FG, Tsujimoto Y, Croce CM. The t(8;14) translocation of the Daudi endemic Burkitt's lymphoma occurred during immunoglobulin gene rearrangement and involve the D_H region. Proc Natl Acad Sci USA 1987; 84: 6835–6839.
20. Haluska FG, Finver S, Tsujimoto Y, Croce CM. The t(8;14) chromosomal translocation occurring in B-cell malignancies results from mistakes in V-D-J joining. Nature 1986; 324: 158–61.
21. Hayday AC, Gillies SD, Saito H, Wood C, Wiman K, Hayward WS, Tonegawa S. Activation of a translocated human c-MYC gene by an enhancer in the Immunoglobulin heavy chain locus. Nature 1984; 307: 334–340.
22. Battey J, Moulding C, Taub R, Murphy W, Stewart T, Potter H, Lenoir G, Leder P. The human c-myc oncogene: structural consequences of translocation into the IgH locus in Burkitt lymphoma. Cell 1983; 34: 779–87.
23. Hamlyn PH, Rabbits TH. Translocation joins c-myc and immunoglobulin γ_1 gene in Burkitt lymphoma revealing a third exon in the c-myc oncogene. Nature 1983; 304: 135–39.
24. Showe LC, Ballantine M, Nishikura K, Erikson J, Kaji H, Croce CM. Cloning and sequencing of a c-myc oncogene in Burkitt's Lymphoma cell line that is translocated to a germ line alpha switch region. Mol Cell Biol 1985; 5: 501–9.
25. Erikson J, Nishikura K, ar-Rushdi, Finan J, Emanuel B, Lenoir G, Nowell PC, Croce CM. Translocation of an immunoglobulin K locus to a region 3' of an unrearranged c-myc oncogene enhances c-myc transcription. Proc Natl Acad Sci USA 1983; 80: 7581–85.
26. Hartl P, Lipp M. Generation of a variant t(2;8) translocation of Burkitt's Lymphoma by site specific recombination via kappa light-chain joining signals. Mol Cell Biol 1987; 7: 2037.
27. Showe LC, Croce CM. The role of chromosomal translocations in B and T cell neoplasia. Ann Rev Immunol 1987; 5: 253–277.
28. Gemmill RM, Coyle-Morris J, Ware-Uribe L, Pearson N, Hecht F, Brown RS, Li PF, Drabkin HA. A 1.5 Megabase restriction map surrounding Myc does not include the translocation breakpoint in familial renal cell carcinoma. Genomics 1989; 4: 28–35.
29. Wiman KG, Clarkson B, Hayday AC, Saito H, Tonegawa S, Hayword WS. Activation of a translocated c-myc gene: Role of structural alterations in the upstream region. Proc Natl Acad Sci USA 1984; 81: 6798–67802.
30. Pelicci PG, Knowles DM, Magrath I, Dalla-Favera R. Chromosomal breakpoints and structural alterations of the c-myc locus differ in endemic and sporadic forms of Burkitt lymphoma. Proc Natl Acad Sci USA 1986; 83: 2984–88.
31. Gelman EP, Psallidopoulos MC, Papas T, Dalla-Favera R. Identification of reciprocal translocation sites within the c-myc oncogene and immunoglobulin μ locus in a Burkitt lymphoma. Nature 1983; 306: 799–803.

32. Sun LK, Showe LC, Croce CM. Analysis of the 3' flanking region of the human c-myc gene in lymphomas with the t(8;22) and t(2;8) chromosomal translocations. Nucleic Acids Res 1986; 14: 4037–50.

33. Henglein B, Synovzik H, Groitl P, Bornkamm GW, Hartl P, Lipp M. Three breakpoints of variant t(2;8) translocation in Burkitt's Lymphoma cell fall within a region 140 kb distal from myc. Mol Cell Biol 1989; 9: 2105–2113.

34. Mengle-Gaw L, Rabbits TH. A human chromosome 8 region with abnormalities in B cell, HTLV-1+T cell and c-myc amplified tumors. EMBO J 1987; 6: 1959–1965.

35. Shtivelman E, Henglein B, Groitl P, Lipp M, Bishop M. Identification of a human transcription unit affected by the variant chromosomal translocation 2;8 and 8;22 of Burkitt lymphoma. Proc Natl Acad Sci USA 1989; 86: 3257–3260.

36. Neri A, Barriga F, Knowles DM, Magrath I, Dalla-Favera R. Different regions of the immunoglobulin heavy chain locus are involved in chromosomal translocations in distinct pathogenetic forms of Burkitt lymphoma. Proc Natl Acad Sci USA 1988; 85: 2748–2752.

37. Haluska FG, Russo G, Kant J, Andreff M, Croce CM. Molecular resemblance of on Aids-associated lymphoma and endemic Burkitt lymphoma: Implications for their pathogenesis. Proc Natl Acad Sci 1989; 86: 8907–8911.

38. Haluska FG, Tsujimoto Y, Croce CM. Oncogene Activation by chromosome translocation in human malignancy. Ann Rev Genet 1987; 21: 321–45.

39. ar-Rushdi A, Nishikura K, Erikson J, Watt R, Rovera G, Croce CM. Differential expression of the translocated and untranslocated c-myc oncogene in Burkitt lymphoma. Science 1983; 222: 390–393.

40. Eick D, Bornkamm GW. Expression of normal and translocated c-myc alleles in Burkitt's lymphoma cells: evidence for different regulation. EMBO J 1989; 8: 1965–1972.

41. Nishikura K, ar-Rushdi A, Erikson J, DeJesus E, Dugan D, Croce CM. Repression of rearranged gene and translocated c-myc in mouse 3T3 cells × Burkitt lymphoma cell hybrids. Science 1984; 224: 399–402.

42. Nishikura K, Murray JM. The mechanism of inactivation of the normal c-myc gene locus in human Burkitt's lymphoma cells. Oncogene 1988; 2: 493–498.

43. Leder P, Battey J, Lenoir G, Moulding C, Murphy W, Potter H, Stewart T, Taub R. Translocations among antibody genes in human cancer. Science 1983; 222: 765–71.

44. Murphy N, Sarid J, Taub R, Vasicek T, Battey J, Lenoir G, Leder P. Translocated human c-myc oncogene is altered in a conserved coding sequences. Proc Natl Acad Sci USA 1986; 83: 2939–43.

45. Rabbitts PH, Forster A, Stinson MA, Rabbits TH. Truncation of exon 1 from the c-myc gene results in prolonged c-myc mRNA stability. EMBO J 1985; 4: 3727–33.

46. Croce CM, Nowell PC. Molecular basis of human B-cell neoplasia. Blood 1985; 65: 1–7.

47. Feo S, Harvey R, Showe L, Croce CM. Regulation of translocated c-myc genes transfected into plasmacytoma cells. Proc Natl Acad Sci USA 1986; 83: 706–9.

48. Richman A, Hayday A. Normal expression of a rearranged and mutated c-myc oncogene after stable transfection into fibroblasts. Science 1989; 246: 494–97.

49. Adams JM, Harris AW, Pinkert CA, Corcoran LM, Alexander WS, Cory S, Palmiter RD, Brinster RL. The c-myc oncogene driven by immunoglobulin enhancer induces lymphoid malignancy in transgenic mice. Nature 1985; 318: 533–38.

50. Langdon WY, Harris AW, Cory S, Adams JM. The c-myc oncogene perturbs B lymphocyte development in Eµ-myc transgenic mice. Cell 1986; 47: 11–18.

51. Leder A, Pattengale PK, Kuo A, Stewart TA, Leder P. Consequences of widespread deregulation of the c-myc gene in transgenic mice: multiple neoplasms and normal development. Cell 1986; 45: 485–95.

52. Schmidt EV, Pattengale PK, Weir L, Leder P. Transgenic mice bearing the human c-myc activated by an immunoglobulin enhancer. A pre B-cell lymphoma model. Proc Natl Acad Sci USA 1988; 85: 6047–6051.

53. Yancopoulos GD, Alt FW. Developmentarity controlled and tissue specific expression of unrearranged V_H gene segments. Cell 1985; 40: 271–81.

54. Yunis JJ, Frizzera G, Oken MM, McKenna J, Theologides A, Arnesen M. Multiple recurrent genomic defects in follicular lymphoma, a possible model for cancer. New England J Med 1987; 316: 79–84.

55. Tsujimoto Y, Finger LR, Yunis J, Nowell PC, Croce CM. Cloning of the chromosomal breakpoint of neoplastic B-cells with t(14;18) chromosome translocation. Science 1984; 226: 1097–94.

56. Tsujimoto Y, Cossman J, Jaffe E, Croce CM. Involvement of the bcl-2 gene in human follicular lymphoma. Science 1985; 228: 1440–43.

57. Cleary ML, Galili N, Sklar J. Detection of second t(14;18) breakpoint cluster region in human follicular lymphomas. J Exp Med 1986; 164: 315–320.

58. Tsujimoto Y, Bashir MM, Givol I, Cossman J, Jaffe E, Croce CM. The DNA rearrangements in human follicular lymphoma can involve the 5' or the 3' region of the bcl-2 gene. Proc Natl Acad Sci USA 1987; 84: 1329–1331.

59. Adachi M, Cossman J, Longo D, Croce CM, Tsujimoto. Variant translocation of the bcl-2 gene to IGλ in chronic lymphocytic leukemia. Proc Natl Acad Sci USA 1989; 86: 2771–2774.

60. Adachi M, Tefferi A, Greipp PR, Kipps TJ, Tsujimoto Y. Preferential linkage of BCL-2 to immunoglobulin light chain gene in chronic lymphocytic leukemia. J Exp Med 1990; 171: 559–564.

61. Cleary ML, Smith SD, Sklar J. Cloning and structural analysis of cDNAs for bcl-2 and a hybrid bcl-2/immunoglobulin transcript resulting from the t(14;18) translocation. Cell 1986; 47: 19–28.

62. Tsujimoto Y, Croce CM. Analysis of the structure, transcripts and protein products of bcl-2, the gene involved in human follicular lymphoma. Proc Natl Acad Sci USA 1986; 83: 5214–5218.

63. Ngan B-Y, Chen-Levy Z, Weiss LM, Warnke RA, Cleary ML. Expression in non Hodgkin lymphoma of the bcl-2 protein associated with the t(14;18) translocation. N Engl J Med 1988; 318: 1638–1644.

64. Chen-Levy Z, Nourse J, Cleary M. The bcl-2 candidate proto-ongogene product is a 24 kd integral-membrane protein highly expressed in lymphoid cell lines and lymphomas carrying the t(14;18) translocation. Mol Cell Biol 1989; 9: 701–710.

65. Haldar S, Beatty C, Tsujimoto Y, Croce CM. The bcl-2 gene encodes a novel G protein. Nature 1990; 342: 195–198.

66. Pezella F, Tse A, Cordell JL, Pulford KAF, Gatter KC, Mason DY. Expression of the bcl-2 oncogene protein is not specific for the 14;18 chromosomal translocation. Am J Pathol 1990; 137 (in press).

67. Monica K, Chen-Levy Z, Cleary M. Small G proteins are expressed ubiquitously in lymphoid cells and do not correspond to Bcl-2. Nature 1990; 346: 184–191.

68. Vaux DL, Cory S, Adams JM. Bcl-2 gene promotes haemopoietic cell survival and cooperates with c-myc in immortalized pre B-cells. Nature 1989; 335: 440–42.

69. Nunez G, Seto M, Seremetic S, Ferrero D, Grignani F, Korsmeyer S, Dalla-Favera R. Growth and tumor promoting effects of deregulates Bcl-2 in human B lymphoblastoid cells. Proc Natl Acad Sci USA 1989; 86: 4589–4593.

70. Tsujimoto Y. Overexpression of the human BCL-2 gene product results in growth enhancement of Epstein-Barr virus immortalized B cells. Proc Natl Acad Sci USA 1990; 86: 1958–1962.

71. McDonnell TJ, Deane N, Platt FM, Nunez G, Jaeger U,

18

Mckearn JP, Korsmeyer SJ. Bcl-2 immunoglobulin transgenic mice demonstrate extended B cell survival and follicular lymphoproliferation. Cell 1989; 57: 74–88.

72. Reed J, Holdar S, Cuddy M, Croce CM, Makover D. Deregulated Bcl-2 expression enhances growth of a human B cell line oncogene 1989; 4: 1123–1127.

73. Reed JC, Cuddy M, Haldar S, Croce CM, Nowell P, Makover D, Bradley K. Bcl-2 mediated tumorogenicity of a human T-lymphoid cell line: Synergy with Myc and inhibition by Bcl-2 antisense. Proc Natl Acad Sci USA 1990; 87: 3660–3664.

74. Reed JC, Haldar S, Croce CM, Cuddy MP. Transformation by complementing oncogenes that encode GTP binding proteins: Bcl-2 and HA-RAS. Mol Cell Biol 1990; (in press

75. Van-Den Bergh H, Vermaelen K, Louwagia A, Criel A, Mecucci C, Vaerman JP. High incidence of chromosome abnormalities in IgG3 myeloma 1984;

76. Erikson J, Finan J, Tsujimoto Y, Nowell P, Croce CM. The chromosome 14 breakpoint in neoplastic B cells with the t(11;14) translocation involves the immunoglobulin heavy chain locus. Proc Natl Acad Sci 1984; 81: 4144–48.

77. Tsujimoto Y, Yunis J, Onorato-Showe L, Erikson J, Nowell P, Croce CM. Molecular cloning of the chromosomal breakpoint of B cell lymphomas and leukemias with the t(11;14) chromosome translocation. Science 1984; 224: 1403–6.

78. Tsujimoto Y, Jaffe E, Cossman J, Gorham J, Nowell P, Croce CM. Clustering of breakpoints on chromosome 11 in human B cell neoplasms with the t(11;14) chromosome translocation. Nature 1986; 315: 340–43.

79. Louie E, Tsujimoto Y, Heubner K, Croce CM. Molecular cloning of the chromosomal breakpoint isolated from a B prolymphocytic leukemia patient carrying t(11;14)(q13;q32). Am J Hum Genet 1987; 41: 131 (suppl).

80. Rabbits P, Douglas J, Fischer P, Nachera E, Karpas A, Catovsky D, Melo J, Baer R, Stinson M, Rabbits T. Chromosome abnormalities at 11q13 in B cell tumors. Oncogene 1988; 3: 99–103.

81. Meeker TC, Grimaldi JC, O'Rourke R, Louie E, Juliusson G, Einhorn S. An additional breakpoint region in the BCL-1 locus associated with the t(11;14)(q13;q32) translocation of B lymphocytic malignancy. Blood 1989; 74: 1801–1806.

82. Bloomfield CD, Arthur DC, Frizzera G, Levine EG, Peterson BA, Gajl-Peczalska KJ. Nonrandom chromosome abnormalities in lymphom. Cancer Res 1983; 43: 2975–2984.

83. Ueshima Y, Bird ML, Vardiman J, Rowley J. A 14;19 translocation in B cell chronic lymphocytic leukemia: A new recurring chromosome aberration. Int J Cancer 1985; 36: 287–290.

84. McKeithan TW, Rowely JD, Shows TB, Diase MO. Cloning of the chromosome translocation breakpoint junction of the t(14;19) in chronic lymphocytic leukemia. Proc Natl Acad Sci USA 1987; 84: 9257–9260.

85. Ohno H, Takimoto G, McKeithan TW. The candidate proto-oncogene bcl-3 is related to genes implicated in cell lineage determination and cell cycle control. Cell 1990; 60: 991–997.

86. Simanis V, Nurse P. Characterization of the fission yeast cdc10⁺ protein that is required for commitment to the cell cycle J. Cell Sci 1989; 92: 51–56.

87. Carroll AJ, Raimondi SC, Williams D, Behm FG, Borowitz M, Castleberry RP, Harris MB, Patterson RB, Pullen DJ, Crist WM. t dic (9;12): A nonrandom chromosome abnormality in childhood B-cell precursor acute Lymphoblastic leukemia: a pediatric oncology group study. Blood 1987; 70: 1962–1965

88. Diaz M, Ziemin S, LeBeau MM, Pitha P, Smith SD, Chilcote RR, Rowley JD. Homozygous deletion of the α and β₁ interferon genes in human leukemia and derived cell lines. Proc Natl Acad Sci USA 1988; 35: 5259–5263.

89. Pellet P, Berger R, Bernheim A, Brouet JC, Tsapis A. Molecular analysis of a t(9;14)(p11;q32) translocation in a case of human heavy chain disease. Oncogene 1989; 4: 653–657.

90. Seligmann M, Danon F, Hurez D, Mihaesco E, Preud'Homme JL. Alpha chain disease: a new immunoglobulin abnormality. Science 1968; 162: 1396–1397.

91. Ohno H, Furukawa T, Fukuhara S, Zong SQ, Kamesaki H, Shows TB, LeBeau M, McKeithan TW, Kawakami T, Honjo T. Molecular analysis of a chromosomal translocation, t(9;14)(p13;q32), in a diffuse large cell lymphoma line expressing the Ki-1 antigen. Proc Natl Acad Sci USA 1990; 87: 628–632.

92. Hogan T, Koss W, Murgo A, Amato R, Fontana J, VanScoy F. Acute lymphoblastic leukemia with chromosomal 5;14 translocation and hypereosinophilia: case report and literature review. J Clin Oncol 1987; 5: 382–390.

93. Tono-oka T, Sato Y, Matsumoto T, Veno N, Ohkawa M, Shikano T, Takeda T. Hypereosinophilic syndrome in acute lymphoblastic leukemia with chromosome translocation t(5q;14q). Med Pediatr Oncol 1984; 12: 33.

94. Grimaldi JC, Meeker TC. The t(5;14) chromosomal translocation in a case of acute lymphocytic leukemia joins the interleukin-3 gene to the immunoglobulin heavy chain gene. Blood 1989; 73: 2081–2085.

95. Croce CM, Isobe M, Palumbo A, Puck J, Ming J, Tweardy D, Erikson J, Davis M, Rovera G. Gene for α-chain of human T cell receptor: location on chromosome 14 region involved in T cell neoplasms. Science 1985; 227: 1044–47.

96. Isobe M, Erikson J, Emanuel BS, Nowell PC, Croce CM. Location of gene for β subunit of human T cell receptor at band 7q35, a region prone to rearrangements in T cells. Science 1985; 228: 580–582.

97. Mure C, Waldmann RA, Morton CC, Bongiovanni KF, Waldmann TA, Showe LC, Seidman JG. Human γ chain gene are rearranged in leukemic T cells and map to the short arm of chromosome 7. Nature 1985; 316: 549–52.

98. Minden MD, Mak TW. The structure of the T cell antigen receptor genes in normal and malignant T cells. Blood 1986; 68: 327–36.

99. Hecht F, Morgan R, Hecht BKM, Smith SD. Common region on chromosome 14 in T cell leukemia and lymphoma. Science 1984; 226: 1445–47.

100. Zech L, Gahrton G, Hammarstrom L, Julisson G, Mellstedt H, Robert KH, Smith CIE. Inversion of chromosome 14 marks human T-cell chronic lymphocytic leukemia. Nature 1984; 308: 858–60.

101. Baer R, Foster A, Rabbitts TH. The mechanism of chromosome 14 inversion in a human T cell lymphoma. Cell 1987; 50: 97–105.

102. Denny CT, Hollis GF, Hecht F, Morgan R, Link MP, Smith SD, Kirsh LR. Common mechanism of chromosomal inversion in B and T cell tumors. Science 1986; 234: 197–200.

103. Stern MH, Lipkowitz S, Aurias A, Griscelli C, Thomas G, Kirsh IR. Inversion of chromosome 7 in ataxia telangiectasia is generated by a rearrangement between T-cell receptor β and T cell receptor γ genes. Blood 1989; 74: 2076–2080.

104. Tycko B, Palmer JD, Sklar J. T cell receptor gene transrearrangements: chimeric γ/δ genes in normal lymphoid tissues. Science 1989; 245: 1242–46.

105. Bear R, Forster A, LaVenir I, Rabbitts TH. Immunoglobulin V_H gene are transcribed by T cells in association with a new 5′ exon. J Exp Med 1988; 167: 2011–2016.

106. Mengle-Gaw L, Albertson DG, Sherrington PD, Rabbits TH. Analysis of a T cell tumor-specific breakpoint cluster at human chromosome 14q32. Proc Natl Acad Sci USA 1988; 85: 9171–9175.

107. Russo G, Isobe M, Gatti R, Finan J, Batuman O, Hubner K, Nowell PC, Croce CM. Molecular analysis of a t(14;14) translocation in leukemic T cells of an ataxia telangiectasia patient. Proc Natl Acad Sci USA 1989; 86: 602–606.

108. Russo G, Isobe M, Pegoraro L, Finan J, Nowell PC, Croce CM. Molecular analysis of a t(7;14)(q35;q32) chromosome translocation in a T cell leukemia of a patient with ataxia telangiectasia. Cell 1988; 53: 137–144.

109. Mengle-Gaw L, Willard HF, Smith CIE, Hammarstrom L, Fischer P, Sherrington P, Lucas G, Thompson PW, Baer R, Rabbitts TH. Human T cell tumors containing chromosome 14 inversion or translocation with breakpoints proximal to immunoglobulin joining region at 14q32. EMBO J 1987; 6: 2273–2280.

110. Baer R, Heppel A, Taylor AMR, Rabbitts PH, Boullier B, Rabbitts TH. The breakpoint of an inversion chromosome 14 in a T cell leukemia: sequences down stream of the immunoglobulin heavy chain locus are implicated in tumorigenesis. Proc Natl Acad Sci USA 1987; 84: 9069–9073.

111. Davey MP, Bertness V, Nakahara K, Johnson JP, McBride DW, Waldman TA, Kirsh IR. Juxtaposition of the T cell receptor α-chain locus (14q11) and region (14q32) of potential importance in leukemogenesisi by a 14;14 translocation in a patient with T cell chronic lymphocytic leukemia and ataxia-telangiectasia. Proc Natl Acad Sci USA 1988; 85: 9287–9291.

112. Bertness VL, Felix CA, McBride OW, Morgan R, Smith SD, Sandberg AA, Kirsh IR. Characterization of the breakpoint of a t(14;14)(q11.2;q32) from the leukemic cells of a patient with T-cell Acute Lymphoblastic Leukemia. Cancer Genet Cytogenet 1990; 44: 47–54.

113. Williams DL, Look AT, Melvin SL, Robertson PK, Dahl G, Flake T, Stass S. New chromosomal translocations correlate with specific immunophenotypes of childhood acute lymphoblastic leukemia. Cell 1984; 36: 101–109.

114. Erikson J, Williams DL, Finan J, Nowell PC, Croce CM. Locus of the α-chain of the T cell receptor is split by chromosome translocation in T cell leukemias. Science 1985; 229: 784–786.

115. Boehm T, Buluwela L, Williams SD, White L, Rabbits TH. A cluster of chromosome 11p13 translocations found via distinct D-D and D-D-J rearrangements of the human T cell receptor δ chain gene. EMBO J 1988; 7: 2011–2017.

116. Foroni L, Bohem T, Lampert F, Kaneko Y, Raimondi S, Rabbitts TH. Multiple methylation-free islands flank a small breakpoint cluster region on 11p13 in the t(11;14)(p13;q11) translocation. Gen Ch and Cancer 1990; 1: 301–309.

117. Dube' I, Raimondi S, Pi D, Kalousek DK. A new translocation, t(10;14)(q24;q11), in T cell. Neoplasia. Blood 1986; 67: 1181–1184.

118. Raimondi S, Behm FG, Roberson PK, Pui CH, Rivera GK, Murphy SB, Williams D. Cytogenetics of childhood T cell leukemia. Blood 1988; 72: 1560–66.

119. Kagan J, Finan J, Letofsky J, Besa EC, Nowell PC. α-chain locus of the T-cell antigen receptor is involved in the t(10;14) chromosome translocation of T cell acute lymphocytic leukemia. Proc Natl Acad Sci USA 1987; 84: 4543–4546.

120. Kagan J, Finger LR, Letofsky J, Finan J, Nowell PC, Croce CM. Clustering of breakpoints on chromosome 10 in acute T cell leukemias with the t(10;14) chromosome translocations. Proc Natl Acad Sci USA 1989; 86: 4161–65.

121. Zutter M, Hockett RD, Roberts CWM, McGuire EA, Bloomstone J, Morton CC, Deaven LL, Crist WM, Carroll AJ, Korsmeyer SJ. The t(10;14)(q24;q11) of T cell acute lymphoblastic leukemia juxtaposes the δ-T cell receptor with TCL-3, a conserved and activated locus at 10q24. Proc Natl Acad Sci USA 1990; 87: 3161–3165.

122. Redondo JM, Hata S, Brocklehurst C, Karangel MS. A T cell-specific transcriptional enhancer within the human T cell receptor δ locus. Science 1990; 247: 1225–29.

123. Boehm T, Mengle-Gaw L, Kees UR, Spurr N, Lavenir I, Forster A, Rabbitts TH. Alternating purine-pyrimidine tracsmay promote chromosomal translocation seen in a variety of human lymphoid tumors. EMBO J 1989; 8: 2621–2631.

124. Raimondi SC, Pui CH, Behm FG, Williams DL 7q32–q36 translocations in childhood T cell leukemia: cytogenetic evidence for involvement of TCR$_\beta$ chain gene. Blood 1987; 69: 131–134.

125. Balaban GB, Herlyn M, Clark WM, Nowell PC. Karyotypic evolution in human malignant melanoma. Cancer Genet Cytogenet 1986; 19: 113–122.

126. Gilbert F, Balaban G, Moorhead P, Bianchi D, Schlesinger H. Abnormalities in chromosome 1p in human neuroblastoma tumors and cell lines. Cancer Genet Cytogenet 1982; 7: 33–42.

127. Finger LR, Kagan J, Christopher G, Kurtzberg J, Hershfield MS, Nowell PC, Croce CM. Involvement of the TCL-5 gene on human chromosome 1 in T cell leukemia and melanoma. Proc Natl Acad Sci USA 1989; 86: 5039–5043.

128. Begley CG, Aplan PD, Davey MP, Nakahara K, Tchorz K, Kurtzberg J, Hershfield MS, Haynes BF, Cohen DI, Waldman TA, Kirsch IR. Chromosomal translocation in human leukemic stem-cell line disrupts the T cell antigen receptor δ-chain diversity region and results in previously unreported fusion transcript. Proc Natl Acad Sci USA 1989; 86: 2031–2035.

129. Bernard O, Guglielmi P, Jonreaux P, Cherif D, Gisselbrecht S, Mauchaufte M, Berger R, Larsen CJ, Mathieu-Mahul D. Two distinct mechanisms for the SCL gene activation in the t(1;4) translocation of T cell leukemias. Genes Ch and Cancer 1990; 1: 194–208.

130. Chen Q, Cheng JT, Tsai LH, Schneider N, Buchanan G, Carroll A, Crist W, Ozanne B, Siciliano MJ, Baer R. The tal gene undergoes chromosome translocations in T cell leukemia and potentially encodes a helix-loop-helix protein. EMBO 1990; 9: 415–424.

131. Begley CG, Aplan PD, Danning SM, Haynes BF, Waldman TA, Kirsh IR. The gene SCL is expressed during early hematopoiesis and encodes a differentiation-related DNA-binding morif. Proc Natl Acad Sci USA 1989; 86: 10128–10132.

132. Mellentin SD, Smith SD, Cleary ML. lyl-1, a novel gene altered by chromosomal translocation in T cell leukemia, codes for a protein with a helix-loop-helix DNA binding motif cell. 1989; 58: 77–83.

133. LeBeau MM, McKeithan TW, Shima FA, Goldman-Leikin RE, Chan SJ, Bell GI, Rowley JD, Diaz MO. T cell receptor α-chain gene is split in a human T cell line with a t(11;14)(p15;q11). Proc Natl Acad Sci USA 1986; 83: 9744–9748.

134. Boehm T, Baer R, Lavenir I, Forster A, Waters JJ, Nacheva E, Rabbitts TH. The mechanism of chromosomal translocation t(11;14) involving the T cell receptor Cδ locus on human chromosome 14q11 and a transcribed region of chromosome 11p15. EMBO J 1988; 7: 385–394.

135. McGuire EA, Hockett RD, Pollock KM, Bartholdi MF, O'Brien SJ, Korsmeyer SJ. The t(11;14)(p15;q11) in a T cell a acute Lymphoblastic leukemia cell line activates multiple transcripts, including Ttg-1, a gene encoding a potential zinc finger protein. Mol Cell Biol 1989; 9: 2124–2132.

136. Boehm T, Greenberg JM, Buluwela L, Lavenir I, Forster A, Rabbitts TH. An unusual structure of putative T cell oncogene which allows production of similar proteins from distinct mRNA. EMBO J 1990; 9: 857–868.

137. Finger LR, Harvey RC, Moore RC, Showe LC, Croce CM. A common mechanism of chromosomal translocation in T and B cell neoplasia. Science 1986; 234: 982–85.

138. Cleary ML, Mellentin JD, Spies J, Smith SD. Chromosomal translocation involving the β T cell receptor gene in acute leukemia J Exp Med 1988; 167: 682–87.

139. Reynolds TC, Smith SD, Sklar J. Analysis of DNA surrounding the breakpoints of chromosomal translocations involving the β T cell receptor gene in human Lymphoblastic Neoplasms. Cell 1987; 50: 107–117.

140. Boehm T, Rabbitts TH. The human T cell receptor genes are targets for chromosomal abnormalities in T cell tumors. FABSEB J 1989; 3: 2344–2359.

141. Mathieu-Mahul D, Sigaux F, Zhu C, Bernheim A, Mauchauffe M, Daniel MT, Berger R, Larsen CJ. A t(8;14)(q24;q11) translocation in a T cell leukemia (L1-ALL) with c-myc and

20

TCR alpha chain locus rearrangements. Int J Cancer 1986; 38: 835–840.

142. McKeithan TW, Shima EA, LeBeau MM, Minowada J, Rowley JD, Diaz MO. Molecular cloning of the breakpoint junction of human chromosomal 8;14 translocation involving the TCRα chain gene and sequence on the 3′ side of Myc. Proc Natl Acad Sci USA 1986; 83: 6636–40.

143. Park JK, McKeithan TW, LeBeau MM, Bitter MA, Franklin WA, Rowley JD, Diaz MD. An (8;14)(q24;q11) translocation involving the T cell receptor α chain gene and the Myc oncogene 3′ region in a B cell lymphoma. Gene Ch and Cancer 1989; 1: 15–22.

144. Shtivelman E, Lifshitz B, Gale RP, Canaani E. Fused transcript of abl and bcr genes in chronic myelogenous leukemia. Nature 1985; 315: 550–4.

145. Shtivelman E, Lifshitz B, Gale RP, Roe BA, Canaani E. Alternative splicing of RNAs transcribed from human abl gene and from the bcr-abl fused gene. Cell 1986; 47: 277–84.

146. Paskind M, Witte ON. Overlapping cDNA clones define the complete coding region for the p210^{c-abl} gene product associated with chronic myelogenenous leukemia cells containing the Philadelphia chromosome. Proc Natl Acad Sci USA 1986; 83: 9768–72.

147. Hermans A, Heisterkamp N, vonLindern M, Van Baal S, Meijer D, vanderPlas D, Wiedemann LM, Groffen J, Bootsma D, Grosveld G. Unique fusion of bcr and c-abl genes in Philadelphia chromosome positive acute lymphoblastic leukemia. Cell 1987; 51: 33–40.

148. Kurzrock R, Shtalrid M, Romero P, Kloetzer WS, Talpas M, Trujillo, Blick M, Beran M, Gutterman J. A novel c-abl protein product in Philadelphia positive acute lymphoblastic leukemia. Nature 1987; 325: 631–635.

149. Fainstein E, Marcelle C, Rosner A, Canaani E, Gale RP, Dreazen O, Smith SD, Croce CM. A new fused transcript in Philadelphia chromosome positive acute lymphocytic leukemia. Nature 1987; 330: 386–88.

150. ar-Rushdi A, Negrini M, Kurzrock R, Huebner K, Croce CM. Fusion of the bcr and the c-abl genes in Ph′-positive acute lymphocytic leukemia with no rearrangement in the breakpoint cluster region. Oncogene 1988; 2: 353–357.

151. Nourse J, Mellentin JD, Galili N, Wilkinson J, Stanbridge E, Smith SD, Cleary M. Chromosomal translocation t(1;19) results in synthesis of a homeobox fusion mRNA that codes for a potential chimeric transcription factor. Cell 1990; 60: 535–345.

152. Kamps M, Murre C, Sun X, Baltimor D. A new homeobox gene contributes the DNA binding domain of the t(1;19) translocation protein in Pre-B ALL. Cell 1990; 60: 547–555.

153. Hagemeijer A, Bartrum CR, Smit EME, van Agthoven AJ, Bootsma D. Is the chromosomal region 9q34 always involved in variants of the Ph′ translocations? Cancer Genet cytogenet 1984; 13: 1–6.

154. Ishihara T, Minamihisamatsu M, Tosuji H. Chromosome 9 in variant Ph′ translocations. Cancer Genet cytogenet 1985; 14: 183–84.

155. Bartram CR, Kleinhauer E, de Klein A, Grosveld G, Teyssier JR, Heisterkamp N, Groffen J. c-abl and bcr are rearranged in a Ph′ negative CML patients. EMBO J 1985; 4: 683–86.

156. Heisterkamp N, Stephenson JR, Groffen J, Hansen PF, de Klein A, Bartram CR, Grosveld G. Localization of the c-abl oncogene adjacent to a translocation breakpoint in chronic myelocytic leukemia. Nature 1983; 306: 239–42.

157. Bernards A, Rubin CM, Westbrook CA, Paskind M, Baltimore D. The first intron in the human c-abl gene is at least 200 kb long and is a target for translocations in chronic myelogenous leukemia. Mol Cell Biol 1987; 7: 3231–6.

158. Ben-Neriah Y, Bernards A, Paskind M, Daley GQ, Baltimore D. Alternative 5′ exons in ce-abl mRNA. Cell 1986; 44: 577–86.

159. Groffen J, Stephenson JR, Heisterkamp N, de Klein A, Bartram CR, Grosveld G. Philadelphia chromosomal breakpoints are clustered within a limited region, bcr, on chromosome 22. Cell 1984; 36: 93–99.

160. Hesterkamp N, Stam K, Groffen J, de Klein A, Grosveld G. Structural organization of the bcr gene and its role in the Ph′ translocation. Nature 1985; 315: 758–61.

161. Hariharan IK, Adams JM. CDNA sequence for human bcr gene that translocates to the abl oncogene in chronic myeloid leukemia. EMBO J 1987; 6: 115–9.

162. Stam K, Heisterkamp N, Reynolds FH, Groffen J. Evidence that the Ph′ gene encodes a 160,000 dalton phosphoprotein with associated kinase activity. Mol Cell Biol 1987; 7: 1955–60.

163. Kloetzer W, Kurzrock R, Smith L, Talpaz M, Spiller M, Gutterman J, Arlinghaus RB. The human cellular abl gene product in the chronic myelogenous leukemia cell line K562 has an associated tyrosine protein kinase activity. Virology 1985; 140: 230–8.

164. Clark SS, McLaughlin J, Crist WM, Champlin R, Wittee ON. Unique forms of the abl tyrosine kinase distinguish Ph′-positive CML from Ph′-positive ALL. Science 1987; 235: 85–88.

165. Kurzrock R, Kloetzer WS, Talpaz M, Blick M, Walters R, Arlinghaus RB, Gutterman JU. Identification of molecular variants of p210$^{bcr-abl}$ in chronic myelogenous leukemia. Blood 1987; 70: 233–236.

166. Whitlock CA, Wittee ON. The complexity of virus-cell interactions in Abelson Virus infection of lymphoid and other hematopoietic cells. Adv Immunol 1985; 37: 73–98.

167. Knopka JB, Wittee ON. Activation of the abl oncogene in murine and human leukemias. Biochim Biophys Acta 1985; 823: 1–17.

168. Williams DL, Look AT, Melvin SL, Roberson PK, Dahl G, Flake T, Stass S. New chromosomal translocations correlate with specific immunophenotypes of childhood acute lymphoblastic leukemia. Cell 1984; 36: 101–109.

169. Carroll AJ, Crist WM, Parmley RT, Roper M, Cooper MD, Finley WM. Pre B cell leukemia associated with chromosome translocation 1 : 19. Blood 1984; 63: 721–724.

170. Michael PM, Garson OM, Collen DF. A review of the t(1;19) breakpoints in acute lymphocytic leukemia. Cancer Genet Cytogenet 1985; 17: 79–80.

171. Murre C, McCaw PS, Baltimore D. A new DNA binding and dimerization motif in immunoglobulin enhancer binding, daughterless Myod and Myc proteins. Cell 1989; 56: 777–783.

172. Henthorn P, Kiledjian M, Kadesch T. Two distinct transcriptional factors that bind the immunoglobulin enhancer μE5/μE2. Motif Science 1990; 247: 467–470.

173. Mellentin JD, Murre C, Donlon TA, McCaw PS, Smith SD, Carroll AJ, McDonald ME, Baltimore D, Cleary ML. The gene for enhancer binding protein E12/EU7 lies at the t(1;19) breakpoint in acute leukemias. Science 1989; 246: 379–382.

174. Galili N, Nourse J, Cleary M. Characterization of a novel homeobox gene on chromosome 19p13 which is structurally altered by the 1;19 translocation in pre B cell ALL. The first meeting on The Molecular basis of human cancer. 1990.

175. Bishop MJ. The Molecular genetics of Cancer. Science 1987; 235: 305–311.

176. Hansen MF, Cavenee WK. Genetics of Cancer predisposition Cancer Res 1987; 47: 5518–5527.

177. Flaron ER, Feinberg AP, Hamilton SH, Vogelstein B. Loss of genes on short arm of chromosome 11 in bladder cancer. Nature 1985; 318: 377–380.

178. Scrabble HJ, Witte DP, Lampkin BC, Cavenee WK. Chromosomal localization of the human rhabdomyosarcoma locus by mitotic recombination mapping. Nature 1987; 329: 645–647.

179. Finger LR, Huebner K, Canizzaro LA, McLeod K, Nowell PC, Croce CM. Chromosomal translocation in T cell leukemia line Hut 78 results in a Myc fusion transcript. Proc Natl Acad Sci USA 1988; 85: 9158–9162.

180. Aghib DF, Bishop JM, Otto lenghi S, Guerrasio A, Serra A, Saglio G. A 3′ truncation of Myc caused by chromosomal

translocation in a human T-cell leukemia increases mRNA stability. Oncogene 1990; 5: 707–711.

181. Gauwerky CE, Huebner K, Isobe M, Nowell PC, Croce CM. Activation of Myc in a masked t(8; 17) translocation results in an aggressive B cell leukemia. Proc Natl Acad Sci USA 1989; 86: 8867–8871.

182. Lee MS, Chang KS, Cabanillas F, Freireich EJ, Trujillo JM, Stass SA. Detection of minimal residual cells carrying the t(14;18) by DNA sequence amplication. Science 1987; 237: 175–178.

183. Kagan J, Finger LR, Besa E, Croce CM. Detection of minimal residual disease in leukemic patients with the t(10;14)(q24;q11) chromosome translocation. Cancer Research 1990; 50: 5240–5244.

Correspondence to:
Carlo M. Croce, M.D.
Fels Institute for Cancer Research
and Molecular Biology
Temple University School of Medicine
3420 North Broad Street
Philadelphia, Pennsylvania 19140, USA

Annals of Oncology, Supplement 2 to Volume 2: 23–28, 1991.
© 1991 *Kluwer Academic Publishers.*

Original article

An epidemiologist's view of the new molecular biology findings in Hodgkin's disease

Nancy Mueller*
Harvard School of Public Health, Boston, Massachusetts, USA

Summary. Recent advances in molecular biology provide new strategies to address the pathogenesis of Hodgkin's disease (HD). Immunophenotyping studies of Reed-Sternberg cells suggest lymphoid cells, 'frozen in a state of activation.' Clonal rearrangement studies find heavy and light chain immunoglobulin and β and Γ T-cell receptor gene changes. Chromosomal studies find a complex but nonrandom mixture of structural rearrangements including many seen in other hematologic disorders. These findings are consistent with a pathogenesis involving chronic antigenic stimulation. This interpretation is supported by the epidemiologic features of HD which suggest that HD may develop as a rare consequence of infection with a common latent virus where risk is increased if infection is delayed until adolescence or young adulthood. Such 'late' infections are generally more clinically severe and may result in more chronicity of virus replication. Serologic and genome probe studies of the Epstein-Barr virus – a candidate agent – in HD specimens support this hypothesis. In summary, the new molecular biology findings in HD converge with the previous epidemiologic, immunologic, and clinical data to support a unifying hypothesis of pathogenesis in which genetic abnormalities occur secondarily to a sustained host response to chronic tissue-based antigenic stimulation.

Key words: epidemiology, Epstein-Barr virus, Hodgkin's disease, molecular biology, pathogenesis

The pathogenesis of Hodgkin's disease (HD) has long been a matter of contention. The admixture of the features of a chronic infectious process and of a complex immune disorder with those of malignancy perplex the clinician, basic scientist, and epidemiologist alike. The continuing saga over the cellular origin of the Reed-Sternberg cell is an earmark of the lack of consensus on the fundamental nature of this disease.

Recent advances in the application of molecular biology have provided new strategies for attacking this question. These include immunophenotyping of Reed-Sternberg cells, immunogenotyping of clonal gene rearrangements, the use of viral-specific genetic probes, all coupled with renewed interest in chromosomal analyses. The purpose of this review is to interpret the recent findings of these new approaches within the framework of the unique epidemiologic features of HD.

In their succinct report from the First International Symposium on Hodgkin's Lymphoma in 1987 concerning the nature of the Hodgkin cell, Drexler and Leber note that 'virtually every cell in the hematopoietic system (the rarer and more obscure, the better) has been blamed: lymphocytes (T, B, or non-T/non-B), macrophages, monocytes, myeloid cells, dendritic cells' [1]. They conclude that genotypically the cells are lymphoid precursors and phenotypically they are lymphoid cells, 'frozen in a state of activation.' Counter arguments in favor of an activated macrophage origin have also been recently put forth [2, 3]. Of note, all agree that the Reed-Sternberg cell reflects immune activation.

More recently, molecular probes for immunoglobulin and T-cell receptor genes became available. Used in immunogenotypic analysis, these probes make it possible not only to distinguish T and B lymphocytes but also to identify clonal rearrangements. These techniques have been widely applied to the analysis of tissue from HD cases. In 1988, Griesser and Mak [4] reviewed the immunogenotypic findings in 112 cases. They reported that clonal rearrangements of T-cell receptor gamma- and beta-chain genes, as well as immunoglobulin heavy- and light-chain genes, were detected in a subset of cases. These findings argue that clonal T or B lymphocytic cell populations are frequently present. However, no one pattern was uniformly found, nor were gene rearrangements detected in all cases. Griesser and Mak also reported that the size of the clonal cell population as estimated by the intensity of the rearranged bands does not correlate with the number of Reed-Sternberg cells in the specimens. Given the mixed cellular environment which is the hallmark of HD, these rearrangements may not necessarily

* Dr. Mueller is a recipient of an American Cancer Society Faculty Research Award.

Table 1. Summary of immunoglobulin gene and T-cell receptor gene rearrangements in tissue from Hodgkin's disease cases.

Study	Number of cases	Immuno-globulin		T-cell receptor	
		Heavy	Light	β	Γ
Griesser *et al.* [5, 6]	22	0.09*		0.18	0.68
Knowles *et al.* [7]	15	0.13		0.07	
Weiss *et al.* [8]	8	0.50	0.75	0	
Brinker *et al.* [9]	11	0.36	0.45	0	
O'Connor *et al.* [10]	35	0.06	0.06	0	
Sundeen *et al.* [11]	8	0.25	0.13	0	
Raghavachar *et al.* [12]	32	0.16	0	0	0
Roth *et al.* [13]	14	0	0	0.07	0.07
Daus *et al.* [14]	13	0.08		0.31	
Herbst *et al.* [15]	39	0.10	0.03	0.15	0.06
	197	0.16**		0.08	

Adapted from Dexler *et al.* [16].
* Proportion positive.
** Proportion positive either or both heavy and light chain genes.

occur in the Reed-Sternberg or Hodgkin's cell populations themselves.

Subsequent studies generally confirmed these findings, although fewer clonal rearrangements of T-cell receptor gamma-chain genes have been reported. Table 1 summarizes the studies to date. Overall, about one in four cases have been found to have a clonal rearrangement. Several investigators have attempted to separate the Reed-Sternberg cells from other cells to show the specificity of association. However, absolute certainty that these rearrangements occur only in the putative malignant cell is not possible. In reviewing all of these data, Drexler et al. [16] reiterate the conclusion that the Reed-Sternberg cell derives from either a T or B lymphocyte, possibly depending on the type of HD.

The data from chromosomal studies are less clear (Table 2). These studies have been fraught with technical difficulties given the overall low mitotic activity of HD tissue. Cabanillas [17] recently reviewed the frequency of detection of structural chromosomal abnor-

malities in five case series involving 44 patients and five cell lines. Of these, there were 35% with abnormalities of 14q, 32% of 11q, 18% of 8q, and 32% of 6q. The most commonly recurring abnormality was 14q32. This is noteworthy, since 14q32 is the location of the immunoglobulin heavy-chain genes, and abnormalities at this site are associated with B-cell lymphoid disorders. The other structural abnormalities also correspond to those seen in other hematologic disorders. For 11q, the most common point of breakage was in region 11q/21–23, which has also been observed in a subset of childhood acute lymphocytic leukemia. The most common point of breakage of chromosome 6 was at 6q23, and for chromosome 8, 8q22/24. Cabanillas points out that deletion of 6q is typical in large-cell lymphoma and translocations of 8q24 are common in Burkitt's lymphoma.

In a later review which partially overlaps with that of Cabanillas, Thangavelu and Le Beau [23] provide some support that the same structural rearrangement sites recur. Again, translocation of 14q32 was the most common (4 of 25). However, other sites were also involved, notably 1p, 1q, 2q, 11p, and 22q. These authors concur that the structural rearrangements are nonrandom.

In sum, not all HD patients show evidence of chromosomal abnormalities, and although structural rearrangements seen in other lymphoid diseases are common, none are universal. The sites of T-cell receptor genes are not evident. The most persistent finding is translocation of 8q24, site of the immunoglobulin heavy-chain genes. These findings suggest that the chromosomal damage may be secondary to enhanced mitotic activity, rather than primary to pathogenesis.

These findings of a phenotype of an activated lymphocyte, clonal rearrangements of immunoglobulin and T-cell receptor genes, and relatively frequent occurrence of chromosomal rearrangements of regions containing immune function genes, are consistent with the complex immunologic profile of HD patients. As extensively reviewed by Romagnani et al. [24], patients show impairment of delayed-type hypersensitivity, en-

Table 2. Summary of studies on the presence of selected structural chromosomal abnormalities in tissue from Hodgkin's disease cases.

Study		Location of structural rearrangements			
		14q	11q	8q	6q
Hossfeld *et al.* [18]	6	0.33	0.50	0.17	0.17
Reeves *et al.* [19]	5	0.40	0	0	0.80
Fleishman [20]	15	0.40			
Fonatsch *et al.* [21]	5	0.40	0.40	0.20	0.20
Cabanillas *et al.* [22]	18	0.28	0.33	0.22	0.28
Total	49	0.35	0.32	0.18	0.32
Thangavelu *et al.* [23]	40	0.13	0.15	0.05	0.23

* Modified from Cabanillas, 1988.
** These data include the first two reports summarized above.

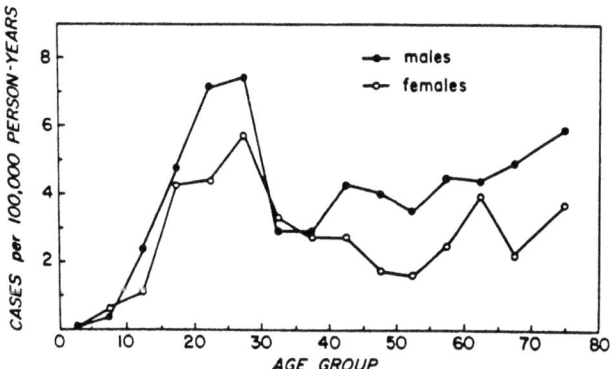

Fig. 1. Age-specific incidence rates of HD in the Boston and Worcester, Massachusetts (USA), standard metropolitan statistical areas from mid-1973 through 1977, by sex, based on the estimated population in 1975. Reprinted with permission of the New England Journal of Medicine [28].

hanced immunoglobulin production, high levels of circulating immune complexes, production of antilymphocyte and anti-Ia antibodies, and a variety of serum factor abnormalities. In vitro, peripheral lymphocytes exhibit spontaneous DNA and IgG synthesis, yet have depressed proliferative response to T-cell mitogen stimulation. Ford et al. [25, 26] have proposed that the primary immune defect is the deficiency of interleukin-2 (IL-2) production by T cells upon activation by macrophage-processed antigen. However, the majority of patients have significantly high serum levels of soluble IL-2 receptors [27]. This suggests that there is a chronic stimulation by IL-2 in these patients, which may result in a down-regulation in IL-2 production.

The picture that emerges from all the biologic evidence is of sustained antigenic stimulation [24]. The question is, how does this fit with the epidemiology of HD? The answer is, rather well. Epidemiologic research on HD has been driven – to a large extent – by the need to explain its unusual age-specific incidence curve. Unlike most malignancies where incidence follows an exponential increase with age beginning in early middle age, HD has a bimodal distribution. Typical of data from economically advantaged populations are those from eastern Massachusetts in the late 1970s (Figure 1) [28]. In such populations there is very low incidence in childhood, a rapid increase of incidence among teenagers which peaks about age 25, followed by a decrease to a plateau through middle age. Beginning about age 50, incidence rates increase with advancing age to the second peak. There is generally a male excess in both peaks. In 1957, MacMahon [29] proposed that this bimodality results from the overlap of two disease distributions with differing peak ages. More specifically, he proposed that among young adults, HD is caused by a biologic agent of low infectivity, while among older persons, the cause is probably similar to those of the other lymphomas [30].

In 1971, Correa and O'Conor [31] noted that among low-income populations, a different age pattern is evident. In such populations, there is an early peak in childhood – especially among boys – with no peak evident among young adults. Intermediate patterns also occur. Longitudinal data have shown transition in population curves in parallel with economic development [32, 33].

These observations, coupled by analogy with the epidemiology of paralytic poliomyelitis in the prevaccine era, led to a hypothesis which could be evaluated by epidemiologic methods concerning the disease in younger persons. This hypothesis proposed that HD may develop as a rare consequence of a common infection with risk increased if infection is delayed until adolescence or young adulthood [32]. This hypothesis was testable, as risk factors associated with age of exposure with common childhood infections could be evaluated in relation to young adult HD. These include sibship size, housing density, and parental social class. Subsequent research has confirmed these associations. Tables 3 and 4 summarize some of the findings from a

Table 3. The relative risk (RR) of Hodgkin's disease associated with sibship size by age group of cases at diagnosis.

Sibship size	15–39 years			40–54 years			≥55 years		
	cases (225)*	ctrls (447)	RR	cases (53)	ctrls (106)	RR	cases (47)	ctrls (93)	RR
1–2	0.34**	0.23	1.0	0.40	0.29	1.00	0.11	0.17	1.0
3–5	0.53	0.58	0.62	0.49	0.45	0.80	0.47	0.51	1.5
≥6	0.13	0.19	0.48	0.11	0.25	0.33	0.43	0.32	2.1
	1.00	1.00		1.00	1.00		1.00	1.00	

* Number.
** Proportion.
From Gutensohn *et al.* [28]; Gutensohn [34].

Table 4. The relative risk (RR) of Hodgkin's disease associated with type of housing in childhood by age group of cases at diagnosis.

Housing type	15–39 years			40–54 years			≥55 years		
	cases (225)*	ctrls (447)	RR	cases (53)	ctrls (106)	RR	cases (47)	ctrls (93)	RR
1 family	0.67**	0.57	1.0	0.38	0.33		0.36	0.48	1.0
2 family	0.16	0.16	0.88	0.30	0.24	1.00	0.21	0.24	
≥3 units	0.17	0.28	0.52	0.32	0.43	0.62	0.43	0.28	1.9
	1.00	1.00		1.00	1.00		1.00	1.00	

* Number.
** Proportion.
From Gutensohn *et al.* [28]; Gutensohn [34].

population-based case-control study conducted in eastern Massachusetts. These findings are reported in detail elsewhere [28, 34].

The most important finding for risk of HD among young adults was a statistically significant twofold inverse association with sibship size. That is, persons who were from a family with six or more children had half the risk of those who were an only child or had a single brother or sister. This finding has been replicated in every study in which sibship size has been evaluated [33]. Since exposure to common childhood infections is often from siblings, this finding supports the hypothesis that susceptibility to 'late' infections, that is following puberty, is a risk factor for young adult HD. This finding was also true for middle-aged cases, suggesting such cases may be associated with infections transmitted by their children. However, among the oldest persons, there was an opposite trend in the relative risk (RR) with sibship size, suggesting that an independent set of factors is associated with HD in this group.

Similar findings concern the type of housing subjects had lived in during childhood, as classified by multiplicity of units. In parallel with the sibship size findings, young adult and middle-aged cases were more likely to have lived in single-family dwellings than the population controls; the reverse was true for the oldest cases. These findings were independent of those for family size. Comparable results were found with parental – especially maternal – education.

Thus, for young adults and middle-aged persons, risk of HD is associated with having had a childhood social environment that fostered protection from early infections. Late infections with common viruses often result in more severe symptoms. With an infection that establishes latency, this may result in an alteration of immunologic control and somewhat more chronic viral expression and antigenic stimulation. Risk for older persons is not related to these epidemiologic factors. However, with a loss of cellular immunity as part of aging, a similar pattern of latent virus activation may occur.

The leading candidate as an infectious agent which fits this hypothesis is the Epstein-Barr virus (EBV). This is because EBV infects B lymphocytes, has known oncogenic potential, and history of infectious mononucleosis (a common manifestation of primary EBV infection in adolescents and young adults) is associated with a threefold increase in risk of HD [33, 35]. Multiple serologic case-control studies repeatedly have found that HD cases have significantly higher titers of antibody against the viral capsid antigen and against the early antigen of the EBV, suggestive of viral activation [36]. Recently, we had the opportunity to evaluate whether this pattern was present prior to the diagnosis of HD. This allowed us to determine whether the elevation of EBV antibodies simply reflects the immune dysfunction of overt HD. This study has been reported in detail elsewhere [37]. Briefly, 43 persons with HD were identified for whom blood had been drawn and stored

for an average of 50.5 months before their diagnosis as part of several large population-based health studies. In comparison to 96 controls identified from the same populations, the cases had elevated levels of IgG and IgA antibodies against the viral capsid antigen; the RR = 2.6 and 3.7, respectively. Cases also had a higher prevalence of elevated titers of antibody against the early antigen (diffuse) (RR = 2.6) and against the nuclear antigen (RR = 4.0), but significantly lower prevalence of IgM against capsid antigen. These findings suggest that in some patients, the occurrence of HD is preceded by enhanced replication of the EBV.

These epidemiologic and serologic associations with EBV have been paralleled by molecular biologic studies on tissue from HD patients. There are now at least six published studies reporting the use of molecular hybridization and polymerase chain reaction to detect EBV genome in HD biopsy material. As summarized in Table 5, the proportion of positive cases ranges from 13% to 29%. In several of these studies [39, 41, 42], in situ hybridization alone or in combination with immunophenotyping demonstrated that the EBV DNA was in the Reed-Sternberg cells and not in lymphocytes. Taken together, these results support the role of EBV in the pathogenesis of a subset of HD cases.

To summarize, the biologic picture of HD is one of a chronically activated immune system where repeated mitogenic stimulation may produce the clonal gene rearrangements, the chromosomal structural rearrangements, and the giant Reed-Sternberg cells. The role of increased activation of latent viral infection is supported by the consistent epidemiologic finding of an inverse association with family size, pointing to late age at infection as a primary modifier of risk. In addition, there is a consistent and specific association with the EBV.

Smithers [43] has proposed a mechanism by which chronic antigenic stimulation could act in the pathogenesis of HD. He stated, 'we are bound to look at the evidence for the effect of prolonged pressures on the cell-mediated arm of the immune system and for feedback failure of restraint in influencing the development of this disease.' It may be that there is an alteration in expression of a gene which controls the production of lymphokines released by antigen-stimulated cells. This alteration results in either greatly amplified message or

Table 5. Summary of studies on the detection of Epstein-Barr viral genome in tissue from Hodgkin's disease cases.

Study	Number of cases	Number positive (%)
Weiss et al. [38]	21	4 (19)
Weiss et al. [39]	16	3 (19)
Staal et al. [40]	28	8 (29)
Herbst et al. [15]*	39	5 (13)
Anagnostopoulos [41]*	42	7 (17)
Uhara et al. [42]*	31	8 (26)

* Overlapping case series.

under-expression of feedback inhibition. Either case could result in an immune system that is frozen in response to a chronic antigen and unable to respond to other antigens. Thus there is a 'malignant immortalization' of a message, rather than of a cellular population. This hypothesis can explain the gene and chromosomal alterations reflecting the underlying genetic change, and the immunologic defects reflecting the unbalanced lymphokine production. Future applications of the new molecular biology may resolve the issues that have held our interest for decades in the etiology of HD.

References

1. Drexler HG, Leber BF. The nature of the Hodgkin cell. Report of the First International Symposium on Hodgkin's Lymphoma, Kohl, FRG, October 2–3, 1987. Blut 1988; 56: 135–137.
2. Hsu S-M, Hsu P-L. Aberrant expression of T cell and B cell markers in myelocyte/monocyte/histiocyte-derived lymphoma and leukemia cells: Is the infrequent expression of T/B cell markers sufficient to establish a lymphoid origin for Hodgkin's Reed-Sternberg cells? Am J Pathol 1989; 134: 203–212.
3. Andreesen R, Brugger W, Lohn GW et al. Human macrophage can express the Hodgkin's cell-associated antigen Ki-1 (CD30). Am J Pathol 1989; 134: 187–192.
4. Griesser H, Mak TW. Immunogenotyping in Hodgkin's disease. Hematol Oncol 1988; 6: 239–245.
5. Griesser H, Feller A, Lennert K et al. Rearrangement of the β chain of the T cell antigen receptor and immunoglobulin genes in lymphoproliferative disease. J Clin Invest 1986; 78: 1179–1184.
6. Griesser H, Feller AC, Mak TW et al. Clonal rearrangements of T-cell receptor and immunoglobulin genes and immunophenotypic antigen expression in different subclasses of Hodgkin's disease. Int J Cancer 1987; 40: 157–160.
7. Knowles II DM, Neri A, Pelicci PG et al. Immunoglobulin and T-cell receptor β-chain gene rearrangement analysis of Hodgkin's disease: Implications for lineage determination and differential diagnosis. Proc Natl Acad Sci USA 1986; 83: 7942–7946.
8. Weiss LM, Strickler JG, Hu E et al. Immunoglobulin gene rearrangements in Hodgkin's disease. Hum Pathol 1986; 17: 1009–1014.
9. Brinker MGL, Poppema S, Buys GHCM et al. Clonal immunoglobulin gene rearrangements in tissues involved by Hodgkin's disease. Blood 1987; 70: 186–191.
10. O'Connor NTJ, Crick JA, Gatterk C et al. Cell lineage in Hodgkin's disease. Lancet 1987; i: 158.
11. Sundeen J, Lipford E, Uppenkamp M et al. Rearranged antigen receptor genes in Hodgkin's disease. Blood 1987; 70: 96–103.
12. Raghavachar A, Binder T, Bartram CR. Immunoglobulin and T cell receptor gene rearrangements in human leukaemias and lymphomas. Cancer Res 1988; 48: 3591–3594.
13. Roth MS, Schnitzer B, Bingham EL et al. Rearrangement of immunoglobulin and T-cell receptor genes in Hodgkin's disease. Am J Pathol 1988; 131: 331–338.
14. Daus H, Schwarze G, Kumel G et al. Immunoglobulin and T-cell receptor gene rearrangements in Hodgkin's disease. Acta Haemat 1989; 82: 110–111.
15. Herbst H, Tippelmann G, Anagnostopoulos I et al. Immunoglobulin and T-cell receptor gene rearrangements in Hodgkin's disease and Ki-1-positive anaplastic large cell lymphoma: Dissociation between phenotype and genotype. Leuk Res 1989; 13: 103–116.
16. Drexler HG, Johns DB, Diehl V et al. Is the Hodgkin cell a T- or B-lymphocyte? Recent evidence from geno- and immunophenotypic analysis and in-vitro cell lines. Hematol Oncol 1989; 7: 95–113.
17. Cabanillas F. A review and interpretation of cytogenetic abnormalities identified in Hodgkin's disease. Hematol Oncol 1988; 271–274.
18. Hossfeld DK, Schmidt CG. Chromosome findings in effusions from patients with Hodgkin's disease. Int J Cancer 1978; 21: 147–156.
19. Reeves BR, Pickup VL. The chromosome changes in non-Burkitt lymphomas. Hum Genet 1980; 53: 349–355.
20. Fleishman T. Reported in Rowley JD. Chromosomes in Hodgkin's disease. Cancer Treat Rep 1982; 66: 639–643.
21. Fonatsch C, Diehl V, Schaadt M et al. Cytogenetic investigations in Hodgkin's disease. I. Involvement of specific chromosomes in marker formation. Cancer Genet Cytogenet 1986; 20: 39–52.
22. Cabanillas F, Pathak S, Trujillo J et al. Cytogenetics of Hodgkin's disease suggest possible origin from a lymphocyte. Blood 1988; 71: 1615–1617.
23. Thangavelu M, LeBeau MM. Chromosomal abnormalities in Hodgkin's disease. Hemat/Oncol Clin N Amer 1989; 3: 221–236.
24. Romagnani S, Ferrini PLS, Rici M. The immune derangement in Hodgkin's disease. Sem Hematol 1985; 22: 41–55.
25. Ford RJ, Tsao J, Kouttab NM et al. Association of an interleukin abnormality with the T cell defect in Hodgkin's disease. Blood 1984; 64: 386–392.
26. Ford RJ, Rajaraman C, Lu M et al. In vitro analysis of cell populations involved in Hodgkin's disease lesions and in the characteristic T cell immunodeficiency. Hematol Oncol 1988; 6: 247–255.
27. Pizzolo G, Chilosi M, Vinante F et al. Soluble interleukin-2 receptors in the serum of patients with Hodgkin's disease. Br J Cancer 1987; 55: 427–428.
28. Gutensohn (Mueller) N, Cole P. Childhood social environment and Hodgkin's disease. N Engl J Med 1981; 304: 135–140.
29. MacMahon B. The epidemiologic evidence on the nature of Hodgkin's disease. Cancer 1957; 10: 1045–1054.
30. MacMahon B. Epidemiology of Hodgkin's disease. Cancer Res 1966; 26: 1189–1200.
31. Correa P, O'Connor GT. Epidemiologic patterns of Hodgkin's disease. Int J Cancer 1971; 8: 192–201.
32. Gutensohn (Mueller) N, Cole P. Epidemiology of Hodgkin's disease in the young. Int J Cancer 1977; 19: 595–604.
33. Mueller N. Hodgkin's disease. In D. Schottenfeld, J. Fraumeni, Jr. (eds). Cancer Epidemiology and Prevention, Second Edition, New York, Oxford University Press (in press).
34. Gutensohn (Mueller) N. Social class and age at diagnosis of Hodgkin's disease: New epidemiology evidence on the 'two-disease' hypothesis. Cancer Treat Rep 1982; 66: 689–695.
35. Evans AS. The Epstein-Barr virus. In A. Evans (ed.) Viral infections in Humans: Epidemiology and Control, Third Edition, New York, Plenum Press (in press).
36. Evans AS, Gutensohn (Mueller) NM. A population-based case-control study of EBV and other viral antibodies among persons with Hodgkin's disease and their siblings. Int J Cancer 1984; 34: 149–157.
37. Mueller N, Evans A, Harris NL et al. Hodgkin's disease and Epstein-Barr virus: Altered antibody patterns before diagnosis. N Engl J Med 1989; 320: 689–695.
38. Weiss LM, Strickler JG, Warnke RA et al. Epstein-Barr viral DNA in tissues of Hodgkin's disease. Am J Pathol 1987; 129: 86–91.
39. Weiss LM, Movahed LA, Warnke RA et al. Detection of Epstein-Barr viral genomes in Reed-Sternberg cells of Hodgkin's disease. N Engl J Med 1989; 320: 502–506.
40. Staal SP, Ambinder R, Beschorner WE et al. A survey of Epstein-Barr virus DNA in lymphoid tissue: Frequent detec-

tion in Hodgkin's disease. Am J Clin Path 1989; 91: 1–5.

41. Anagnostopoulos I, Herbst H, Niedobitek G et al. Demonstration of monoclonal EBV genomes in Hodgkin's disease and Ki-1 positive anaplastic large cell lymphoma by combined southern blot and in situ hybridization. Blood 1989; 74: 810–816.

42. Uhara H, Sato Y, Mukai K et al. Detection of Epstein-Barr virus DNA in Reed-Sternberg cells of Hodgkin's disease using the polymenase chain reaction and in situ hybridization. Jpn J Cancer Res 1990; 81: 272–278.

43. Smithers D. On some general concepts in oncology with special references to Hodgkin's disease. Int J Radiation Oncol Biol Phys 1983; 9: 731–738.

44. Gutensohn (Mueller) NM. The epidemiology of Hodgkin's disease: Clues to Etiology. In RJ Ford, LM Fuller and FB Hagemeister (eds.) Ut M.D. Anderson Clinical Conference on Cancer, Vol. 27, Raven Press, New York, 1984, pp 3–9.

Correspondence to:
Nancy Mueller, Sc.D.
677 Huntington Avenue
Boston, MA 02115, USA

Annals of Oncology, Supplement 2 to Volume 2: 29–31, 1991.
© 1991 *Kluwer Academic Publishers.*

Original article ─────────────────────────────

The continuing challenge of Hodgkin's disease*

Saul A. Rosenberg

Stanford University School of Medicine, Stanford, California, USA

Summary. Patients with Hodgkin's disease, treated at most major medical centers, enjoy a cure rate on the average of approximately 75 percent. An additional 5 or 10% will not die of Hodgkin's disease, because of the success of secondary treatments or because their deaths result from other related or unrelated causes. There are subgroups of patients who fare better or worse than this average, depending on prognostic factors such as age, stage, bulk, or site of disease and on the primary management program.

Substantial improvements in these curability and survival statistics will be difficult to achieve and demonstrate. The major efforts of clinical investigators of Hodgkin's disease in 1990 are to identify and reduce the serious long-term morbidities of treatment programs and to assure that the excellent outcome results achieved at major centers can be accomplished more widely throughout the world.

The emerging challenge for investigators of Hodgkin's disease in the next decade is not only to refine treatment methods but to gain a better understanding of the nature, etiology, and pathogenesis of the disease.

There are very important data and observations that suggest that Hodgkin's disease is not a single disease entity, based on epidemiologic, histologic, and immunologic characteristics. Despite the heterogeneity of the disease, familial clustering and HLA correlations give strong evidence that there is a genetic basis for at least a component of the pathogenesis.

The new tools and concepts of the molecular geneticist combined with the recognition of more homogeneous disease subgroups give great promise that the genetic basis of Hodgkin's disease will soon be understood.

Then, as with other diseases identified as genetic in origin, the challenge will be to know whether a single gene or multiple genes are involved, what the role of environmental factors may be, which gene products (or the absence of which products) are responsible for the disease, and finally, how to prevent or reverse the disorder on a rational, rather than empiric, basis.

Hodgkin's disease is no longer a fatal disease. In major medical centers throughout the world, a majority of patients are cured of the disease. As many as 75% of all patients are curable by their initial management program, and approximately 10% of the remaining patients will not die of the disease (Fig. 1).

Classical prognostic factors for patients with Hodgkin's disease, such as histologic subtype and stage of the disease, are no longer major variables for survival and curability (Figs 2 and 3). Other prognostic variables have emerged as significant, including patient age (Fig. 4), site, and bulk of disease.

As patients are surviving for many years after treatment for Hodgkin's disease, the long-term complications and morbidity of therapy have become more clear and of major concern. These complications are listed in Table 1. The challenge to physicians and clinical investigators of the next decade is to recognize and acknowledge the importance of these complications and refine and modify management programs to reduce them as much as possible.

For patients with favorable settings of the disease and good prognoses, it is essential to reduce the acute toxicity and long-term effects of chemotherapy and irradiation programs. Radiation field sizes and doses may be gradually reduced, especially if combined with relatively well-tolerated chemotherapy regimens

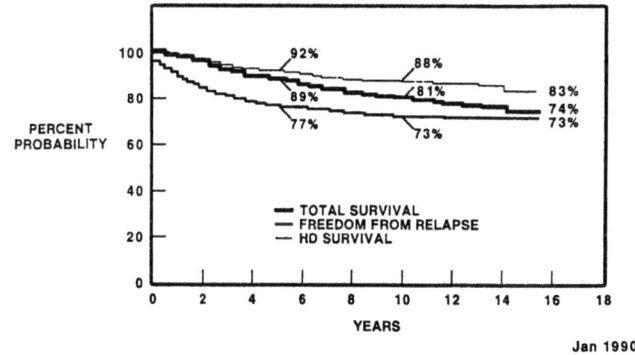

Fig. 1. Actuarial freedom from relapse and survival of Hodgkin's disease and overall survival for 1344 consecutive patients managed at Stanford University from 1974–1989.

* Studies reported herein were supported in part by grant CA-34233 from the National Cancer Institute, Bethesda, MD, USA.

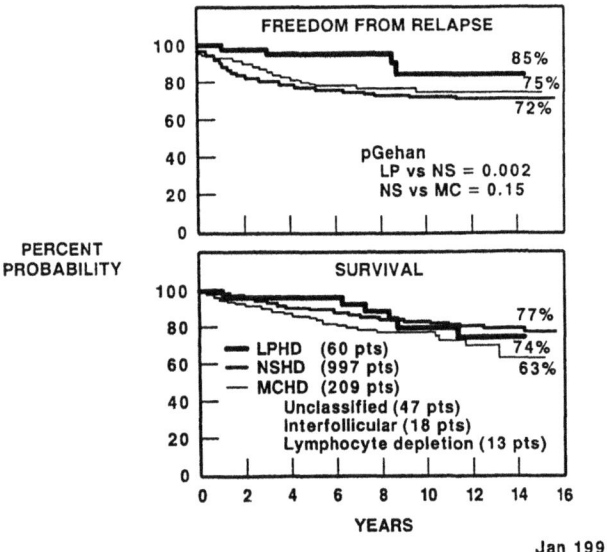

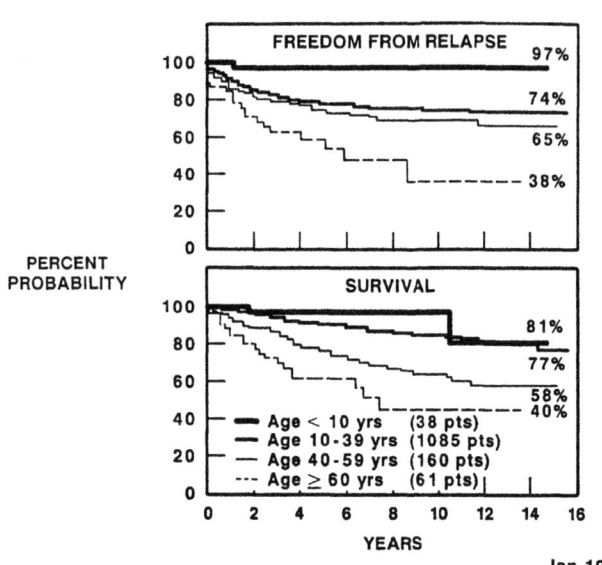

Fig. 2. Actuarial freedom from relapse and overall survival of 1344 consecutive patients from 1974–1989, according to histologic subtype of Hodgkin's disease.

Fig. 4. Actuarial freedom from relapse and overall survival of 1344 consecutive patients with Hodgkin's disease from 1974–1989 according to age at onset.

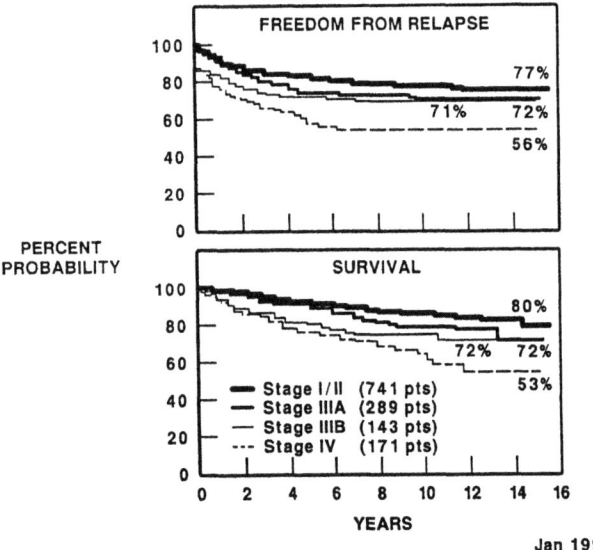

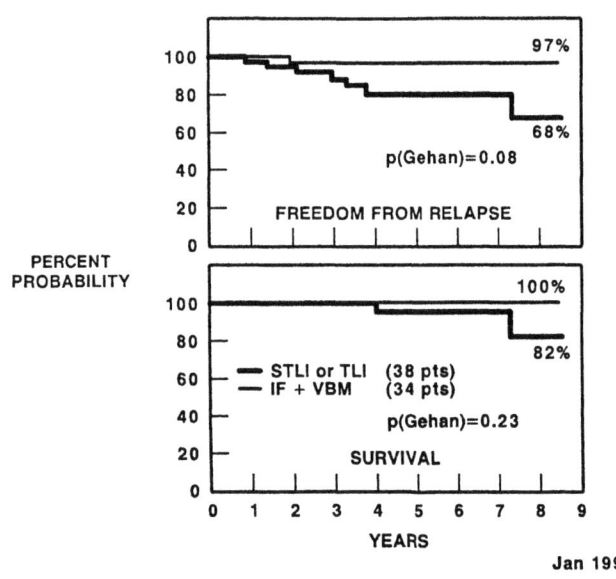

Fig. 3. Actuarial freedom from relapse and overall survival of 1344 consecutive patients from 1974–1989 according to stage of Hodgkin's disease.

Fig. 5. Actuarial freedom from progression and overall survival of a randomized study comparing subtotal or total lymphoid irradiation (STLI or TLI) and involved-field irradiation with adjuvant vinblastine, bleomycin, methotrexate chemotherapy (IF + VBM) in pathologically staged favorable I-II and IIIA patients with Hodgkin's disease.

(Fig. 5). Agents and regimens which induce sterility and acute leukemia should be avoided in the initial treatment of favorable patients.

Diagnostic laparotomy and splenectomy should be utilized only in selected instances and primarily for younger patients (i.e., under the age of 40 years) who may be effectively treated with irradiation alone. The bipedal lymphogram remains the most accurate method of identifying retroperitoneal Hodgkin's disease and following this important, often occult, site of the disease.

Patients with initially poor prognoses and those who

recur after primary management will require more effective chemotherapy programs. Regimens with increased dose intensity, preferably of shorter duration (12 weeks) should be developed and tested. Irradiation should be incorporated in the primary management of patients with bulky disease.

Clinical investigators during the next decade will be preoccupied with selection of patients, at the onset of disease or after first recurrence, for the application of autologous bone marrow transplantation as a curative management approach. Hematopoietic growth factors will become available to allow greater dose intensity,

Table 1. Hodgkin's disease treatment complications.

Major
- Acute myelogenous leukemia (chemotherapy induced)
- Secondary cancers (irradiation induced)
- Secondary non-Hodgkin's lymphoma.

Significant
- Chemotherapy- and radiation-induced sterility.

Other
- Postsplenectomy sepsis
- Opportunistic infections
- Radiation pulmonary and cardiac dysfunction
- Radiation bone and soft tissue abnormalities
- Hypothyroidism
- Psychosocial problems

and probably eliminate bone marrow tolerance as a limiting factor in treating patients who present or recur with poor-prognosis disease.

As important as these refinements of the management of Hodgkin's disease may be today, they are not the most important challenge that faces the clinical investigators of the next decade.

It is necessary to clarify the apparent heterogeneity of Hodgkin's disease. There is clear and accumulating evidence, histologic, immunologic, epidemiologic, and genetic, that Hodgkin's disease is heterogeneous.

Very important studies are being carried out and reported utilizing modern methods of molecular biology and genetics which offer the real probability of understanding the etiology and pathogenesis of Hodgkin's disease. The basic scientists and epidemiologists must be provided with clinical data and materials from homogeneous subtypes of the disease if their studies are to be successful and meaningful.

The clinical investigators of the recent past (Peters, Kaplan, Smithers, Rappaport, Lukes, De Vita, Bonadonna, and others) deserve great credit for transforming Hodgkin's disease from a usually fatal disease to a highly curable one. Many thousands of patients have lived normal lives, many of them parenting normal children, as a result of these investigators' efforts.

But we cannot be satisfied. The treatment required for high cure rates remains empirical, difficult, and costly. Specific therapy based on the knowledge of the cause and pathogenesis of the disease must be the goal of investigators, and it is realistic to believe that goal can be achieved during the next decade.

Acknowledgement

The results of Stanford clinical studies reported herein were obtained with the collaboration of Richard Hoppe, Sandra Horning, Steven Hancock, Ronald Dorfman, the late Henry S. Kaplan and others.

Correspondence to:
Saul A. Rosenberg, MD
Stanford Medical Center
Stanford, CA 94305, USA

Annals of Oncology, Supplement 2 to Volume 2: 33–38, 1991.
© 1991 *Kluwer Academic Publishers*.

Original article ━━━━━━━━━━━━━━━━━━━━━━━━━━━━━━━━━━━━

The nature of Hodgkin and Reed-Sternberg cells, their association with EBV, and their relationship to anaplastic large-cell lymphoma*

Harald Stein, Hermann Herbst, Ioannis Anagnostopoulos, Gerald Niedobitek, Friederike Dallenbach & Hans-Christoph Kratzsch
Institute of Pathology, Steglitz Medical Center, Free University of Berlin, Berlin, Germany

Summary. This review focuses on the cellular origin of Hodgkin and Reed-Sternberg (HRS) cells, their association with the Epstein-Barr virus (EBV), and their relation to Ki-1+ anaplastic large-cell (ALC) lymphoma. The tingibility of HRS cells in paraffin sections for polyclonal immunoglobulin represents a staining artifact and thus can no longer serve as an argument for the histiocytic nature of HRS cells. Immunolabeling studies do not support the putative relationship of HRS cells to cell types such as macrophages or interdigitating reticulum cells, but instead suggest: a) that lymphocyte-predominant (LP) Hodgkin's disease (HD) represents a B-cell neoplasm which is distinct from non-LP HD, and b) that non-LP HD constitutes a syndrome rather than a disease entity, with the existence of T-cell types and B-cell types. HRS cells (and the tumor cells in ALC lymphomas) frequently display an immature genotype in association with late activation markers, leading to the assumption that the tumor cells in many cases of HD (and some cases of ALC lymphoma) may be derived from immature lymphoid cells that are infected by a virus that superimposes characteristics of mature activated lymphocytes on these cells. Southern blotting, in situ hybridization, and polymerase chain reaction (PCR) experiments revealed an association of EBV with HRS cells in a significant proportion of HD cases, suggesting that EBV may be responsible for the dissociation between genotype and phenotype in HRS cells, because EBV is a strong inducer of the activation antigens CD30 and CDw70. While clear-cut morphological and immunohistological differences between Ki-1+ ALC lymphoma and HD have not yet been found, the comparison of chromosomal aberrations observed in Ki-1+ ALC lymphoma and HD disclosed differences supporting the view that these two tumors are separate entities.

Although 150 years have passed since Thomas Hodgkin described the disease that later bore his name, several questions remain unanswered, or have not been answered to everybody's satisfaction: (1) What is the cellular origin of Hodgkin and Reed-Sternberg cells? (2) Is Hodgkin's disease (HD) an entity, or rather a syndrome? (3) What is the reason for the presence of the many nonmalignant cells in Hodgkin's disease? and (4) How closely are the Ki-1+ anaplastic large-cell (ALC) lymphomas related to Hodgkin's disease?

The nature of Hodgkin and Reed-Sternberg (HRS) cells

Significance of IgG-κλ staining of HRS cells

In 1973, Garvin et al. described the staining of HRS cells with anti-IgG antibodies in routinely processed paraffin sections [1]. This reactivity was regarded by some authors as an indication for a B-cell derivation of these tumor cells. Shortly thereafter, however, when it was reported [2, 3] that the same staining can be produced with both anti-κ and anti-λ sera in the same individual HRS cells, this labeling was interpreted as a result of phagocytosis of serum IgG by the tumor cells [4]. Now the stainability of HRS cells was taken as strong evidence for their macrophage or histiocytic origin. When highly sensitive immunodetection systems were adapted for application in frozen sections in the beginning of the 1980s, it became evident that HRS cells in cryostat sections did not react – with very rare exceptions – with antibodies to IgG, κ or λ [5]. This included those HRS cells which were stainable with these anti-Ig antibodies in paraffin sections. This discrepancy between immunohistological reactions seen in paraffin and frozen sections was interpreted either as the result of a fixation artifact or as the result of inaccessibility of the Ig chains in frozen sections. We therefore studied Ig light chain expression on the transcription level by in situ hybridization [6]. With the exception of four cases, Ig light chain-specific mRNA was not detectable in any of the 22 cases studied (Table 1). The four exceptional cases showed clear type restriction in their Ig light chain-specific mRNA expression. These results indicate the following: (1) The staining of HRS cells for IgG

* This work was supported by the Deutsche Krebshilfe, Mildred-Scheel-Stiftung.

Table 1. Ig light chain staining and IgL-mRNA in HSR cells in Hodgkin's disease.

No. of cases	Paraffin sections		Frozen sections		mRNA	
	κ	λ	κ	λ	κ	λ
11	–	–	–	–	–	–
7	+	+	–	–	–	–
1	+	+	–	+	–	+
3	–	–	–	–	+	–

κ and λ in paraffin sections represents a fixation artifact in most instances, probably due to passive penetration of serum immunoglobulins into the tumor cells during formol fixation. (2) Monoclonal expression of Ig light chains can be masked by passive uptake of serum poly-clonal IgG during fixation. (3) The stainability of HRS cells in paraffin sections for κ and λ can no longer serve as an argument for their histiocytic nature. (4) Restriction of IgLmRNA to one IgL type suggests a B cell-derivation of the HRS cells, at least in those HD cases where this was observed.

Absence of macrophage-associated antigens in HRS cells

Several groups have performed studies to demonstrate macrophage antigens on HRS cells [5, 7, 8, 9, 10]. All these studies gave negative results. In extension of these studies, we applied monoclonal antibodies directed against four new macrophage-associated antigens to 58 cases of HD. None of the four antibodies (three of them effective in routinely processed paraffin sections) showed a staining in HRS cells in any of the 58 cases studied, whereas macrophages present in the same tissue were strongly labeled (Table 2). This result, in conjunction with the previous studies, excludes a close relationship between HRS cells and histiocytes.

Relation of HRS cells to interdigitating cells

In the last 10 years, a close relationship between HRS cells and interdigitating reticulum cells has been repeat-

Table 2. Constant absence of four new macrophage markers in HRS cells of Hodgkin's disease.

Type of cells	KP1[1] (CD68)	KiM1P[2]	PG-M1	Ber-MAC3[4]
Granulopoiesis	++	+	–	–
Macrophages	+++	+++	+++	+++
Resting B or T cells	–	–	–	–
Activated B or T cells	–*	–	–	–
HSR cells (n = 58)	–	–	–	–

* Some are positive in frozen sections, but not in paraffin sections.
[1] (34)
[2] Generated by Pawaresch *et al.* (not yet published).
[3] Generated by Falini *et al.* (not yet published).
[4] (35, 36).

Table 3. Absence of antigenic relationship between HSR cells and interdigitating cells (IDC).

Marker/ molecule	Pre-treatment with neura-minidase	IDC	HSR cells	Macro-phages	Germinal center cells
CD15	–	–	+(–)	–(+)	–
CD15	+	+	+		
IRAC*	–	+	+(–)	+(–)	+
S100	–	+	–	–	–
CD1a	–	+	–	–(+)	–
CD30 (Ki-1)	–	–	+	–	–
CDw70 (Ki-24)	–	–	+	–	–(+)
CD25 (IL-2R)	–	–	+(–)	–(+)	–

* Generated by Hsu *et al.* [14].

edly suggested [11, 12, 13]. Recently, Hsu and col-leagues re-emphasized this putative cellular relation-ship, basing their argument on the demonstration of the CD15 molecule on both interdigitating reticulum cells and HRS cells, as well as on the reactivity of the newly established monoclonal antibody IRAC, which was re-ported to react selectively with both interdigitating cells and HRS cells in 10–20% of HD cases [14]. However, CD15 antibodies only stain interdigitating cells after pretreatment of the sections with neuraminidase (Table 3). Such an enzymatic pretreatment of sections is not necessary to label HRS cells. The IRAC antibody proved to be unrestricted in its specificity to inter-digitating cells. This antibody also stains macrophages, germinal center cells, and other lymphoid cells. Furthermore, antigens expressed at a high density on interdigitating cells, such as CD1a and S-100, are ab-sent from HRS cells, and conversely, antigens associat-ed with HRS cells, such as CD30, CDw70, and CD25, are consistently missing in IDC (Table 2). Thus, there appears to be no reasonable indication of a link be-tween HRS cells and interdigitating cells.

Relation of HRS cells to B cells and T cells

For confirmation that HRS cells should be allocated to the lymphoid lineage, three antibodies proved to be of considerable value. The first antibody is βF1, which is directed at a formol-resistant epitope on the constant region of the β chain of the T-cell receptor (TCR) [15].

Table 4. The T-cell receptor β-chain, the B-cell marker CD20, and the CD3 molecule in HRS cells of Hodgkin's disease as identified with the monoclonal antibodies βF1, L26, and polyclonal anti-CD3 antiserum.

HD type	TCR-β	CD20	CD3
Lymphocyte-predominant	0/14	19/22	3/9
Nodular sclerosing	14/41	5/41	13/41
Mixed cellularity	6/35	6/45	4/11
Lymphocyte depleted	1/5	3/7	
Totals	**21/95**	**33/115**	**20/61**

Thus, the monoclonal antibody βF1 recognizes a structure which defines T cells. The second antibody is a polyclonal anti-CD3 antibody effective on paraffin sections [16]. The third important antibody is L26, which was shown by Mason et al. to be directed against the B cell-specific CD20 molecule [17]. The staining results obtained with these antibodies on a large series of HD cases are summarized in Table 4. These data show that in lymphocyte-predominant HD, the B-cell antigen CD20 is expressed at a high density, and there is no expression of the TCR β chain [18, 19]. This varies from results seen in other types of HD, which showed a heterogenous pattern of reactivity [19]. These studies show that lymphocyte-predominant HD represents a B-cell neoplasm, and is distinct from the non-lymphocyte-predominant types of HD. The heterogenous reactivity seen in non-lymphocyte-predominant HD cases is consistent with results of previous studies using other monoclonal antibodies, suggesting that non-lymphocyte-predominant HD represents a syndrome rather than a disease entity, with the existence of T-cell types and B-cell types.

Epstein-Barr virus and HRS cells

In the search of HRS cell-specific markers, two molecules (designated Ki-1/CD30 and Ki-24/CDw70) were detected. In HD-affected tissue, the expression of these antigens is restricted to HRS cells [5, 7, 20]. In normal lymphoid tissue and in vitro experiments, it was shown that these antigens are also expressed in activated B cells and T cells, but not on resting B or T cells, nor on precursor B or T cells. We proposed that HRS cells represent neoplastic counterparts to activated T or B cells [7]. However, the observation that the Epstein-Barr virus (EBV) can induce the expression of CD30 and CDw70 in peripheral T cells and B cells [7] suggests that the expression of CD30 and CDw70 molecules by HRS cells may also be interpreted differently; their expression may also be a result of EBV infection of HRS cells. Following these lines of thought, we investigated extracted DNA of 42 cases of HD for the presence of EBV genomes using the Southern blot technique. Seven cases proved to be positive. Weiss and colleagues, pursuing the same approach, obtained nearly identical results [21]. Subsequent in situ hybridizations revealed the presence of the EBV genome in the tumor cells, but not in any of the admixed non-malignant cells [22, 23]. Using gene probes specific for terminal regions of the EBV genome, it was possible to extract additional information regarding the clonal origin of these viral genomes from Southern blot analyses [24]. The principle of this approach is explained in Figure 1. In all EBV+ cases of HD studied by Weiss et al. [23] and our group [22], the EBV genome indeed proved to be monoclonal. Therefore, it follows that the tumor cells harboring EBV must be monoclonal as well and that the virus entered the tumor cells prior to clonal expansion.

Since the sensitivity of direct filter hybridization techniques is limited, and since the EBV-harboring HRS cells constitute only a small percentage of the total number of cells in HD-afflicted tissue, it is conceivable that EBV escaped detection in many cases. We therefore extended our investigations to enzymatic DNA amplification by polymerase chain reaction (PCR) [25]. Using a set of nested primers specific for sequences within the long internal repetitive region of the EBV genome, we investigated 198 cases of HD as well as 191 specimens from non-Hodgkin's lymphomas and normal lymphoid tissues for the presence of EBV. Of the 198 cases of HD, 57% were EBV+ (Table 5). This is in clear contrast to the results obtained in the non-Hodgkin's lymphomas and normal lymphoid tissues, in which the percentage of positive signals was considerably lower. Corroborative evidence was obtained by subjecting 30 HD cases seen to be EBV+ with the PCR to in situ hybridization. Of these cases, 22 presented with a distinct autoradiographic signal over the HRS cells. These data indicate that the tumor

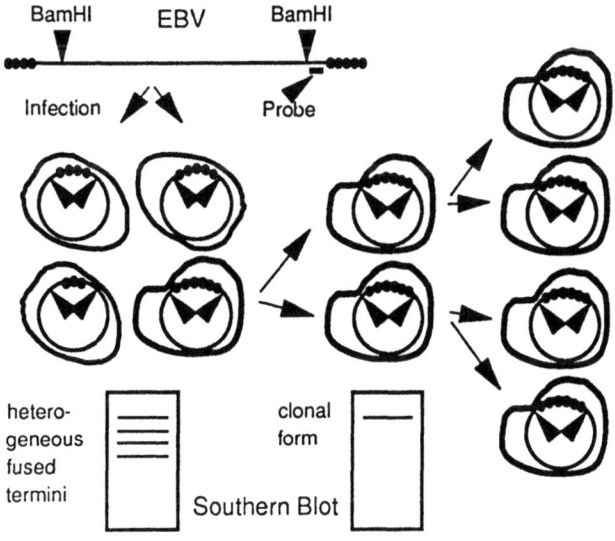

Fig. 1. Schematic representation of the principle of EBV genome clonality analysis modified according to Raab-Traub and Flynn [24]. After infection, the termini of linear DNA fuse intracellularly, forming episomal (circular) viral DNA. Due to the variable number of terminal repeats, the precise configuration of fused termini varies for each genome after episome formation. Multiple identical episomes are maintained in the progeny of each effector cell. Differences in the configuration may be revealed by Southern blot analysis, which produces several bands in the event of infection of several different cells ('polyclonal pattern') (left), or one band in the event of clonal expansion of one particular infected cell ('monoclonal pattern') (right).

Table 5. Detection of EBV-specific DNA by PCR in lymph node biopsies.

Hodgkin's disease	114/198	(57%)
Ki-1+ ALC lymphomas	6/23	(26%)
Non-Hodgkin's lymphomas	21/128	(16%)
B-CLL	1/20	(5%)
Normal lymph nodes	2/20	(10%)

cells in HD are associated with EBV in a high percentage of cases. This frequent association between EBV and HD fits with other serological and epidemiological studies [26] showing an increased risk of developing HD in patients with previous infectious mononucleosis and high titers of IgG antibodies to viral capsid antigen and other viral structures.

Dissociation between phenotype and genotype in HRS cells

Whereas the studies on EBV produced straightforward results, the findings obtained by Ig and TCR gene rearrangement investigations varied considerably among the different laboratories and were difficult to interpret. Rearrangements of Ig and TCR β chain have been detected in 5–20% of the cases studied. Since one would expect lymphoid tumors to be rearranged in all instances, it was hypothesized that rearrangements escaped detection in many cases because of the scarcity of tumor cells. A correlation between detectable gene rearrangements and the number of tumor cells, as well as corresponding studies on DNA extracted from cell suspensions enriched in HRS cells, clearly showed that tumor cell scarcity is responsible for the apparent absence of rearrangement in many, but not all instances [27, 28]. The comparison of Ig heavy and light chain gene rearrangement showed that the first was detected more frequently than the latter. It is extremely unlikely that this is the result of a technical artifact, because the detection of light chain gene rearrangement usually does not require more sensitive techniques for detecting Ig heavy chain rearrangement in the same specimen. Similar results were seen in the HD-derived cell lines [27, 29]. Rearrangement of the Ig heavy chain locus in the absence of rearranged Ig light chains is characteristic of precursor (pre-B) B cells. Thus, the gene rearrangement data indicate an early genotype of HRS cells in most instances. This is surprising, because the phenotype, i.e., expression of activation markers, is that of late lymphoid cells. One clue for an understanding of this dissociation between genotype and phenotype is provided by experiments in which progenitor B cells (without any gene rearrangement) and pre-B cells (rearranged heavy chain genes in the absence of rearranged light chain genes) were infected with EBV in vitro, leading to the establishment of permanent cell lines with the germ-line configuration of Ig and TCR genes, and cell lines with rearranged heavy chain and nonrearranged light chain genes [30]. Phenotypical characterizations of these cell lines revealed reactivity with CD30 and CDw70, and thus these cell lines are phenotypically identical to the EBV⁺ lymphoblastoid cell lines with both rearranged Ig heavy chains and Ig light chains. This experiment shows that genotypically early B cells can develop into phenotypically late B cells. Therefore, it may well be that HRS cells are derived from early (i.e., precursor) lymphoid cells that are infected by a virus such as EBV prior to or during Ig

gene or, possibly, TCR gene rearrangements. The virus, a powerful inducer of the activation differentiation program, may superimpose an activated phenotype on the genotypically early cells.

Relationship between Hodgkin's disease and Ki-1 (CD30) positive ALC lymphoma

The application of the Ki-1 (CD30) monoclonal antibody on tumors previously diagnosed as malignant histiocytosis, undifferentiated carcinomas, malignant fibrous histiocytoma, melanomas, and other sarcomas led to the identification of a novel tumor entity: Ki-1 (CD30)⁺ ALC lymphomas [7]. Because these Ki-1⁺ ALC lymphomas exhibit considerable morphological and phenotypical resemblance to HRS cells (Table 6), the question as to the relationship between these two diseases became of interest. All attempts to find morphological and immunohistological criteria to distinguish between these two diseases – especially between Ki-1⁺ ALC lymphomas containing a proportion of HRS-like cells and lymphocyte-depleted variants of HD – have failed. These studies did, however, lead to the separation of borderline cases of Ki-1⁺ ALC lymphoma, i.e., those that exhibit features of both Ki-1⁺ ALC and Hodgkin's lymphomas (designated *HD-related ALC lymphomas*).

The assessment of the Ig and TCR gene rearrangement status revealed that Ki-1⁺ ALC lymphomas are genotypically heterogeneous, comprising cases with and without gene rearrangements, in a manner similar to the genotypical heterogeneity seen in HD [27]. Therefore, the justification of classifying ALC lymphomas as a distinct, separate entity has been repeatedly questioned. However, comparison of the chromosomal aberrations observed in HD (Table 7) and ALC lymphomas clearly supports the view that at least primary Ki-1⁺ T-ALC lymphomas are different from HD, because the 5q35 breakpoint associated with Ki-1⁺ ALC lymphomas of T-cell origin [31, 32] has not yet been observed in HD [33]. The relation of the non-T-ALC

Table 6. Comparison of Ki-1⁺ ALC lymphoma types and Hodgkin's disease and definition of borderline groups.

	Common ALC	Hodgkin-related ALC	Hodgkin's disease
Capsule thickening	−/+	+	+
Diagnostic RS cells	−/(+)	+	+
Lacunar cells	−	+/−	+/−
Nodular sclerosis	−	−/	−/
Marked fibrosis	−	+/−	+/−
Marked eosinophilia	−/+	+/−	+/−
Sinusoidal growth pattern	+/−	+/−	−
Epithelial membrane antigen (EMA) expression	+	+/−	−
CD15	−	−/+	+/−

Table 7. Localization of non-random chromosome aberrations in Hodgkin's disease*.

Primary Hodgkin tumor tissue	Hodgkin-derived cell lines	Hodgkin-derived large cell lymphomas
1p21–22	1p22	
1q		
2q	2q33	2p23/25
		3q27/29
5p15		
6q11–21, 24		
	7q11–36	7q22–36
8q22–24		8q24
		9q34
11p13		
11q13		
11q23	11q21–23	
14q32	14q32	
	15p12	
		16q22/24
18p		
	21q21–22	

* Data from Diehl *et al.* [33].

lymphomas (especially the so-called HD-related ALC lymphoma type) to HD remains to be determined. The chromosomal breakpoints seen in three cases of Ki-1$^+$ ALC lymphomas of B-cell type were also encountered in some cases of HD (Table 7).

Acknowledgment

The authors thank Mr. B. Young for help preparing the text.

References

1. Garvin AJ, Spicer SS, Parmley RT, Munster AM. Immuno-histochemical demonstration of IgG in Reed-Sternberg and other cells in Hodgkin's disease. J Exp Med 1974; 139: 1077–1083.
2. Taylor CR. Immunohistological study of lymphoma. Eur J Cancer 1976; 12: 61.
3. Papadimitriou CS, Stein H, Lennert K. The Complexity of im-munohistochemical staining pattern of Hodgkin and Sternberg-Reed cells. Demonstration of immunoglobulin, albumin, anti-alpha 1-chymotrypsin, and lysozyme. Int J Cancer 1978; 21: 531–541.
4. Kadin M, Stites DP, Levy R, Warnke R. Exogenous im-munoglobulin and the macrophage origin of Reed-Sternberg cells in Hodgkin's disease. New Engl J Med 1978; 299: 1208–1214.
5. Stein H, Gerdes J, Schwab U, Lemke H, Mason DY, Ziegler A, Schienle W, Diehl V. Identification of Hodgkin and Sternberg-Reed cells as a unique cell type derived from a newly detected small cell population. Int J Cancer 1982; 30: 445–459.
6. Herbst H, Kratzsch HC, Niedobitek G, Anagnostopoulos I, Dienemann D, Falini B, Stein H. Immunoglobulin light chain gene transcripts and protein in Hodgkin's disease (submitted).
7. Stein H, Gerdes J. Phänotypische und genotypische Marker bei malignen Lymphomen. Ein Beitrag zum zellulären Ursprung des Morbus Hodgkin und der malignen Histiozytose sowie Im-plikationen für die Klassifikation der T-Zell and B-Zell-Lym-phome. Verh Dtsch Ges Path 1986; 70: 127–151.
8. Stein H, Mason DY, Gerdes J, O'Connor N, Wainscoat J, Pallesen G, Gatter K, Falini B, Delsol G, Lemke H, Schwarting R, Lennert K. The expression of the Hodgkin's disease-asso-ciated antigen Ki-1 in reactive and neoplastic lymphoid tissue. – Evidence that Reed-Sternberg cells and histiocytic malig-nancies are derived from activated lymphoid cells. Blood 1985; 66: 848–858.
9. Strauchen JA, Dimitriu-Bona A. Immunopathology of Hodg-kin's disease: Characterization of Reed-Sternberg cells with monoclonal antibodies. Am J Pathol 1986; 123: 293–300.
10. Casey TT, Olson SJ, Cousar JB, Collins RD. Immunopheno-types of Reed-Sternberg cells: A study of 19 cases of Hodgkin's disease in plastic-embedded sections. Blood 1989; 74: 2624–2628.
11. Kadin ME. Possible origin of the Reed-Sternberg cell from an interdigitating reticulum cell. Cancer Treat Rep 1982; 66: 601.
12. Hansmann ML, Kaiserling E. Electron microscopic aspects of Hodgkin's disease. J Cancer Res Clin Oncol 1981; 101: 135–148.
13. Hsu SM, Yang K, Jaffe ES. Phenotypic expression of Hodgkin and Reed-Sternberg cells in Hodgkin's disease. Am J Pathol 1985; 118: 209–217.
14. Hsu PL, Hsu SM. Identification of an M$_r$ 70 000 antigen asso-ciated with Reed-Sternberg cells and interdigitating reticulum cells. Cancer Res 1990; 50: 350–357.
15. Brenner MB, McLean J, Scheft H, Warnke RA, Jones N, Strominger JL. Characterization and expression of the human alpha-beta T cell receptor by using a framework monoclonal antibody. J Immunol 1987; 138: 1502–1509.
16. Cibull ML, Stein H, Gatter KC, Mason DY. The expression of the CD3 antigen in Hodgkin's disease. Histopathol 1989; 15: 599–605.
17. Mason DY, Comans-Bitter WM, Cordell JL, Verhoeven MA, van Dongen JJ. Antibody L26 recognizes an intracellular epi-tope on the B-cell-associated CD20 antigen. Am J Pathol 1990; 136: 1215–1222.
18. Pinkus GS, Said JW. Hodgkin's disease, lymphocyte predomi-nance type, nodular – further evidence for a B cell derivation. Am J Pathol 1988; 133: 211–217.
19. Dallenbach FE, Stein H. Expression of T-Cell-Receptor β-Chain in Reed-Sternberg Cells. Lancet 1989; ii: 828–830.
20. Stein H, Gerdes J, Schwab U, Lemke H, Diehl V, Mason DY, Bartels H, Ziegler A. Evidence for the detection of the normal counterpart of Hodgkin's and Sternberg-Reed cells. Haematol Oncol 1983; 1: 21–29.
21. Weiss LM, Strickler JG, Warnke RA, Purtilo DT, Sklar J. Epstein-Barr viral DNA in tissues of Hodgkin's disease. Am J Pathol 1987; 129: 86.
22. Anagnostopoulos I, Herbst H, Niedobitek G, Stein H. Demon-stration of monoclonal EBV genomes in Hodgkin's disease and Ki-1 positive large cell anaplastic lymphoma by Southern Blot and in situ Hybridization. Blood 1989; 74: 810–816.
23. Weiss LM, Movahed LA, Warnke RA, Sclar J. Detection of Epstein-Barr viral genomes in Reed-Sternberg of Hodgkin's disease. New Eng J Med 1989; 320: 502–506.
24. Raab-Traub N, Flynn K. The structure of the termini of the Epstein-Barr virus as a marker of clonal cellular proliferation. Cell 1986; 47: 883–889.
25. Herbst H, Niedobitek G, Kneba M, Hummel M, Finn T, Anagnostopoulos I, Bergholz M, Krieger G, Stein H. High inci-dence of Epstein-Barr virus genomes in Hodgkin's disease. Am J Pathol 1990; 137: 13–18.
26. Mueller N, Evans A, Harris NL, Comstock GW, Jellum E, Magnus K, Orentreich N, Polk F, Vogelman J. Hodgkin's dis-ease and Epstein-Barr virus: Altered antibody pattern before diagnosis. New Engl J Med 1989; 320: 689–695.
27. Herbst H, Tippelmann G, Anagnostopoulos I, Gerdes J, Schwarting R, Boehm T, Pileri S, Jones DB, Stein H. Im-

munoglobulin and T-cell receptor gene rearrangements in Hodgkin's disease and Ki-1 positive anaplastic large cell lymphoma: Dissociation between phenotype and genotype. Leukemia Research 1989; 13: 103–116.

28. Sundeen J, Lipford E, Uppenkamp M, Sussman E, Wahl L, Raffeld M, Cossman J. Rearranged antigen receptor genes in Hodgkin's disease. Blood 1987; 70: 96–103.

29. Falk MH, Stein H, Tesch H, Diehl V, Jones DB, Fonatsch C, Bornkamm GW. Phenotype versus immunoglobulin and T cell receptor genotype of Hodgkin-derived cell lines: Activation of immature lymphoid cells in Hodgkin's disease. Int J Cancer 1987; 40: 262–269.

30. Gregory CD, Kirchgens C, Edwards CF, Young LS, Rowe M, Forster A, Rabbitts TH, Rickenson AB. Epstein-Barr virus-transformed human precursor B cell lines: Altered growth phenotype of lines with germline or rearranged but non-expressed heavy chain genes. Eur J Immunol 1987; 17: 1199.

31. Mason DY, Bastard C, Rimokh R, Dastugue N, Huret JL, Kristoffersson U, Magaud JP, Nezelof C, Tilly H, Vannier JP, Hemet J, Warnke R. CD30-positive large cell lymphomas (Ki-1 lymphoma) are associated with a chromosomal translocation involving 5q35. Brit J Haematol 1990; 74: 161–168.

32. Bitter MA, Franklin WA, Larson RA, McKeithan TW, Rubin CM, Le Beau MM, Stephens JK, Vardiman JW. Morphology in Ki-1 (CD30)-positive non-Hodgkin's lymphoma is correlated with clinical features and the presence of a unique chromosomal abnormality, t(2;5)(p23;q35). Am J Surg Pathol 1990; 14: 305–316.

33. Diehl V, von Kalle C, Fonatsch C, Tesch H, Schaadt M. The Cell Biology of Hodgkin's disease (in press).

34. Micklem K, Cordell J, Rigney E, Simmons D, Pulford K, Stross P, Mason DY. A macrophage-associated antigen defined by five mAb. In: Knapp W et al.: Leucocyte Typing IV, Oxford University Press, Oxford, 1990; pp. 843–846.

35. Backé E, Schwarting R, Gerdes J, Ennen J, Stein H. Ber-MAC3: A new monoclonal antibody that defines a monocyte/macrophage activation antigen (submitted).

36. Gadd S. Report on unclustered antibodies. In: Knapp W et al.: Leucocyte Typing IV. Oxford University Press, Oxford, 1990; pp. 846–850.

Correspondence to:
Prof. Dr. H. Stein
Institut für Pathologie
Klinikum Steglitz
Hindenburgdamm 30
D-1000 Berlin 45
Germany

Annals of Oncology, Supplement 2 to Volume 2: 39–42, 1991.
© 1991 *Kluwer Academic Publishers*.

Original article

Quantitative magnetic resonance studies of lumbar vertebral marrow in patients with refractory or relapsed Hodgkin's disease

S. R. Smith, C. E. Williams, R. H. T. Edwards & J. M. Davies
Magnetic Resonance Research Centre and Department of Haematology, Liverpool University, P.O. Box 147, Liverpool, L69 3BX, UK

Summary. Lumbar vertebral (LV) bone marrow proton relaxation times were measured from midline sagittal magnetic resonance images of the lumbar spine of 20 patients with refractory or relapsed Hodgkin's disease (HD) referred for autologous bone marrow transplantation (ABMT) and 18 aged-matched normal volunteers.

Two patients with positive bone marrow biopsies had markedly elevated mean LV marrow T_1 and T_1 variation. Elevated mean LV marrow T_1 or T_1 variation, consistent with bone marrow involvement with HD, was also seen in four other patients with negative bilateral posterior iliac crest bone marrow biopsies.

Four patients with abnormal quantitative MR studies were examined serially following treatment. Mean LV marrow T_1 and T_1 variation normalised post ABMT, consistent with a good response to treatment.

Quantitative MR studies of LV marrow may improve the detection of bone marrow involvement with lymphoma and be a complementary examination to bone marrow biopsy. Serial studies allow an objective and non-invasive assessment of treatment response.

Key words: autologous bone marrow transplantation, bone marrow, Hodgkin's disease, magnetic resonance imaging, proton relaxation times

Introduction

Bone marrow involvement in Hodgkin's disease is diagnosed histologically from bone marrow biopsy specimens, usually obtained from the posterior iliac crest [1]. As marrow involvement by lymphoma is often focal, bone marrow biopsy is subject to sampling errors [1]. Although detection rates may be improved by performing bilateral iliac crest biopsies, only a relatively small volume of marrow is sampled [2], and again sampling errors may exist.

Magnetic resonance (MR) imaging is a totally non-invasive technique that is suited to studying relatively large volumes of bone marrow [3], and has been shown to be of value in detecting bone marrow infiltrates in lymphoma [4, 5]. Elevated proton relaxation times (T_1 and T_2), which can be measured from MR images, have been reported in various bone marrow disorders [6–8], and potentially provide an objective means of detecting focal bone marrow abnormalities and assessing response to treatment. The clinical role of quantitative MR imaging in lymphoma is, however, unclear.

A means of improving the detection of bone marrow involvement by lymphoma would have important therapeutic implications. MR imaging of bone marrow may improve the accuracy of staging of some patients. In addition, techniques that allow dose escalation, such as autologous bone marrow transplantation (ABMT), are only suitable for patients with noninvolved marrow [9].

As alternative means of dose escalation for patients with involved marrow exist [10], a method of improving the documentation of bone marrow involvement may improve patient selection for such procedures.

The aim of this study was to evaluate the role of quantitative MR imaging in patients with refractory or relapsed Hodgkin's disease referred for autologous bone marrow transplantation.

Materials and methods

Patients

Twenty patients (11 male, age range 19–46 years) referred to a Haematology unit with refractory or relapsed Hodgkin's disease underwent quantitative MR imaging studies of the lumbar vertebral (LV) bone marrow as part of their assessment prior to ABMT. All patients also had bilateral posterior iliac crest bone marrow biopsies.

Patients referred for ABMT had failed two modalities of treatment; either two different chemotherapeutic regimens or combination chemotherapy and radiotherapy schedules. Twelve patients had received radiotherapy, two having radiotherapy fields that included the lumbar vertebrae.

Eighteen patients with no biopsy evidence of bone marrow involvement with HD subsequently had bone marrow harvested and cryopreserved. This group then received an autologous transplant following conditioning with a regimen based on cyclophosphamide, carmustine, and etoposide [11]. Two patients with positive bone marrow biopsies did not proceed to ABMT but received further chemotherapy and a peripheral stem cell autograft.

MR studies

MR studies were performed on a 1.5-Tesla General Electric Signa system using a receive rectangular surface coil placed under the lumbar vertebrae. From a gradient echo coronal localising scan, a single 10-mm midline sagittal slice of the lumbar vertebrae was imaged. A T_1 data set consisting of six images of this midline slice obtained with varying repetition times (TR) from 2400 to 250 msec and a T_2 data set consisting of four images with echo times (TE) of 25–100 msec (TR 2000 msec) were then acquired. Details of the imaging protocol have been given elsewhere [8]. The reproducibility of the protocol had previously been ascertained by studies of test objects and longitudinal studies of normal volunteers [8, 11].

Two rectangular region of interest (ROI) cursors

were placed in each of the five lumbar vertebrae (Fig. 1), and computer-derived T_1 and T_2 values for these regions obtained. A mean T_1 or T_2 value for the lumbar bone marrow was obtained, and the degree of variation in relaxation times over the 10 ROI cursors estimated by the standard deviation (SD)/mean × 100. Confidence intervals (95% CI) for the LV bone marrow T_1 and T_2 values and relaxation time variation of the controls were estimated.

Results

Normal volunteers

T_1 and T_2 data for the controls are shown in Figures 2 and 3, respectively. The mean LV bone marrow T_1 of controls was 783 msec (SD = 155; 95% CI 705–860), and mean T_1 variation 11.9% (SD = 3.7, 95% CI

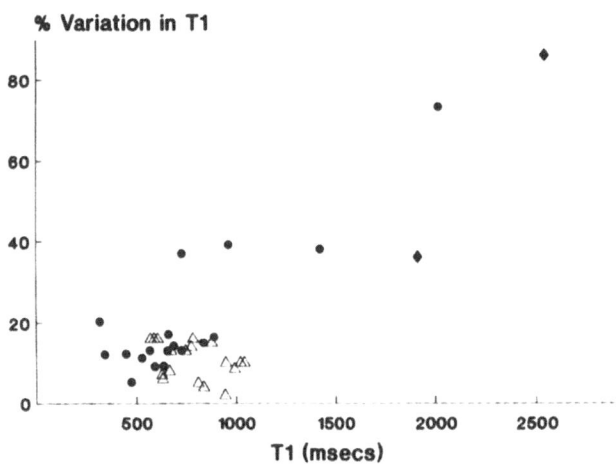

Fig. 2. Scatter diagram showing mean lumbar vertebral marrow T_1 and percent T_1 variation for controls (△), patients with Hodgkin's disease (HD) and positive bone marrow biopsies (◆), and patients with HD and negative bone marrow biopsies (●).

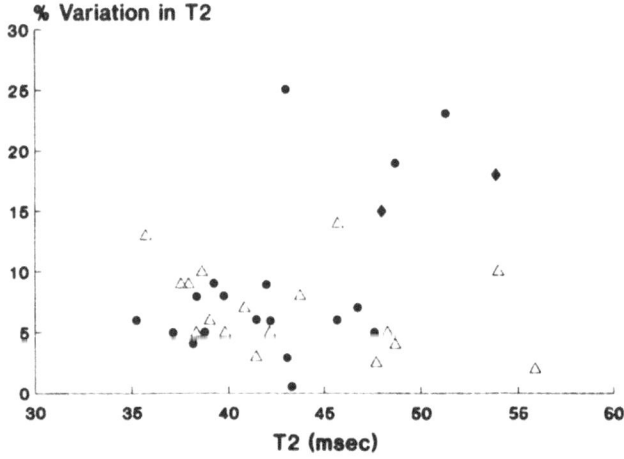

Fig. 3. Scatter diagram showing mean lumbar vertebral marrow T_2 and percent T_2 variation for controls (△), patients with HD and positive bone marrow biopsies (◆), and patients with HD with negative bone marrow biopsies (●).

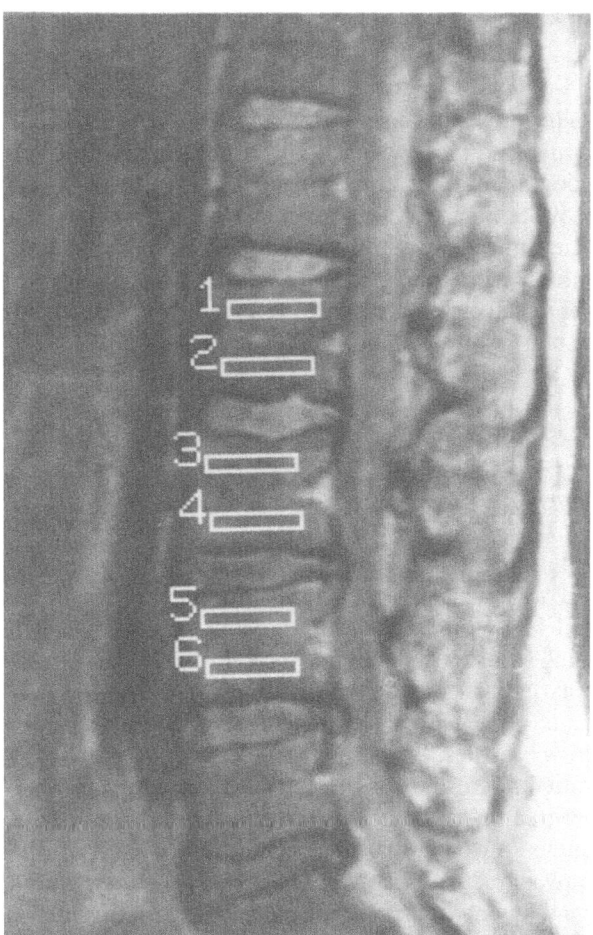

Fig. 1. T_1 weighted midline sagittal image of lumbar spine of a normal volunteer showing use of region of interest cursors in second, third, and fourth lumbar vertebrae.

10–13.8%). Mean LV marrow T_2 was 43.1 msec (SD = 5.82, 95% CI 40.0–46.2), and T_2 variation 6.8% (SD = 3.3, 95% CI 5.1–8.6%). T_2 data for one of the controls were not available.

Biopsy-positive Hodgkin's disease

Two of the 20 patients had positive bone marrow biopsies. Both had qualitative abnormalities of the lumbar spine that have been previously reported [11]. Elevated mean LV bone marrow T_1 values were present in both cases with markedly increased T_1 variation (Fig. 2). The alterations in T_2 were less marked. T_2 variation was slightly increased in the two patients with positive bone marrow biopsies, but mean LV bone marrow T_2 overlapped with controls (Fig. 3).

Biopsy-negative Hodgkin's disease

Eighteen patients had no evidence of bone marrow involvement by lymphoma on bilateral iliac crest bone marrow biopsy. Four of these 18 patients had quantitative abnormalities of the LV bone marrow, either elevated mean LV bone marrow T_1 and/or increased T_1 variation. In three cases both mean T_1 and T_1 variation were increased whilst in the fourth case mean T_1 was within the 95% confidence intervals of controls but T_1 variation was significantly increased (Fig. 2).

No consistent alterations in mean LV marrow T_2 were seen in the four patients with elevated mean T_1 or T_1 variation, although three had increased T_2 variation (Fig. 3).

In only two of these patients were qualitative abnormalities discernible. In both cases these were focal areas of decreased signal intensity on T_1 weighted (TR/TE 500/25 msec) images.

Serial studies

Four of the six patients with quantitative MR abnormalities underwent serial studies after treatment. Three of these patients had undergone an autologous bone marrow transplantation and were reexamined approximately 10 weeks after the procedure when full haematopoietic recovery had taken place. The other patient, who had positive bone marrow trephines, was reexamined after receiving a peripheral stem cell autograft.

Three of the patients with elevated mean LV bone marrow T_1 values showed normalisation of T_1 post treatment. In the fourth patient no change in mean T_1 was seen (Fig. 4). Patients with increased pretreatment T_1 variation showed marked reduction and/or normalisation of T_1 variation following chemotherapy (Fig. 5). Reassessment by bone marrow biopsy of the patient with previously documented bone marrow involvement now showed the marrow to be free of lymphoma.

No consistent alteration in mean LV bone marrow T_2 was seen following treatment, although reduction or

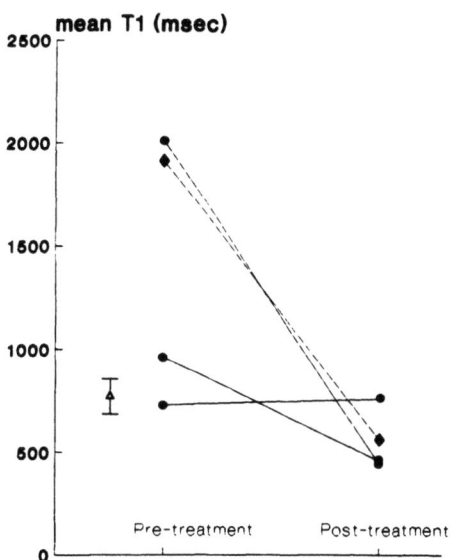

Fig. 4. Pre- and post-treatment mean lumbar vertebral marrow T_1 of patients studied serially. The 95% confidence intervals for controls of lumbar vertebral marrow T_1 are shown ($\triangle$).

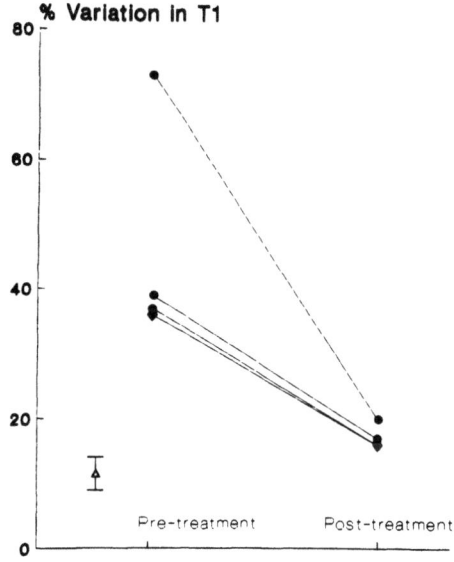

Fig. 5. Pre- and post-treatment percent T_1 variation of patients studied serially. The 95% confidence intervals for controls of lumbar vertebral marrow T_1 variation are shown ($\triangle$).

normalisation of T_2 variation was seen in three of the four patients studied serially.

Discussion

Conventional magnetic resonance imaging is of value in detecting malignant marrow infiltrates [3, 5, 12] and has been shown to be superior to bone marrow scintigraphy in the evaluation of bone marrow status [5]. A quantitative approach, however, allows an objective assessment of the presence of marrow abnormalities to be made and, importantly, provides a means of assessing treatment response.

Quantitative MR imaging studies have shown that the T_1 of LV bone marrow reflects alterations in bone marrow cellularity (the more cellular the marrow the higher the T_1). Elevated T_1, however, is not specific to any particular infiltrative pathology [6, 8]. The abnormal areas of elevated T_1 detected in these patients with HD probably reflect generalised or focal increases in bone marrow cellularity and/or fibrosis due either to malignant infiltration by HD or possibly to areas of hypercellular reactive bone marrow.

Quantitative MR detected bone marrow involvement correctly in the two patients with positive bone marrow biopsies but also detected marrow abnormalities in four other patients with normal bone marrow biopsies. Focal areas of significant T_1 elevation were seen in these four patients which produced either an elevated mean LV bone marrow T_1 value, or perhaps more importantly in disorders of a focal nature, increased T_1 variation across the tissue of interest. The increased variation in relaxation times presumably reflected aspects of tissue heterogeneity and the often focal nature of bone marrow involvement by HD. There are grounds for confidence that these high T_1 areas correspond to areas of bone marrow infiltration by HD, as postmortem studies of a patient who died following ABMT confirmed the presence of areas consistent with partially treated HD in abnormal lumbar vertebrae identified from MR studies [11].

Serial studies allowed an objective assessment of treatment response to be made by following alterations in T_1 with treatment. Mean LV bone marrow T_1 and/or T_1 variation normalised following treatment in patients with abnormal pretreatment MR studies. In the patient with abnormal bone marrow histology who was studied serially, normalisation of relaxation times was associated with elimination of histological evidence of bone marrow infiltration with HD. These alterations in mean LV marrow T_1 mirror changes that have been reported in acute leukaemia after the attainment of remission [13, 14].

Improved methods of investigating T_1 variation in bone marrow on a pixel-by-pixel basis may increase the sensitivity of quantitative MR imaging techniques and allow aspects of the documentation of residual disease to be assessed [15]. In addition, abnormal areas of bone marrow identified by elevated T_1 may possibly be targeted for guided biopsy.

The documentation of areas of bone marrow infiltrated with HD by quantitative MR imaging in patients with refractory lymphoma is clinically important, as only patients with noninvolved bone marrow are suitable for procedures such as autologous bone marrow transplantation, and alternative means of dose escalation exist for patients with involved marrow. Quantitative MR imaging may be a complementary technique to bone marrow biopsy in assessing bone marrow status when the presence of bone marrow involvement limits or dictates therapeutic options.

Acknowledgement

This work was supported by a grant from the North West Cancer Research Fund.

References

1. Kapadia SB, Krause JR. Hodgkin's Disease. In: Krause JR (ed), Bone Marrow Biopsy. 1981; pp. 146–155. Churchill Livingstone, Edinburgh.
2. Brunning RD, Bloomfield CD, McKenna RW et al. Bilateral trephine bone marrow biopsies in lymphoma and other neoplastic diseases. Ann Intern Med 1975; 83: 365–366.
3. Vogler JB, Murphy WA. Bone marrow imaging. Radiology 1988; 168: 679–693.
4. Shields AF, Porter BA, Churchley S et al. The detection of bone marrow involvement by lymphoma using magnetic resonance imaging. J Clin Oncol 1987; 5: 225–230.
5. Linden A, Zankovich R, Theissen P et al. Malignant lymphoma: Bone marrow imaging versus biopsy. Radiology 1989; 173: 335–339.
6. Nyman R, Rehn S, Glimelius B et al. Magnetic resonance imaging in diffuse malignant bone marrow disease. Acta Radiol 1987; 28: 199–205.
7. Richards MA, Webb JAW, Jewell SE et al. Low field strength magnetic resonance imaging of bone marrow in patients with lymphoma. Br J Cancer 1988; 57: 412–415.
8. Smith SR, Williams CE, Davies JM et al. Bone marrow disorders: Characterisation with quantitative MR imaging. Radiology 1989; 172: 805–810.
9. Jagannath S, Armitage JO, Dicke KA et al. Prognostic factors for response and survival after high dose cyclophosphamide, carmustine and etoposide with autologous bone marrow transplantation for relapsed Hodgkin's disease. J Clin Oncol 1989; 7: 179–185.
10. Kessinger A, Armitage JO, Dicke KA et al. Autologous peripheral haemopoietic stem cell transplantation restores haemopoietic function following marrow ablative therapy. Blood 1988; 71: 723–727.
11. Smith SR, Williams CE, Edwards RHT et al. Quantitative magnetic resonance imaging in autologous bone marrow transplantation for Hodgkin's disease. Br J Cancer 1989; 60: 961–965.
12. Trillet V, Revel D, Combaret V et al. Bone marrow metastases in small cell lung cancer: detection with magnetic resonance imaging and monoclonal antibodies. Br J Cancer 1989; 60: 83–88.
13. Moore SG, Gooding CA, Brasch RG et al. Bone marrow in children with acute lymphocytic leukaemia: MR relaxation times. Radiology 1986; 160: 237–240.
14. Thomsen C, Sorensen PG, Karle H et al. Prolonged bone marrow T_1-relaxation in acute leukaemia. In vivo tissue characterisation by magnetic resonance imaging. Mag Reson Imag 1987; 5: 251–257.
15. Roberts N, Smith SR, Edwards RHT. Characterisation of bone marrow disorders using quantitative magnetic resonance imaging and image analysis techniques. European Congress of NMR in Medicine and Biology, Strasbourg, France. May 2–5th 1990. Works in Progress, Abstract No 412.

Correspondence to:
Dr. S. R. Smith
Magnetic Resonance Research Centre
Pembroke Place, P.O. Box 147,
Liverpool, L69 3BX, United Kingdom

Annals of Oncology, Supplement 2 to Volume 2: 43–47, 1991.
© 1991 *Kluwer Academic Publishers*.

Original article ——————————————————————————

Low serum interleukin-2 receptor levels correlate with a good prognosis in patients with Hodgkin's lymphoma*

Angela Gause, Volker Roschansky, Astrid Tschiersch, Kleri Smith, Dirk Hasenclever,
Rudolf Schmits, Volker Diehl & Michael Pfreundschuh
Laboratories of Immunology and Tumor Biology, Medizinische Klinik, University of Cologne, Cologne, Germany

Summary. In order to evaluate the clinical significance of soluble interleukin-2 receptor (sIL-2R) levels in the serum of patients with Hodgkin's disease (HD), we tested the pretreatment sera of 82 patients. The HD patients had significantly higher sIL-2R levels than normal controls (4787 U/ml versus 290 U/ml; P < 0.001). In patients presenting with B-symptoms, the median sIL-2R levels were significantly higher than in patients without B-symptoms (7978 versus 2128 U/ml; P < 0.01). Patients in stage IVB had the highest sIL-2R levels (10 450 U/ml). Of 77 patients evaluable for response, all patients with sIL-2R levels <1000 U/ml achieved complete remission and no relapses occurred in this group after a median of 20 months. The fact that sIL-2R levels dropped after therapy, even in patients who suffered from progressive disease, suggests that Hodgkin and Reed-Sternberg cells are only a minor source of sIL-2R in HD. Therefore sIL-2R levels are of limited value as a marker of disease activity. However, pretreatment sIL-2R levels <1000 U/ml define a subgroup of adult HD patients with an excellent prognosis, and this fact might be helpful for the design of more custom-tailored therapy programs.

Key words: Hodgkin's lymphoma, interleukin-2 receptors, prognostic factors

Introduction

Interleukin-2 is a potent modulator of immune responses. To exert its biological effects, it must interact with a specific receptor on cell membranes. This interleukin-2 receptor (IL-2R) is a molecule composed of two distinct polypeptide chains [1], the larger alpha chain (molecular mass 75 kd) and a smaller beta chain (molecular mass 55 kd). High-affinity binding of interleukin-2 occurs only when both alpha and beta chains are expressed simultaneously. The beta chain was first characterized by the monoclonal CD25 antibody anti-Tac [2]. The IL-2R is expressed by normal lymphocytes upon activation, and activated lymphocytes release a truncated soluble form of the beta chain of IL-2R with a molecular mass of 40–45 kd [3].

A number of recent reports have described increased sIL-2R levels in several lymphoproliferative disorders, such as adult T-cell leukemia/lymphoma [4], B-cell chronic lymphocytic leukemia [5], hairy cell leukemia [6], and lymphoblastic lymphoma/leukemia [7, 8].

Knowing that the neoplastic cells of Hodgkin's disease (HD), the Hodgkin and Reed-Sternberg cells, express Il-2R [9] and that Hodgkin's-derived cell lines release sIL-2R into the supernatant in vitro [10], we in-

vestigated sIL-2R in the sera of untreated patients with HD. We report that sIL-2R levels are elevated in patients with HD, especially in patients who present with B symptoms, and that patients with low sIL-2R levels have a good prognosis.

Patients and methods

Patients

Between January 1987 and March 1988, 147 untreated patients were registered for the multicenter therapeutic trials of the German Hodgkin Study Group. Before the start of treatment, 82 of these patients (56%) had frozen serum samples taken which were used to determine sIL-2R levels. Their ages ranged from 16 to 60 years (median 32). The stages according to the Ann Arbor classification were: IA: 10; IB: 0; IIA: 17; IIB: 7; IIIA: 15; IIIB: 14; IVA: 4; IVB: 15. Staging was based on findings in the physical examination, diagnostic imaging (chest x-ray, abdominal sonograms, and CT scans in all, and lymphangiogram in some patients), and bone marrow and liver biopsy. Staging laparotomy with splenectomy was performed in those cases where clinical staging revealed clinical stage (CS) I or II with-

* This work was supported by BMFT grant 01GA3315/7.

out risk factors. Risk factors were defined as massive mediastinal mass (>1/3 of the maximal thoracic diameter), extranodal disease, or massive splenic involvement. Thirty-two patients (39%) were staged with laparotomy (4 stage IA, 9 stage IIA, 3 stage IIB, 10 stage IIIA, 1 stage IIIB, 2 stage IVA, 3 stage IVB).

Patients in pathological stages I and II without risk factors (n = 14) were treated with extended-field radiotherapy (40 Gy). Patients in CS/PS IIIA and CS/PS I and II with risk factors (n = 35) were treated according to the HD1 protocol [11] and received two double cycles of COPP + ABVD followed by extended-field radiotherapy (20 Gy versus 40 Gy). Patients in CS/PS IIIB/IV (n = 33) were treated according to the HD-3 protocol [11] and received three double cycles of COPP + ABVD, and in cases of complete remission (CR) were randomized into either another double cycle of COPP + ABVD or 20 Gy involved-field radiotherapy; in cases of non-CR, patients received involved-field radiotherapy for persisting nodal disease or the CEVD-protocol [12] or autologous bone marrow transplantation for persisting systemic disease. Informed consent was obtained for all patients, and the study had been approved by the clinical trials review committee of the Medical Association of North Rhine Westphalia.

Sera

The sera were stored at −70 °C until use. They were coded and tested blind. The sera of 50 healthy persons served as controls.

Soluble IL-2R assay

Two monoclonal antibodies recognizing different epitopes of the IL-2R molecule were used in a sandwich ELISA test kit (Cellfree™ IL-2R test kit, T-Cell Science, Cambridge, Mass.). Briefly, sIL-2R in the test samples or standards were bound to the polysterene microtiter wells which had been coated with 100 μL anti-IL2R monoclonal antibody (100 μg/mL). This was followed by incubation of a horseradish peroxidase-conjugated anti-IL-2R monoclonal antibody directed against a second epitope on the IL-2R molecule. After washing the plates with phosphate-buffered saline to remove unbound enzyme-conjugated antibody, O-phenlyenediamine was added for development of the reaction product. The reaction was stopped

with 2N H_2SO_4, and the degree of substrate conversion was determined at 492 nm using a Titertek ELISA reader (Flow Laboratories). A standard curve was created using different concentrations of a standard preparation of 1000 U/mL of supernatant from phytohemagglutinin-stimulated peripheral blood lymphocytes. Normal values of sIL-2R levels, as detected in the serum of 50 healthy controls, ranged from 80 to 420 U/mL, and the mean value (± SEM) was 295 (± 17) (Table 1).

Statistical methods

The χ^2 test was used to compare sIL-2R levels among different subgroups of patients. Correlation between IL-2R and erythrocyte sedimentation rate, albumin, lactate dehydrogenase (LDH), serum alkaline phosphatase, leukocyte and lymphocyte counts were calculated by Spearman's rank correlation coefficient. The influence of potentially significant prognostic factors on complete remission rates and freedom from treatment failure (FFTF) was estimated with the Cox regression model, which permits comparison of treatment outcome for two or more subsets of patients while simultaneously adjusting for the effect of other factors (covariates) in the model. FFTF curves were constructed by the Kaplan-Meier method. FFTF was defined as the time interval between the start of treatment and the failure to achieve a complete remission (CR) or to relapse after CR. A serum IL-2R level of 1000 U/mL was chosen as the dividing point based on the maximum ratio of the estimated hazard for the two groups. All patients received stage- and risk-factor-directed therapy, and those with the same extent of the disease were treated uniformly, precluding analysis of treatment as a prognostic factor.

Results

Pretreatment sera

The summary of the results is shown in Table 1 and Figure 1. In all of the 82 untreated patients included in this study the IL-2R levels were higher than in normal controls, with values ranging from 540 to 21 750 U/mL. The median sIL-2R level of all patients was 4787 (± 760) U/mL. The median level was 7978 (± 1218) U/mL in patients who presented with B-symptoms (range 710–21 750 U/mL). This is significantly higher (P < 0.001) than in patients without B-symptoms, who had median levels of 2129 (± 404) U/mL (range 540–13 650).

There was no clear-cut correlation with stage for patients who did not have systemic symptoms, while in patients with B-symptoms, the levels increased significantly from stages IIIB (3359 U/mL) through IIIB (7814 U/mL) to stage IVB (10 450 U/mL), where the highest levels were observed (Fig. 1).

Table 1. sIL-2R levels in the sera of patients with Hodgkin's lymphoma and healthy controls.

	n	sIL-2R U/mL (± s.e.m.)	
All patients	82	4787 ± 760	
Stages I–IVA	46	2128 ± 404	P < 0.001
Stages I–IVB	36	7978 ± 1218	
Controls	50	295 ± 17	

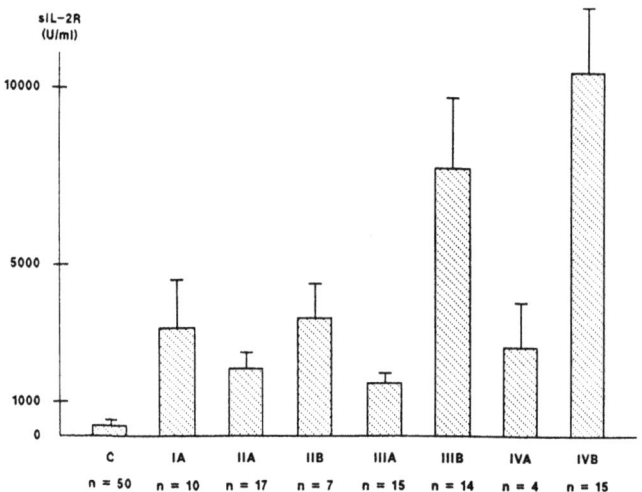

Fig. 1. sIL-2R levels in the pretreatment sera of 82 newly diagnosed patients with Hodgkin's lymphoma.

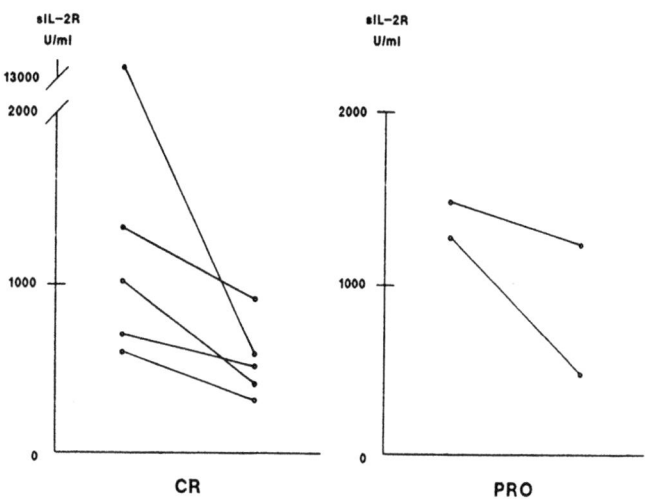

Fig. 2. sIL-2R levels before and after therapy. CR = patients achieving complete remission; PRO = patients suffering from progressive disease. sIL-2R levels drop even in patients with progressive disease, suggesting that the neoplastic Hodgkin and Reed-Sternberg cells are only a minor source of sIL-2R in the serum of patients with Hodgkin's lymphoma.

Correlation with other parameters

The correlation of pretreatment sIL-2R with other clinical and laboratory parameters is shown in Table 2. Levels of sIL-2R were strongly correlated with B-symptoms. Using Spearman's correlation coefficient, there was also a correlation with erythrocyte sedimentation rate, LDH, and alkaline phosphatase, while the correlation with albumin and leukocyte and lymphocyte counts was weak.

Table 2. Correlation of sIL-2R with other parameters.

ESR*	0.41
LDH*	0.40
Alkaline phosphatase*	0.32
Albumin*	−0.26
sCD30*	0.19
Leukocytes (total)*	0.13
Lymphocytes (total)*	−0.12
B-Symptoms**	0.52

* Spearman's correlation coefficient.

** x^2 test.

Follow-up sera

To study the value of sIL-2R levels as a marker for disease activity, the available sera of 52 patients taken after the end of therapy were studied. The representative results of eight patients are shown in Figure 2. In nearly all patients, sIL-2R levels declined after therapy; however, this was also the case in some patients who suffered from progressive disease. Thus, IL-2R levels are not very helpful for monitoring disease activity.

Results of therapy

The results of 77 patients who are evaluable for response are shown in Table 3. The complete response rate was 84% for all patients; 13% suffered from progressive disease. The complete response rate of patients with IL-2R levels below 1000 U/mL was 100%. This is significantly higher (P < 0.03) than in patients with intermediate levels (1000–10 000 U/mL) and patients with very high levels (>10 000 U/mL), who had complete remission rates of 83% and 67%, respectively.

When looking at FFTF (Fig. 3), different prognostic subgroups can be defined by the pretreatment sIL-2R levels. After a median of 20 months, the FFTF was 100% in the 20 patients with sIL-2R levels <1000 U/mL. This is significantly better (P < 0.02) than in patients with intermediate (1000–10 000) or high (>10 000 U/mL) sIL-2R levels.

Table 3. Results of therapy in 77 patients treated for Hodgkin's lymphoma.

	ALL	sIL-2R <1000 U/mL	sIL-2R 1000–10 000 U/mL	sIL-2R >10 000 U/mL
Evaluable for response	77	20	42	15
Complete remissions	65 (84%)	20 (100%)*	35 (83%)*	10 (67%)*
Partial remissions	2	0	1	1
Progressing disease	10 (13%)	0	6	4

* P < 0.03.

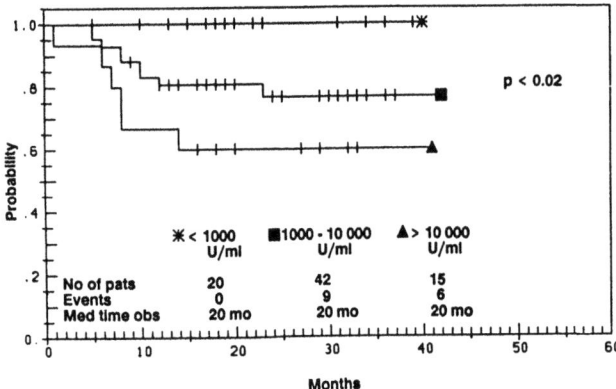

Fig. 3. Comparison of freedom from treatment failure (FFTF) according to sIL-2R levels for 77 patients evaluable for response. There is no event in the 20 patients with sIL-2R levels <1000 U/mL. FFTF is significantly better (P < 0.02) than in patients with intermediate (1000–10 000 U/mL) and high (>10 000U/mL) sIL-2R levels.

The characteristics of the patients with low sIL-2R levels (<1000 U/mL) are shown in Table 4. Five of the 20 patients had B-symptoms, and five were in the advanced stages IIIB and IV. This suggests that their good prognosis cannot be explained by low stage or the absence of systemic symptoms alone. In a univariate analysis of prognostic factors associated with treatment failure (Table 5), only stage IIIB/IV and sIL-2R levels showed a significant correlation with FFTF. B-symptoms showed a weak correlation, and other factors such as age, sex, histology, erythrocyte sedimentation rate, alkaline phosphatase, LDH, albumin, white blood cell count, and total lymphocyte count showed no correlation with treatment failure. However, in a multivariate analysis using the Cox regression model, only advanced stages IIIB/IV retained significance (P = 0.01) as an independent parameter for the prediction of treatment failure.

Discussion

Whereas soluble tumor-associated antigens are widely used as serum markers for solid tumors, serum tumor markers play only a limited role in hematological malignancies. To date, the erythrocyte sedimentation

Table 4. Characteristics of 20 patients with sIL-2R < 1000 U/mL.

All patients	n
	20
Stage	
IA	5
IIA	5
IIB	2
IIIA	3
IIIB	2
IVA	2
IVB	1

Table 5. Prognostic factors for freedom from treatment failure in Hodgkin's lymphoma.

1. Univariate analysis	
IIIB/IV	P = 0.002
sIL-2R	P = 0.02
B-symptoms	P = 0.1
Age (>50)	P > 0.1
Sex (m)	P > 0.1
Histology (MC, LD)	P > 0.1
ESR (>80 mm/hr)	P > 0.1
Alk. phosphatase	P > 0.1
LDH	P > 0.1
Albumin	P > 0.1
Hemoglobin	P > 0.1
WBC	P > 0.1
Lymphocytes	P > 0.1
*2. Multivariate analysis**	
IIIB/IV	P = 0.01
sIL-2R	P = 0.18

* Cox Regression Model.

rate (ESR), which is rather unspecific, is the only widely used marker for disease activity in Hodgkin's lymphoma. The erythrocyte sedimentation rate has been shown to have prognostic significance for both limited and advanced disease [13, 14], and its evolution is useful in the follow-up of patients in remission [15].

In this study, sIL-2R levels were strongly associated with B-symptoms, and moderately with erythrocyte sedimentation rate, LDH, and alkaline phosphatase. Most importantly, sIL-2R levels <1000 U/mL were associated with an excellent prognosis. Similar findings have been reported in a small study of adult patients with HD by Pizzolo et al. [16] and in children by Pui et al. [17]. While Pizzolo et al. [16] were not able to find a correlation of sIL-2R with treatment outcome (probably because of the low number of patients included in their study), Pui et al. [17] observed a poor prognosis in children with sIL-2R levels >5000 U/mL. In contrast to the latter study, sIL-2R was not an independent variable predicting treatment failure in the adult patients included in our study; moreover, in our study only stages IIIB/IV were of significance in a multivariate analysis, while in the study of Pui et al. [17], sex was an additional independent factor. These differences may be due to different treatment strategies in the two patient populations or to a different biology of HD in children and adults.

The functional role of sIL-2R in patients with HD is unknown. Since the soluble receptor is capable of binding interleukin-2 [18], it might compete with normal lymphocyte cellular IL-2R for the ligand. In this respect, increased serum levels of sIL-2R could enhance neoplastic growth by suppressing host antitumor immunity [18]. The fact that sIL-2R levels dropped even in patients who suffered from progressive disease suggests that most of the sIL-2R in the serum of HD patients is released by reactive cells and not by the neoplastic

Hodgkin and Reed-Sternberg cells. The release of sIL-2R into the serum of HD patients mainly by reactive cells and only to a minor degree by the neoplastic Hodgkin and Reed-Sternberg cells may also be the reason that sIL-2R levels do not correlate with disease activity and may be influenced by nonspecific events such as intercurrent infections or (as observed in one of our patients; data not shown) by radiation pneumonitis.

References

1. Teshigawara K, Wang HM, Kato K, Smith KA. Interleukin-2 high affinity receptor expression requires two distinct binding proteins. J Exp Med 1987; 165: 223–238.

2. Robb RJ, Greene WC. Direct demonstration of the identity of the T cell growth factor binding protein and the Tac antigen. J Exp Med 1983; 158: 1332–1337.

3. Rubin LA, Kurman CC, Fritz ME et al. Soluble interleukin-2 receptors are released from activated human lymphoid cells in vitro. J Immuno 1985; 135: 3172–3177.

4. Greene WC, Leonard WJ, Depper JM, Nelson DL, Waldmann TA. The human interleukin-2 receptor: normal and abnormal expression in t cells and in leukemias induced by the human T-lymphotropic retroviruses. Ann Intern Med 1986; 105: 560–572.

5. Semenzato G, Foa R, Agostini C et al. High levels of soluble interleukin-2 receptor in patients with B chronic lymphocytic leukemia. Blood 1987; 70: 396–400.

6. Chilosi M, Pizzolo G, Semenzato G, Cetto GL. Detection of a soluble form of the receptor for interleukin-2 in the serum of patients with hairy cell leukaemie. Int J Biol Markers 1986; 1: 101–104.

7. Wagner DK, Kiwanuka J, Edwards BK, Rubin LA, Nelson DL, Magrath IT. Soluble interleukin-2 receptor levels in patients with undifferentiated and lymphoblastic lymphomas: correlation with survival. J Clin Oncol 1987; 1262–1274.

8. Pui CH, Ip SH, Iflah S et al. Serum interleukin receptor levels in childhood acute lymphoblastic leukemia. Blood 1988; 71: 1135–1137.

9. Sheibani K, Winberg CD, van de Veld S, Blayney DW, Rappoport H. Distribution of lymphocytes with interleukin-2 receptors (Tac antigens) in reactive lymphoproliferative processes, Hodgkin's disease, and non-Hodgkin's lymphomas: an immunohistologic study of 3000 cases. Am J Pathol 1987; 127: 27–37.

10. Pfreundschuh M, Pohl C, Berenbeck C, Schroeder J, Diehl V, Gause A. Detection of soluble CD30 antigen in the sera of patients with malignant lymphomas, adult T-cell leukemia and infectious mononucleosis. Int J Cancer (in press).

11. Pfreundschuh M, Löffler M, Rühl U, Hiller G. Wilmanns W, Kirchner H. Therapy of Hodgkin's Lymphomas. Results of the German Hodgkin Study Group. Onkologie 1988; 11: 48–52.

12. Pfreundschuh M, Schoppe WD, Fuchs R, Pflueger KH, Loeffler M, Diehl V. Lomustine, etoposide, vindesine, and dexamethasone (CEVD) for Hodgkin's lymphoma refractory to COPP and ABVD. A multicenter trial of the German Hodgkin Study Group. Cancer Treatment Reports 1987; 71: 1207.

13. Tubiana M, Henry-Amar M, van der Werf-Messing B, Henry J, Abbatucci J, Burgers M, Hayat M, Somers R, Laugier A, Carde P. A multivariate analysis of prognostic factors in early stage Hodgkin's disease. Int J Rad Oncol Biol Phys 1985; 11: 23–29.

14. Löffler M, Pfreundschuh M, Hasenclever D et al. Prognostic risk factors in advanced Hodgkin's lymphoma. Blut 1988; 56: 949–955.

15. Friedman S, Henry-Amar M, Cosset JM, Carde P, Hayat M, Dupouy N, Tubiana M. Evolution of erythrocyte sedimentation rate as predictor of early relapse in posttherapy early stage Hodgkin's disease. J Clin Oncol 1988; 6: 596–601.

16. Pizzolo G, Chilosi M, Semenzato G et al. Immunohistological analysis of Tac antigen expression i tissues involved by Hodgkin's disease. Br J Cancer 1984; 50: 415–419.

17. Pui CH, Ip SH, Thompson E, William J, Brown M et al. High serum interleukin-2 receptor levels correlate with a poor prognosis in children with Hodgkin's disease. Leukemia 1989; 3: 481–484.

18. Rubin LA, Kurman CC, Fritz ME, Biddison WE, Boutin B, Yarchoan R, Nelson DL. Soluble interleukin-2 receptors are released from activated lymphoid cells in vitro. J Immunol 1985; 135: 3172–3177.

Correspondence to:
Michael Pfreundschuh, M.D.
Medizinische Universitaetsklinik I
Josef-Stelzmann-Str. 9
D-5000 Koeln 41
Germany

Annals of Oncology, Supplement 2 to Volume 2: 49–54, 1991.
© 1991 *Kluwer Academic Publishers.*

Original article ———————————————————

A randomised study of adjuvant MVPP chemotherapy after mantle radiotherapy in pathologically staged IA-IIB Hodgkin's disease: 10-year follow-up

H. Anderson,[1] D. Crowther,[1] D. P. Deakin,[2] W. D. J. Ryder[3] & J. A. Radford[1]

[1] *CRC Department of Medical Oncology,* [2] *Department of Radiotherapy and* [3] *Department of Medical Statistics, Christie Hospital, Manchester, UK*

Summary. One hundred fifteen untreated patients with supra-diaphragmatic, pathologically staged (PS) IA–IIB Hodgkin's disease (HD) were entered into a randomised study comparing treatment using mantle radiotherapy followed by adjuvant treatment with mustine, vinblastine, prednisolone, and procarbazine (MVPP) with mantle radiotherapy alone.

Fifty-six patients were randomised to receive radiotherapy alone (RT) and 59 to radiotherapy followed by six cycles of adjuvant MVPP (RT + MVPP). One hundred fourteen patients achieved a complete remission (CR) with radiotherapy. One patient achieved a partial remission. The overall 10-year survival after correction for inter-current death was 92% with no difference between the two treatment groups (90% for RT alone and 95% for RT + MVPP P = 0.66). There were 9 (8%) deaths from HD (5 patients had received RT alone), and 10 (9%) intercurrent deaths. Eight (7%) patients have developed a second malignancy, and two of them are alive. No patient has developed secondary acute myelogenous leukaemia.

The 10-year relapse-free survival (RFS) was 79% overall, 67% in the RT group, and 91% in the RT + MVPP group (P = 0.0004). There were 25 relapses; 20 patients had received RT alone and 5 had received adjuvant MVPP. Of the relapsed patients, 13 (52%) have received successful salvage therapy and are in CR. In the RT alone group, 45 (80%) patients are alive in CR, 5 (9%) died of HD, and 6 (11%) died of intercurrent causes. In the adjuvant MVPP group, 51 (86%) are alive in CR, 4 (7%) died of HD, and 4 (7%) died of intercurrent causes.

Univariate analysis showed that the following factors adversely influenced survival: pruritus P = 0.0014, night sweats P = 0.0016, B symptoms P = 0.0023, bulk P = 0.0002, monocytes >0.5 × 10⁹/L P = 0.0059, increasing stage P = 0.0191, mixed cellularity P = 0.0227, and lymphocyte count ≤1.7 × 10⁹/L P = 0.0385. Univariate analysis showed that the following factors adversely influenced RFS: treatment with RT alone P = 0.0004, lymphocyte count ≤1.7 × 10⁹/L P = 0.0013, bulk P = 0.0208, and B symptoms P = 0.025.

Multivariate analysis was performed only to determine prognostic factors for relapse. With only 9 deaths from HD it was not possible to analyse prognostic factors for survival by multivariate analysis. Analysis of 24 variables showed that only three variables (treatment with RT alone P < 0.0001, log lymphocyte count P < 0.0001, and albumin ≤43 g/L P = 0.0193) predicted relapse.

Key words: PSIA-IIB HD, adjuvant MVPP, 10yr results

Introduction

This paper presents the 10-year follow-up of a randomised study designed to assess the role of adjuvant chemotherapy with mustine, vinblastine, prednisolone, and procarbazine (MVPP) in the treatment of pathologically staged (PS) IA–IIB Hodgkin's disease. The study commenced in 1974 and was closed in 1981. The five-year results were reported in 1984 and showed that the relapse-free survival (RFS) was significantly better for the group of patients who received adjuvant MVPP (RFS 93% versus 69% for those treated by mantle radiotherapy (RT) only) [1]. A multivariate analysis showed that RT alone, bulk, and B symptoms were ad-

verse prognostic variables for relapse. There was no significant difference in survival between the group treated with RT alone and the group treated with adjuvant chemotherapy. Since there were so few deaths from Hodgkin's disease, a multivariate analysis of prognostic factors for survival was inappropriate. A univariate analysis of prognostic factors for survival showed that bulk, B symptoms, and increasing stage had a statistically significant adverse effect on survival.

Patients and methods

Between October 1974 and August 1981, 115 patients

were entered into this randomised trial comparing treatment using mantle radiotherapy followed by adjuvant MVPP with mantle radiotherapy alone for PS IA–IIB Hodgkin's disease (HD). Patients were excluded from entry if massive mediastinal disease precluded laparotomy staging, if their age was outside the range 16–65 years, or if they had received prior therapy.

Staging was according to the Ann Arbor classification [2]. Prior to laparotomy and splenectomy investigations included routine haematology, bone marrow examination, serum biochemical profile, plain radiology of the chest and either abdominal lymphangiography (before 1976) or abdomino-pelvic CT scan (after 1976). In all cases the pathology was reviewed and classified according to the Rye classification [3].

Bulk disease was defined as a mass of lymph nodes outside the chest measuring $\geqslant 5$ cm in any one axis. Mediastinal bulk was considered to be present if the ratio of the maximum width of mediastinal disease to the chest diameter at T5/6 was $\geqslant 0.33$ [4]. Response to mantle radiotherapy was defined according to standard criteria [5]. Patients were then randomised to receive adjuvant MVPP for six cycles or no further treatment.

Treatment

Mantle radiotherapy (RT)

Anterior and posterior opposed 4-MeV fields were used to encompass the major node areas in the upper half of the body. The fields extended from the external auditory meatus to the eleventh thoracic vertebra, covering the axillae laterally. The dose delivered at the midplane was 3500 cGy in 20 fractions over four weeks. From the onset of therapy, the lungs were shielded by individually fashioned blocks. The spinal cord was shielded for half the posterior treatments, and a compensatory anterior mediastinal field was used to deliver 600 cGy on the final treatment day. There was a dose gradient of 2900 cGy in the posterior mediastinum to 3900 cGy in the anterior mediastinum.

MVPP

Mustine (6 mg/m^2; maximal dose 10 mg) and vinblastine (6 mg/m^2; maximal dose 10 mg) were given intravenously on days 1 and 8. On days 1–14 patients were given oral prednisolone, 50 mg, and procarbazine, 100 mg/m^2. Cycles of MVPP were given every six weeks if the leukocyte count was $\geqslant 3 \times 10^9$/L and the platelet count $\geqslant 100 \times 10^9$/L.

Statistical methods

The effects of variables on survival and RFS have been analysed by calculating Kaplan-Meier curves which were then compared using the log-rank test [6]. Cox's proportional hazards model [6] was used to determine the most significant variables that affect RFS.

Results

Fifty-six patients were randomised to receive RT alone and 59 to RT followed by adjuvant MVPP. Patient characteristics were similar in the two treatment groups (Table 1). The median duration of follow-up was 131 months. Of the 115 patients, 114 achieved a CR. One patient in the adjuvant MVPP group achieved only a partial remission and died of progressive HD without achieving a CR.

Since the previous analysis, some of the data have altered. One patient with PS IA non-bulky disease who had been lost to follow-up has been traced and remains well in first CR. There have been six additional relapses: four patients had RT only, none had B symptoms at presentation, and only one had bulky mediastinal disease. Review of the bulk category has shown one patient was incorrectly classified as having mediastinal bulk, and two patients have now been reclassified as having mediastinal bulk disease. One patient previously thought to have achieved CR has been reclassified as having a partial remission, since the CR lasted for less than one month.

Table 1. Patient characteristics.

	RT alone	RT + MVPP
Number	56	59
Male	39	39
Female	17	20
Stage IA	25	23
IB	2	2
IIA	19	25
IIB	10	9
Age (mean)	32	31
range	17–62	16–63
KP < 60	6	5
> 70	48	53
unknown	2	1
No bulk disease	37	34
Extrathoracic bulk	8	14
Mediastinal bulk	6	6
Both	5	5
Histology LP	16	20
NS	22	24
MC	18	15
Number of sites 1	23	20
2	12	14
3	12	10
4+	9	15

Relapse-free survival

The overall RFS at 10 years was 79% (confidence interval [CI] 72–87%), 67% (CI 54–80%) in the RT alone group, and 91% (CI 84–99%) in the adjuvant MVPP group (P = 0.0004; Fig. 1). Twenty-five patients have relapsed with HD – 20 (36%) of 56 patients who received RT alone have relapsed, whereas only 5 (9%) of 58 randomised to receive radiotherapy plus adjuvant MVPP have relapsed. In the latter group, two patients received full-dose adjuvant MVPP, but three received no adjuvant MVPP. (One had hepatitis and two had problems with venous access.) Thus, of the 55 patients in the adjuvant group who received chemotherapy, only two have relapsed.

It can be seen from Tables 2 and 3 that the relapse rate increased with stage and the amount of bulky disease. In patients treated with radiotherapy alone, the relapse rate was 60% in stage IIB disease and 64% in patients with mediastinal bulk at presentation.

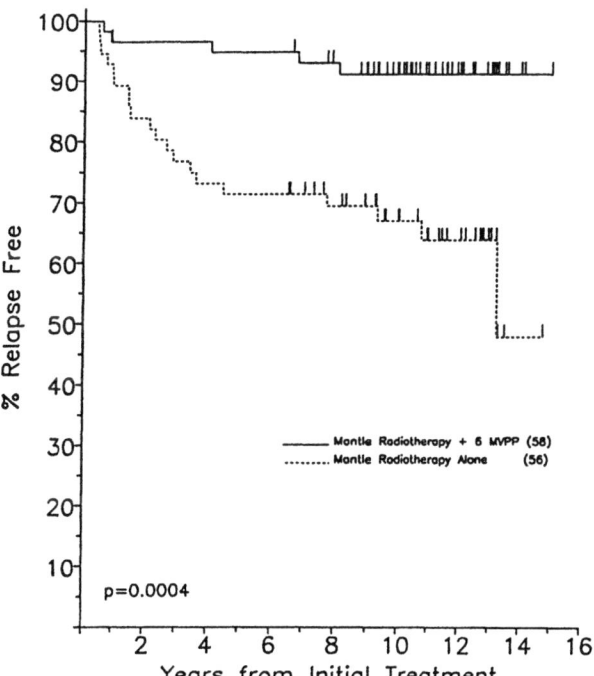

Fig. 1. Relapse-free survival according to treatment group.

Table 2. Relapse rate according to pathological stage and treatment given.

Stage	RT only		RT + MVPP	
	No. (%) relapsed	O/E ratio	No. (%) relapsed	O/E ratio
IA	6/25 (24)	0.63	1/23 (4)	0.49
IB	1/2 (50)	1.18	0/2	0.00
IIA	7/19 (37)	1.00	3/25 (12)	1.36
IIB	6/10 (60)	2.21	1/8 (12.5)	1.72

O/E = observed/'expected' ratio of relapses calculated from the log-rank test under the null hypothesis of no differences. Stratified by treatment.

Table 3. Relapse rate according to amount of disease at presentation and treatment given.

	RT only		RT + MVPP	
	No. (%) relapsed	O/E ratio	No. (%) relapsed	O/E ratio
No bulk disease	11/37 (30)	0.79	1/33 (3)	0.34
Extrathoracic (ET) bulk	2/8 (25)	0.72	2/14 (14)	1.68
Mediastinal ± ET bulk	7/11 (64)	2.13	2/11 (18)	2.39

O/E = observed/'expected' ratio of relapses calculated from the log rank test under the null hypothesis of no differences. Stratified by treatment.

Treatment of relapse

Two patients received no therapy for relapse, one progressed and died during adjuvant chemotherapy, and one patient who had received mantle radiotherapy died of *Escherichia coli* septicaemia and acute renal failure at the time of mediastinal recurrence.

Of the 23 patients who received chemotherapy with or without additional radiotherapy for relapse, 19 (83%) achieved a CR and the other four patients progressed and died of disease. Of the 19 CR patients, three died of HD in second relapse, three died of intercurrent disease, and 13 (68%) continue in CR free from second relapse.

Univariate analysis showed that only four variables were important for predicting relapse: treatment with RT only (P = 0.0004), lymphocyte count $\leqslant 1.7 \times 10^9$/L (P = 0.0013), the presence of bulky disease (P = 0.0208), and B symptoms (P = 0.025). For the purposes of this analysis, values of the peripheral blood lymphocyte count were taken above or below the median of 1.7×10^9/L.

Multivariate analysis was performed using all the variables irrespective of their significance in the univariate analysis (Table 4). Continuous variables were analysed both as continuous variables and as categorical data with two groups divided at the median value for the entire group. The natural logarithm of the lymphocyte count was taken to standardise its distribution.

Table 4. Factors analysed in multivariate analysis for RFS.

Age	Haemoglobin
Sex	Leukocyte count
Karnofsky performance	Lymphocyte count
Pathological stage	Neutrophil count
Treatment	Platelet count
Bulk	Monocyte count
B symptoms	ESR
Sweating	Bilirubin
Number of involved sites	Globulin
Weight loss	Albumin
Pruritus	Aspartate transaminase
Histology	Alkaline phosphatase

NB. Routine serum lactate dehydrogenase not done.

The most important variables for predicting relapse were RT alone (P < 0.0001), log lymphocyte count (P < 0.0001) (low values), and albumin ⩽43 g/L (P = 0.0193). Repeating the analysis for patients treated with RT alone showed that only two variables, log lymphocyte count and serum albumin, predicted relapse.

Survival

The 10-year survival, corrected for intercurrent deaths, was 92% for all patients (CI 88–98%), 90% (CI 81–98%) in the RT group, and 95% (CI 89–100%) in the RT + MVPP group (P = 0.66) (Fig. 2). In the RT alone arm, 45 (80%) of 56 patients are alive and relapse-free, 5 (9%) have died from HD, and 6 (11%) have died from intercurrent causes. In the adjuvant MVPP arm, 51 (86%) of 59 are alive and relapse-free, 4 (7%) have died of HD, and 4 (7%) have died from intercurrent causes.

In the RT alone group the deaths from HD occurred at 0.5, 2.3, 7, 8, and 10 years after diagnosis. Two patients with active HD died of disseminated herpes zoster infection. All patients who died in this group had presented with bulky disease. (The sites of bulk were cervical [1 patient], mediastinal and cervical [2 patients], mediastinum alone [1 patient], and axilla and cervical region [1 patient].) In the adjuvant MVPP group, the deaths from HD occurred at 0.75, 1.2, 7, and 10.5 years from diagnosis. Three patients had bulk at presentation. (The sites of bulk were mediastinum [1 patient], infraclavicular fossa and mediastinum [1 patient] and cervical region [1 patient].) The patient who died at 10.5 years did not receive adjuvant MVPP

(poor venous access). The patient who died at 1.2 years failed to achieve a CR during RT and adjuvant MVPP and died of progressive disease involving the skin and left lung hilum. The patient who died at 0.75 years relapsed during adjuvant MVPP.

Univariate analysis of prognostic factors for survival showed that the following had an adverse effect on survival: pruritus (P = 0.0014), night sweats (P = 0.0016), B symptoms (P = 0.0023), bulk (P = 0.0002), monocyte count >0.5×10^9/L (P = 0.0059), stage (P = 0.0191), mixed cellularity (P = 0.0227), and lymphocyte count ⩽1.7×10^9/L (P = 0.0385). A multivariate analysis for prognostic factors affecting survival was not possible owing to the small number of deaths from HD during the study.

Intercurrent deaths

There were 10 deaths from intercurrent causes; six patients had been randomised to receive RT alone, but two subsequently received salvage chemotherapy for relapse. Four patients who died were randomised to adjuvant MVPP, but one did not receive chemotherapy as he had hepatitis following his radiotherapy. Six patients died from a second malignancy, two had a myocardial infarction, one died from a pulmonary embolism (on oral contraceptives), and one died of pneumococcal septicaemia.

Second malignancy

There have been no cases of secondary acute myelogenous leukaemia. Eight patients developed a second malignancy 1–13 years after the diagnosis of HD, and six of these have died. Two patients are alive with sarcoma. There have been two patients with bronchial carcinoma, two with carcinoma of unknown primary site, one with non-Hodgkin's lymphoma, and one with gastric carcinoma.

Discussion

This study has shown that although adjuvant MVPP was associated with a significantly lower relapse rate there was no significant improvement in survival. Most patients who did relapse were successfully treated by chemotherapy with an 83% CR rate. It is of note that of the 9 deaths from HD, 5 occurred seven years after the original diagnosis was made.

Several studies have been performed using adjuvant chemotherapy after radiotherapy for PS IA–IIB [1, 7–10]. None of these studies have reported an overall survival advantage for the adjuvant chemotherapy group. Survival was 84–93% following RT alone and was 84–100% following adjuvant chemotherapy. On the other hand, RFS was significantly improved by adjuvant chemotherapy: 50–77% for RT alone and 84–95% with adjuvant chemotherapy. In these series, as in ours,

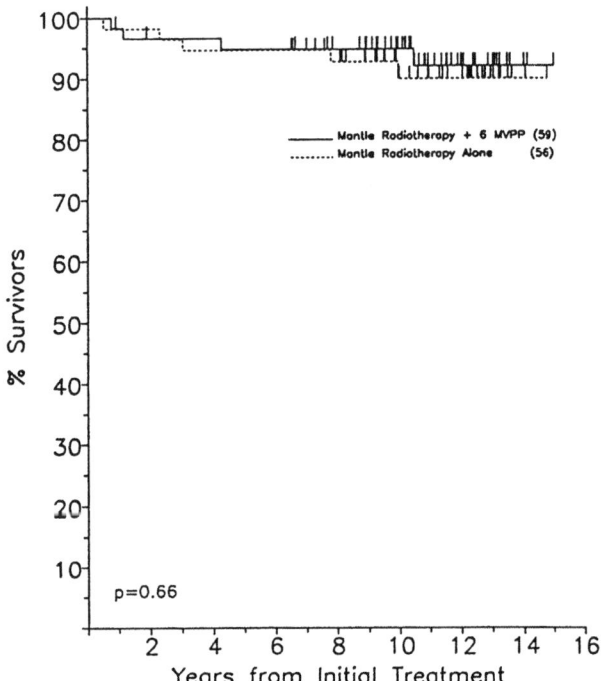

Fig. 2. Survival according to treatment group.

salvage therapy was successful for relapse, and with follow-up of 10 or more years no survival advantage is apparent for patients receiving adjuvant chemotherapy [7, 11].

This study commenced in 1974. Since then it has been shown that patients treated with MOPP chemotherapy have a risk of developing second malignancies [12, 13] and infertility [14–16]. The risk of second malignancy increases with increasing age [11, 17]. The incidence of second malignancy (solid tumours) in our study was 7% at 10 years. Valagussa et al. [12] reported an actuarial risk of $8.9 \pm 2.4\%$ at 12 years after RT alone and $9.9 \pm 4.9\%$ after RT plus MOPP. No cases of secondary acute myelogenous leukaemia were seen in our study.

The aim of the oncologist is to give the minimum amount of therapy that gives the patient the best chance of long-term survival. Prognostic factors should be sought to identify those patients for whom radiotherapy alone would be sufficient treatment. Patients at a high risk of relapse should be offered initial adjuvant chemotherapy, avoiding the physical and psychological morbidity associated with relapse.

The univariate analysis of prognostic factors for death from HD showed that pruritus, night sweats, B symptoms, bulk, monocyte count $>0.5 \times 10^9/L$, increasing stage, mixed cellularity, and lymphocyte count $\leqslant 1.7 \times 10^9/L$ adversely affected survival. There were too few deaths to analyse prognostic factors for survival using multivariate analysis.

Other centres have reported on the results of multivariate analysis. Haybittle et al. [18] analysed ten variables and found that age, mediastinal involvement, erythrocyte sedimentation rate, and gender were prognostic variables for survival in stage I–II patients. Pavlovsky et al. [22] reported that age and bulk were the only prognostic factors of the eight analysed that affected survival in their multivariate analysis of stage I and II patients, all of whom received chemotherapy with or without radiotherapy. Gobbi et al. [20] found that of nine variables, ESR, stage, histology, and age were the best prognostic factors in their group of 586 patients with stage IA–IVB HD.

Our multivariate analysis included 24 variables and showed that there were only three significant factors that predicted relapse: treatment with radiotherapy alone, a low lymphocyte count, and serum albumin $<43 \, g/L$. The multivariate analysis was repeated for patients in the radiotherapy alone group, and there were only two factors that predicted relapse: the lymphocyte count and serum albumin. These results are quite different from our first analysis that showed that treatment with radiotherapy alone was the most important factor, followed by bulk and then B symptoms [1]. In the initial paper only nine variables (age, gender, histology, pathological stage, A/B symptoms, number of sites involved, the result of the chest radiograph, bulk, and treatment) were analysed. Lymphocyte count and serum albumin were not included in the analysis. Lym-

Table 5. Risk factors for relapse in PS IA–IIB HD based on prognostic factors from multivariate analysis.

Variable	Adverse factor	B	Standard error	Relative + risk of relapse	Confidence interval
A. Prognostic factors from 1984 analysis					
Treatment ET bulk	RT only	1.62	0.503	5.0 ×	1.88–13.51
vs no bulk Mediastinal	ET bulk	0.295	0.585	1.3 ×	0.43–4.23
vs no bulk	Mediast. bulk	1.027	0.466	2.8 ×	1.12–6.96
Stage A/B	B	0.627	0.452	1.9 ×	0.77–4.54
B. Prognostic factors from 1990 analysis					
Treatment	RT only	1.89	0.531	6.6 ×	2.34–18.73
Lymphocyte count $(\log)_e$	Low values	−2.018	0.456	*7.5 ×	3.08–18.41
Albumin	$\leqslant 43 G/L$	1.023	0.451	2.8 ×	1.15–6.73

+ 'Risk' of relapse in adverse group compared to reference group.
* Per unit decrease in log lymphocyte count.

phocytopaenia was also shown to be an important adverse prognostic factor for survival in 301 patients with stage III–IV HD treated with MVPP [21]. The variables from the 1984 and 1990 multivariate analysis have been applied to the latest data to give the relative risks of relapse for the adverse variables (Table 5).

There is controversy over the relative importance of prognostic factors reported in multivariate analyses from various centres. There is an argument for a meta-analysis of pooled data to determine the relative importance of prognostic factors for patients with stage I–II HD. From these data a prognostic index could be produced which would allow therapy to be tailored to the patient allowing for the prognostic score.

Adjuvant chemotherapy studies have used either MOPP or MVPP chemotherapy regimens, but others could be used, e.g., ABVD (Adriamycin, bleomycin, vinblastine, and dacarbazine). ABVD is reported to be as effective as MOPP in the treatment of advanced HD [22]. It does cause vomiting and alopecia, but has a lower risk of second malignancy. Valagussa et al. [12] reported that the risk of second malignancy was 5.8% at 12 years after ABVD therapy. An Adriamycin-containing regimen without alkylating agents could be used as adjuvant therapy in patients at high risk of relapse with less risk of sterility and second malignancy.

In conclusion this study has shown that although patients treated with adjuvant chemotherapy following mantle radiotherapy for PS IA–IIB disease had significantly fewer relapses, there was no survival advantage. We propose that only patients with adverse prognostic factors should receive adjuvant chemotherapy.

References

1. Anderson H, Deakin DP, Wagstaff J et al. A randomised study of adjuvant chemotherapy after mantle radiotherapy in supra-

diaphragmatic Hodgkin's disease PS IA–IIB: A report from the Manchester Lymphoma Group. Brit J Cancer 1984; 49: 695–702.

2. Carbone PP, Kaplan HS, Musshoff K et al. Report of the committee of Hodgkin's disease staging classification. Cancer Res 1971; 31: 1860.

3. Lukes RJ, Craver LF, Hall TC et al. Report of the nomenclature committee. Cancer Res 1966; 26: 1311.

4. Anderson H, Jenkins JPR, Brigg D et al. The prognostic significance of mediastinal bulk in patients with stage IA–IVB Hodgkin's disease: a report from the Manchester Lymphoma Group. Clin Radiol 1985; 36: 449–454.

5. Miller AB, Hoogstraten B, Staquet M, Winkler A. Reporting the results of cancer treatment. Cancer 1981; 47: 207–214.

6. Cox DR. Regression models and life tables. J R Stat Soc B 1972; 34: 187.

7. Hoppe RT, Coleman NC, Cox RS et al. The management of stage I–II Hodgkin's disease with irradiation alone or combined modality therapy: The Stanford experience. Blood 1982; 59: 455–465.

8. Nissen NI, Nordentoft AM. Radiotherapy versus combined modality treatment of stage I and II Hodgkin's disease. Cancer Treat Rep 1982; 66: 799–803.

9. Wiernik PH, Gustafson J, Schimpff SC, Diggs C. Combined modality treatment of Hodgkin's disease confined to the lymph nodes. Results eight years later. AJM 1979; 67: 183–193.

10. Coltman CA, Fuller LA, Fisher R, Frei E. Extended field radiotherapy versus involved field radiotherapy plus MOPP in stage I and II Hodgkin's disease. In: Adjuvant therapy of cancer II. Eds: Joned and Salmon. New York. Grune and Stratton 1979; 129–144.

11. Coltman CA, Dahlberg S, Fuller L, Frei E. Localised (Stage I & II, A & B), Hodgkin's disease treated with extended field radiotherapy vs involved field radiotherapy plus MOPP with 16 year followup: a Southwest Oncology Group study. ASCO 1989 Abst 981, 252.

12. Valagussa P, Santoro A, Fossati-Bellani F et al. Second leukaemia and other malignancies following treatment for Hodgkin's disease. J Clin Oncol 1986; 4: 830–837.

13. Coleman CN. Second malignancy after treatment of Hodgkin's disease: an evolving picture. J Clin Onc 1986; 4: 821–824.

14. Chapman RM, Sutcliffe SB, Malpas JS. Cytotoxic-induced ovarian failure in women with Hodgkin's disease 1: Hormone function. JAMA 1979; 242: 1877–1881.

15. Chapman RM, Sutcliffe SB, Rees LH et al. Cyclical combination chemotherapy and gonadal function. Retrospective study in males. Lancet 1979; 1: 285–289.

16. Whitehead E, Shalet SM, Blackledge G et al. The effects of Hodgkin's disease and combination chemotherapy on gonadal function in the adult male. Cancer 1982; 49: 418–422.

17. Mauch PM, Canellos GP, Rosenthal DS, Hellman S. Reduction of fatal complications from combined modality therapy in Hodgkin's disease. J Clin Onc 1985; 3: 501–505.

18. Haybittle JL, Hayhoe FGJ, Easterling MJ et al. Review of the British National Lymphoma Investigation studies of Hodgkin's disease and development of prognostic index. Lancet 1985; 1: 967–972.

19. Pavlovsky A, Maschio M, Santarelli MT et al. Randomised trial of chemotherapy vertus chemotherapy plus radiotherapy for stage I–II Hodgkin's disease. JNCI 1988; 80: 1466–1473.

20. Gobbi PG, Cavalli C, Federico M et al. Hodgkin's disease prognosis: a directly predictive equation. Lancet 1988; 1: 675–678.

21. Wagstaff JW, Gregory WM, Swindell R et al. Prognostic factors for survival in stage IIB and IV Hodgkin's disease: a multivariate analysis comparing two specialist treatment centres. BJC 1988; 58: 487–492.

22. Bonadonna G, Santoro A. ABVD chemotherapy in the treatment of Hodgkin's disease. Cancer Treat Rev 1982; 9: 21–35.

Correspondence to:
Dr. Heather Anderson
CRC Department of Medical Oncology
Christie Hospital and Holt Radium Institute
Wilmslow Road
Withington
Manchester M20 9BX, UK

Annals of Oncology, Supplement 2 to Volume 2: 55–62, 1991.
© 1991 *Kluwer Academic Publishers.*

Original article _____

Alternating versus hybrid MOPP-ABVD in Hodgkin's disease: The Milan experience

S. Viviani, G. Bonadonna, A. Santoro, M. Zanini, R. Zucali, E. Negretti & P. Valagussa
Divisions of Medical Oncology, and Radiation Therapy, Istituto Nazionale Tumori, Milan, Italy

Summary. The long-term therapeutic results achieved in a previous randomized study on stage IV Hodgkin's disease confirm the superiority of MOPP monthly alternated with ABVD compared to MOPP alone. To more closely meet the requirements of the Goldie and Coldman hypothesis, we activated a randomized study testing MOPP-ABVD through two different sequences in July 1982. One arm consisted of monthly alternating one cycle of MOPP and one cycle of ABVD; in the other arm, one half cycle of MOPP was alternated with one half cycle of ABVD within a one-month period (hybrid regimen). Each regimen was given to complete remission plus two consolidation cycles (minimum six cycles). After maximal tumor shrinkage, moderate doses of radiotherapy (25–30 Gy) were delivered to the lymphoid region(s) if bulky at the start of chemotherapy. A total of 300 patients with stage IB, IIA bulky, IIB, III (A + B) and IV Hodgkin's disease previously untreated with chemotherapy or failing after extensive irradiation were evaluated. At a median follow-up of five years, alternating and hybrid regimens yielded superimposable treatment outcomes: complete remission 89 versus 88%, freedom from first progression 65 versus 70%; relapse-free survival 72 versus 78%, overall survival 81 versus 80%, respectively. Tumor cell burden expressed as number of involved nodal sites and presence of pulmonary hilus involvement were the prognostic variables able to significantly influence treatment outcome. Conversely, stage, constitutional symptoms, and histology had no impact on the five-year results. Since the majority of patients with stages II and III who failed after attainment of complete remission recurred in nodal sites only, present data suggest that both the role and the extent of radiotherapy combined with chemotherapy should be reconsidered.

Key words: alternating chemotherapy, Hodgkin's disease, hybrid regimen, MOPP-ABVD

Introduction

In 1974, about 10 years after the initial studies of mechlorethamine, vincristine, procarbazine, and prednisone (MOPP), we began to test the cyclical delivery of two non-cross-resistant combinations as primary chemotherapy for stage IV Hodgkin's disease [1, 2]. ABVD (doxorubicin [Adriamycin], bleomycin, vinblastine, and dacarbazine) was specifically designed in our Institute for MOPP-resistant patients [1] and was able to achieve second durable complete remissions in 46% of patients with Hodgkin's disease failing during primary MOPP or in complete remission for less than 12 months [3]. Knowing that about 20% of patients treated with MOPP do not enter complete remission and that about 40% of initial complete responders relapse within the first years from the end of treatment, we decided to test the administration of MOPP and ABVD alternating monthly to overcome the problem of drug-resistant cells. Our long-term results confirmed the superiority of alternating chemotherapy compared to MOPP alone [4, 5]. Our clinical study design preceded the mathematical model of Goldie and Coldman [6, 7]. According to this hypothesis, to overcome the resistant

subpopulations within the tumor it will be necessary to sequence and deliver the drugs in such a way as to minimize the growth of the partially resistant phenotypes. To more closely meet the requirements for this assumption to work, we have prospectively tested the delivery of MOPP-ABVD through a more rapid rotation of the two drug combinations.

Patients and methods

Trial design

From July 1982, patients with Hodgkin's disease previously untreated with chemotherapy and classified as stage IB, IIA bulky, III (A + B), and IV according to the Ann Arbor criteria [8] were enrolled into a prospective, randomized study comparing alternating versus hybrid administration of MOPP and ABVD. Patients with progressive lymphoma during or after total or subtotal nodal irradiation were also entered into the study. Before randomization, patients were stratified according to stage. Knowing the close relation between tumor volume and primary drug resistance [9, 10, 11], we de-

Table 1. Main patient characteristics.

	Alternating		Hybrid		Total series	
	No.	%	No.	%	No.	%
Total	152		148		300	
Sex						
Males	73	48	88	59	161	54
Females	79	52	60	41	139	46
Age						
≤40 yr	110	72	108	73	218	73
>40 yr	42	28	40	27	82	27
Histopathology						
Nodular sclerosis	119	78	104	69	223	74
Others	33	22	44	30	77	26
Symptoms						
Absent	57	38	69	47	126	42
Present	95	62	79	53	174	58
Disease extent						
Nodal only	108	71	102	69	210	70
Extra ± nodal	44	29	46	31	90	30
≤3 nodal sites	74	49	81	55	155	52
>3 nodal sites	78	51	67	45	145	48
Bulky disease						
No	82	54	85	57	167	56
Yes	70	46	63	43	133	44

Table 2. Hybrid drug combination.

Agent	Dose	Route	Time
Nitrogen mustard	6 mg/m^2	iv	day 1
Vincristine	1.4 mg/m^2	iv	day 1
Procarbazine	100 mg/m^2	po	days 1–7
Prednisone*	40 mg/m^2	im	days 1–7
Adriamycin	25 mg/m^2	iv	day 15
Bleomycin	10 mg/m^2	iv	day 15
Vinblastine	6 mg/m^2	iv	day 15
Dacarbazine	375 mg/m^2	iv	day 15

* On cycles 1, 4, (7), (10).
Repeat every 28 days.

livered moderate doses of irradiation (25–30 Gy) in complete responders or following maximal tumor shrinkage to the lymph node-bearing region(s) only if bulky at the start of chemotherapy.

Patient population

Between July 1982 and April 1990, a total of 410 consecutive patients were entered into the study. For the purpose of present analysis, only patients enrolled before December 1987, that is, with a minimum follow-up of 27 months, were considered. A total of 8 patients were not evaluable owing to refusal of treatment after the first cycle of chemotherapy (2 patients), concomitant AIDS (1 patient), and histologic diagnosis at re-

view (non-Hodgkin's lymphoma in 5 patients). Therefore, a total of 300 patients were considered evaluable for treatment comparison: 152 in the alternating regimen and 148 in the hybrid regimen. The median age in both groups was 32 years (median 31, ranges 17 to 69 in the alternating regimen; median 33, ranges 16 to 69 in the hybrid regimen). The main patient characteristics are reported in Table 1. Nodular sclerosis was the single most frequent histologic subset in both treatment arms, accounting for 74% of the case series. Stages of disease were well balanced between the two treatment groups. Overall, only 2% of patients presented with stage IB lymphoma, 11% with stage IIA bulky lymphoma, 30% with stage IIB, 29% with stage III, and 14% with stage IV disease. Primary radiotherapy failures accounted for 40 patients (13%), and 13 of them presented with extranodal disease. Massive involvement [12] of one or more lymphoid regions was documented in 133 patients (44%). In particular, bulky mediastinal involvement (mass:thoracic ratio >0.33 between the largest transverse diameter of mediastinal mass and the transverse diameter of the thorax at the level of T5 or T6 on a standing posteroanterior chest radiograph) accounted for 87 patients (alternating regimen: 46; hybrid regimen: 41). Half the patients presented with up to three involved nodal sites, and only 30% had extranodal disease. Presence of constitutional symptoms, female sex, nodular sclerosis histology, and involvement of more than three nodal sites were more frequent in the alternating regimen. The median follow-up period from starting therapy was 60 months.

Staging procedure

Clinical staging consisted of physical examination, complete blood cell count (CBC), liver and renal function tests, posteroanterior and lateral chest roentgenogram, and bipedal lymphangiography. Additional roentgenograms and radioisotopic studies were performed only in the presence of given clinical situations. In addition to biopsy of peripheral lymph nodes, invasive tests for pathologic staging included two needle bone marrow core biopsies from bilateral iliac crests in 278 patients (93%) and a single bone marrow biopsy in the remaining 22 patients. The abdominal extent of disease was evaluated through the classical staging laparotomy in 45 patients, whereas 238 patients (79%) underwent staging laparoscopy with multiple liver biopsies to detect or rule out hepatic involvement.

Treatment plan

The alternating regimen (the control arm) consisted of the administration of one full monthly cycle of MOPP followed by one full monthly cycle of ABVD at the classical dose schedules previously reported [1, 2, 4, 13]. The hybrid regimen (the experimental arm) consisted of the administration of a half cycle of MOPP and a half cycle of ABVD within a one-month period

(Table 2). In both regimens, in the presence of myelosuppression on the day of intravenous drug administration, we preferred to delay treatment until full doses could be administered rather than reducing doses of mechlorethamine, procarbazine, Adriamycin, and vinblastine. In the presence of severe paresthesias and/or constipation, the dose of vincristine and vinblastine was reduced by 50%. In the presence of adynamic ileus, both drugs were almost always permanently discontinued.

In the absence of tumor progression, treatment with either alternating or hybrid regimen was continued to the achievement of complete remission plus two consolidation cycles. In all responding patients, a minimum of six treatment cycles had to be administered. Moderate doses of irradiation (25–30 Gy) were delivered through cobalt 60 teletherapy or 6-meV linear accelerator to the site(s) of initial bulky nodal involvement once complete remission or maximal tumor shrinkage was achieved by primary chemotherapy. The interval before starting irradiation ranged from three to five weeks.

Evaluation of treatment response

In the absence of progressive lymphoma during treatment, response was assessed either at the end of chemotherapy regimen or at the completion of both chemotherapy and irradiation for patients with bulky disease. A patient was considered to be in complete remission when all symptoms and signs of disease had disappeared for a minimum of one month. Repeat biopsies were performed in patients presenting with either liver or bone marrow involvement to rule out the presence of lymphoma. Patients were then followed every three months during the subsequent two years and every six months thereafter. Biochemical tests, hemogram, chest roentgenogram, and abdominal flat plate were repeated at these intervals. All patients not achieving complete remission were considered as treatment failures.

Second-line treatments

Patients who failed to attain complete remission or who relapsed within 12 months from complete remission were considered resistant to primary chemotherapy. Patients who achieved only a partial response were initially given salvage irradiation to the site(s) of residual lymphoid disease. All other patients were to be treated with the CEP (CCNU [lomustine], etoposide, and prednimustine) combination [14] ± irradiation. Starting from 1985, selected patients (those aged <40 years, with no bone marrow involvement, Karnofsky performance status >70, and no or limited prior irradiation) were entered into a program of high-dose chemotherapy followed by autologous bone marrow transplant and total body irradiation [15]. Patients who could not be entered into this program, either received high-dose chemotherapy regimens or were treated with CEP with or without irradiation. Patients who showed relapse more than 12 months after achievement of complete remission were to be retreated with the initial regimen.

Statistical analysis

The statistical significance of differences in the frequency of complete response in various subsets was calculated by the chi-square test with correction for continuity. The probabilities of freedom from first progression (FFP) for all patients or relapse-free survival (RFS) in complete responders and of surviving were computed by the life-table method, starting from the date of treatment. In the analysis of FFP and RFS, progressive lymphoma was the only event considered; whereas in the survival analysis, all causes of death were included. The statistical analysis of observed differences was assessed by the log rank test [16].

Results

Comparative five-year analysis

The comparative frequency of complete remission related to the main patient characteristics is reported in Table 3. A total of 267 patients (89%) achieved complete response, 136 of 152 (89%) in the alternating regimen and 131 of 148 (88%) in the hybrid regimen. In all subgroups, there was no difference in the attain-

Table 3. Comparative complete remission rates (Data are in %).

	Alternating	Hybrid	Total series
Total	89	88	89
Sex			
Males	86	86	86
Females	92	92	92
Age			
≤40 yr	89	90	89
>40 yr	90	85	88
Histopathology			
Nodular sclerosis	89	87	88
Others	91	93	92
Symptoms			
Absent	95	90	92
Present	86	87	87
Disease extent			
Nodal only	92	89	90
Extra ± nodal	84	87	86
≤3 nodal sites	96	94	95
>3 nodal sites	83	82	83
Bulky disease			
No	95	91	93
Yes	83	86	84

Table 4. Comparative 5-year results (data are in %).

	Alternating		Hybrid		Total series	
	FFP	RFS	FFP	RFS	FFP	RFS
Total	65	72	70	78	67	75
Sex						
Males	64	73	70	79	68	76
Females	65	72	69	75	67	73
Age						
≤40 yr	65	73	70	78	67	75
>40 yr	65	72	71	78	67	74
Histopathology						
Nodular sclerosis	63	71	68	78	66	75
Others	69	76	74	77	71	76
Symptoms						
Absent	65	69	67	72	66	70
Present	64	74	72	83	68	78
Disease extent						
Nodal only	67	73	72	80	70	76
Extra ± nodal	59	72	65	75	62	73
≤3 nodal sites	73	76	73	78	73	77
>3 nodal sites	58	70	66	77	62	73
Bulky disease						
No	64	68	71	76	68	72
Yes	66	78	69	80	67	73

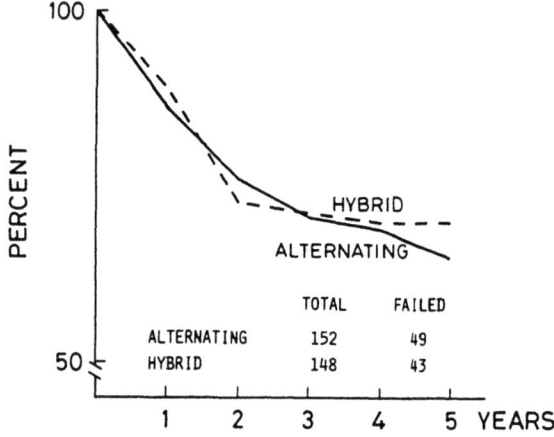

(A) Freedom from first progression

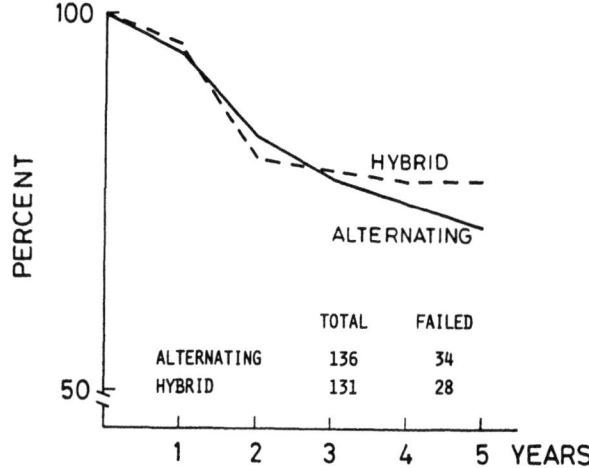

(B) Relapse-free survival.

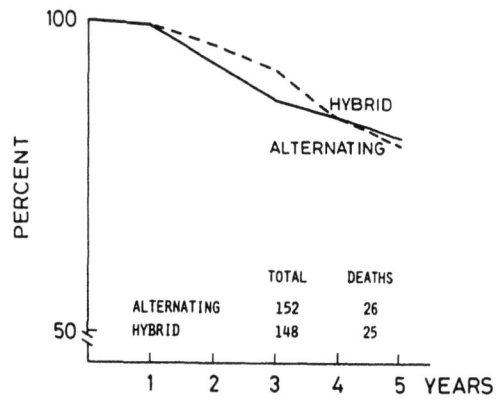

(C) Overall survival.

Fig. 1. Comparative 5-year results after alternating versus hybrid regimen.

ment of complete remission related to the two different rotations of MOPP and ABVD. Median number of cycles required to achieve complete remission was four. A total of 59% of complete responders were given six cycles of either regimen, and only 4% required more than eight cycles to complete their treatment program. One hundred and twelve patients with bulky lymphoma achieved complete remission (84%). In 93 of them, involved-field radiotherapy was delivered after completion of chemotherapy; whereas 17 received irradiation before the last two consolidation cycles, and in two patients radiotherapy was not delivered. A total of 25 of 300 patients (8%) showed progressive lymphoma while on treatment, and in 8 additional patients (3%) primary chemotherapy was able to induce only a partial response.

The comparative five-year results for the entire series are reported in Figure 1 and detailed in Table 4. Overall, 67% of 300 patients remained alive and disease-free within five years from starting primary chemotherapy. No difference was evident between the two treatment regimens, the relative figures for freedom from first progression being 65% in the alternating arm and 70% in the hybrid regimen (Fig. 1a). Similar results were also achieved in terms of relapse-free (72% versus 78%, Fig. 1b) and overall survival (81% versus 80%, Fig. 1c).

Five-year results relative to prognostic variables

Because of the substantial lack of differences between the two treatment regimens, we attempted to assess the relative impact of known prognostic variables on treatment outcome through a univariate analysis. Presence

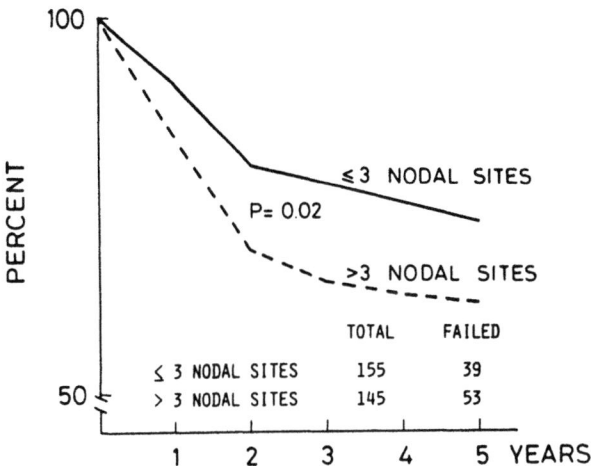

Fig. 2. Freedom from first progression related to the number of involved nodal sites.

Table 5. Influence of mediastinal and pulmonary hilus involvement.

	No. cases	CR %	FFP %
Mediastinal involvement			
Absent	131	92	73*
Nonbulky	82	87	56*
Bulky	87	86	69*
Pulmonary hilus			
Not involved	194	91	71**
Involved	106	85	61**
Nonbulky mediastinum			
P. hilus negative	42	90	63
P. hilus positive	40	82	49
Bulky mediastinum			
P. hilus negative	29	90	74
P. hilus positive	58	84	66

* P = 0.024.
** P = 0.04.

Table 6. Influence of number of involved nodal sites and pulmonary hilus involvement (data are in %).

	No. cases	CR	FFP	RFS	Survival
≤3 nodal sites, no p. hilus	121	94	77	81	87
>3 nodal sites, and/or p. hilus	179	85	61	70	75
P value		0.02	0.002	0.01	0.01

of constitutional symptoms failed to influence either attainment of complete remission ('B' 87% versus 'A' 92%) or freedom from first progression (68% versus 66%, respectively). Also age (≤40 years versus >40 years) had no impact on the five-year freedom from progression (Table 4), but older patients had a significantly lower total survival (64%) compared to younger patients (86%, P < 0.01). This was probably due to a higher frequency of second fatal cancers in patients older than 40 years (see Second Malignancies).

The single most important prognostic variable was represented by tumor cell burden expressed as number of involved nodal sites (three or fewer versus more than three). Patients presenting with minimal tumor cell burden (≤3 nodal sites) experienced a better treatment outcome compared to their counterparts with more than three nodal sites. This held true so far as complete remission (95 versus 83%, P = 0.001), freedom from first progression (Fig. 2, 73 versus 62%, P = 0.02) and total survival rates (86 versus 74%, P = 0.02) were concerned.

The influence of mediastinal and pulmonary hilus involvement on treatment outcome is detailed in Table 5. Briefly, the presence of mediastinal and/or pulmonary hilus involvement negatively influenced the five-year results. Patients with bulky mediastinal adenopathy experienced a better freedom from first progression (69%) compared to patients with only minimal mediastinal involvement (56%). It is worth stressing that, in complete responders, moderate doses of irradiation were delivered only to the site(s) of initial bulky adenopathy, and this could have influenced the final treatment outcome. In fact, in 39 complete responders with initial mediastinal involvement who eventually relapsed, intrathoracic relapses were documented in 28 (72%), and in 20 of the 28 (71%) radiotherapy was not delivered to the mediastinal region because of nonbulky adenopathy. The presence of concomitant involvement of pulmonary hilus contributed to worsening the five-year freedom from first progres-

sion, regardless of the extent of mediastinal adenopathy (Table 5).

The presence of more than three involved nodal sites and/or of pulmonary hilus involvement negatively influenced treatment outcome (Table 6), regardless of whether or not massive adenopathy was present. In fact, in the present case series, patients presenting with three or fewer nodal sites in the absence of pulmonary

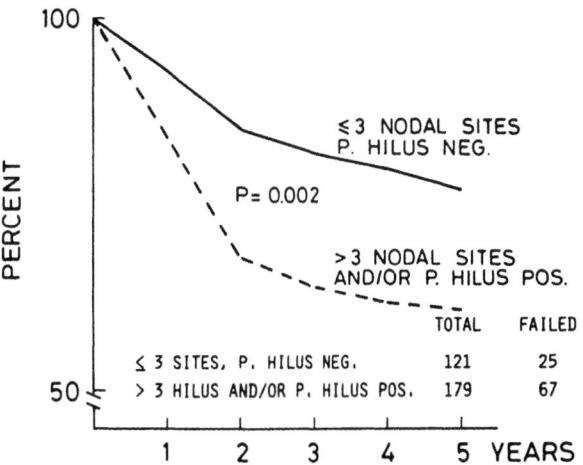

Fig. 3. Freedom from first progression related to the number of involved nodal sites and presence of pulmonary hilus involvement.

hilus involvement experienced the best freedom from first progression (Fig. 3; P = 0.002), relapse-free (P = 0.01) and overall survival (P = 0.01).

Salvage treatment

A total of 69 patients were considered resistant to primary chemotherapy. We also included in this category 6 of the 8 partial responders who were given radiotherapy to the region(s) of residual disease and subsequently manifested disease progression within a median of nine months from completion of irradiation. Overall, 58% of 69 patients were able to enter complete remission with different salvage regimens, with a median duration of 20 months. Table 7 details treatment results according to the modalities utilized. High-dose chemotherapy followed by autologous bone marrow transplant and total body irradiation was able to achieve an impressively high complete remission rate (75%) in 12 selected patients considered resistant to first-line chemotherapy. Twenty-two of the 23 patients whose first complete remission exceeded 12 months are evaluable, and a second complete response was achieved in 82%. Seventeen patients were re-treated with the same regimen utilized as first-line chemotherapy, and the duration of their second complete remission is estimated to be in excess of 22 months.

Table 7. Salvage regimens in relapsing Hodgkin's disease treated with MOPP and ABVD.

Results of primary chemotherapy	No. cases	CR %	Median duration (months)
Failure or CR <12 mo.	69	58	20
CEP ± radiotherapy	44	52	15
High-dose chemotherapy + ABMT and TBI	12	75	>21
Other treatment	13	62	>20
CR >12 months	22	82	>21
MOPP/ABVD	17	76	>22
CEP ± radiotherapy	5	100	>14

CR = complete remission.
ABMT = autologous bone marrow transplant.
TBI = total body irradiation.

Treatment compliance

Both alternating and hybrid regimens were fairly well tolerated and only 7 patients refused to complete their treatment program after achievement of complete remission. The median percentage of optimal dose administered during the first six cycles was 92% for the alternating regimen and 93% for the hybrid regimen. In spite of optimal dose delivered, median relative dose intensity (expressed as doses received during the first six cycles and actual days of treatment divided by planned doses and treatment duration) was only 0.79 for the alternating regimen and 0.78 for the hybrid regi-

men. This was due to the fact that, in the presence of myelosuppression on the day of intravenous drug administration, we preferred delaying treatment for a few days rather than reducing the dose. Leukocyte counts <2500/μL were documented in 70% of patients, and platelet counts <75 000/μL in 8%. No patient required hospital admission for infectious disease. Pulmonary lung fibrosis due to bleomycin administration was documented in two patients. One patient received the hybrid regimen after failure from primary irradiation and the administration of bleomycin contributed to the aggravation of paramediastinal fibrosis; bleomycin was discontinued after the second administration, and the patient died because of pulmonary failure five years from the last administration of chemotherapy while in complete remission from Hodgkin's disease. The other patient never received irradiation; bleomycin was discontinued after the fourth dose, and she is presently alive and well, three years from treatment discontinuation. No cases of congestive heart failure attributable to Adriamycin administration have been so far documented.

Second malignancies

A total of 15 second malignancies were observed within five years from starting primary chemotherapy. Of these 9 patients (median age 45 years, range 19–56) developed acute nonlymphocytic leukemia within a median of 43 months (range 22–53) from the start of primary chemotherapy, and 7 of them died within a few months. Of 2 patients who developed leukemia while in complete remission, 1 had received prior irradiation and 1 had received concomitant irradiation because of bulky adenopathy. In the remaining 7 patients, leukemia developed after they received CEP chemotherapy plus extensive irradiation because of progressive lymphoma. One patient developed high-grade non-Hodgkin's lymphoma while in second complete remission after re-treatment with the alternating regimen followed by irradiation and died of progressive non-Hodgkin's lymphoma. Five second solid tumors were documented, all in patients aged >40 years. Four patients developed lung cancer while in complete remission; only 1 of them received prior irradiation to the mediastinal region, and a history of smoking was reported for 2 other patients. All patients who developed solid tumors died, except 1 patient who developed lung cancer (T_1 lesion) and is presently alive more than three years from the diagnosis of second tumor.

Discussion

The five-year results presented in this paper strongly suggest that our hybrid regimen is not superior to the alternating regimen. However, since more than 400 patients were entered on study, there is a possibility that future evaluations based on a higher number of patients and a longer follow-up may disclose some differences in given prognostic subsets. The correct interpretation of current findings appears very difficult. Considering our previous clinical data [3] as well as those recently reported by the Cancer and Leukemia Group B [17], it is conceivable that MOPP and ABVD may actually not be quantitatively equivalent, i.e., they do not exert the same log kill on the drug-sensitive component and same log kill on the resistant component. If the assumption about lack of symmetry between MOPP and ABVD is correct, then it is not surprising that a more rapid rotation (hybrid) of two unequally effective regimens failed to yield superior results compared to their 'relaxed' administration, i.e., monthly alternation [18]. The advantage of the alternating schedule over MOPP or ABVD alone was found to be significant in disseminated (stage IV) Hodgkin's disease, as previously reported by our group [4, 5] and by investigators of Cancer and Leukemia Group B [17].

The evaluation of our large group of patients as a whole allowed us to reemphasize the importance of some of the known prognostic indicators. Tumor volume expressed by number of sites, extranodal lymphoma, or bulky adenopathy showed a slight but consistent unfavorable influence on the complete remission rate. The same applied to the presence of 'B' symptoms. Freedom from progression was mainly affected by the number of involved nodal sites but not by bulky adenopathy, possibly as a consequence of radiotherapy following chemotherapy in this particular subset. The presence of a radiologically positive pulmonary hilus affected treatment outcome regardless of whether irradiation was or was not delivered post chemotherapy.

The high percentage of first relapse in nodal sites should stimulate the reconsideration of involved-field radiotherapy once complete or almost complete remission is achieved. The irradiation doses should not be less than 25 to 30 Gy; since minimal postchemotherapy doses, as delivered by other investigators [19, 20], failed to influence treatment outcome over combination chemotherapy alone. Although the delivery of high relative dose intensity rather than full doses through treatment delays may be expected to more favorably affect treatment outcome, it is important to stress that present results were achieved in both arms utilizing a lesser number of cycles than in our previous study designed to include a total of 12 cycles [4].

The effectiveness of salvage regimens was related to the duration of first remission, as detailed in another publication [3]. Two points deserve a brief consideration. First, in patients failing on primary MOPP/ABVD or relapsing within 12 months from complete remission, high-dose chemotherapy plus autologous bone marrow transplantation (ABMT) yielded a higher frequency (75%) of second complete response compared to other treatments. Most probably, in these prognostic categories, ABMT should become the treatment of choice when primary chemotherapy is MOPP/ABVD

regardless of the sequence applied. The second consideration regards iatrogenic morbidity. Patients given CEP and extensive radiotherapy for nodal relapse manifested the well-known incidence of fatal secondary acute nonlymphocytic leukemia. Leukemia occurred preferentially in patients older than 40 years of age and was responsible for the lower total survival of this age group compared to younger patients. Thus, the attempt to decrease the percentage of nodal relapses by postchemotherapy involved-field radiation delivered at moderate doses should reduce the necessity of administering salvage regimens including further alkylating agents.

In conclusion, the results of our randomized study should stimulate further discussion about treatment sequences, asymmetry, and uncertainty about protocol strategies for combination chemotherapy in Hodgkin's disease. From the clinical point of view, current findings reiterate the effectiveness of Adriamycin-based combinations and the importance of tumor volume in assessing prognosis.

References

1. Bonadonna G. Chemotherapy strategies to improve the control of Hodgkin's disease. The Richard and Hinda Rosenthal Foundation Award Lecture. Cancer Res 1982; 42: 4309–20.
2. Santoro A, Bonadonna G, Bonfante V et al. Alternating drug combinations in the treatment of advanced Hodgkin's disease. New Engl J Med 1982; 306: 770–5.
3. Bonadonna G, Santoro A, Gianni AM et al. Primary and salvage chemotherapy in Hodgkin's disease. The experience of the Milan Cancer Institute. Ann Oncol 1990 (in press).
4. Bonadonna G, Valagussa P, Santoro A. Alternating non-cross-resistant combination chemotherapy or MOPP in Stage IV Hodgkin's disease. A report of 8-year results. Ann Intern Med 1986; 104: 739–46.
5. Bonadonna G, Valagussa P. The influence of clinical trials on current treatment strategy for Hodgkin's disease. Int J Radiat Oncol Biol Phys 1990; 19: 209–18.
6. Goldie JH, Coldman AJ. A mathematical model for relating the drug sensitivity of tumors to their spontaneous mutation rate. Cancer Treat Rep 1979; 63: 1727–33.
7. Goldie JH, Coldman AJ, Gudauskas GA. Rationale for the use of alternating non-cross resistant chemotherapy. Cancer Treat Rep 1982; 66: 439–49.
8. Carbone PP, Kaplan HS, Musshoff K et al. Report of the committee on Hodgkin's disease staging classification. Cancer Res 1971; 31: 1860–1.
9. De Vita VT Jr. The relationship between tumor mass and resistance to chemotherapy: implication for surgical adjuvant treatment of cancer. Cancer 1983; 51: 1209–20.
10. Goldie JH, Coldman AJ. The genetic origin of drug resistance in neoplasms: implication for systemic therapy. Cancer Res 1984; 3643–53.
11. Skipper HE, Schabel FM Jr. Tumor stem cell heterogeneity: implication with respect to classification of cancers by chemotherapeutic effect. Cancer Treat Rep 1984; 68: 43–61.
12. Bonadonna G, Valagussa P, Santoro A. Prognosis of bulky Hodgkin's disease treated with chemotherapy alone or combined with radiotherapy. Cancer Surveys 1985; 4: 438–58.
13. De Vita VT Jr, Serpick AA, Carbone PP. Combination chemotherapy in the treatment of advanced Hodgkin's disease. Ann Intern Med 1970; 73: 881–95.

14. Bonadonna G, Viviani S, Valagussa P et al. Third-line salvage chemotherapy in Hodgkin's disease. Semin Oncol 1985; 12 (suppl 2): 23–5.
15. Gianni AM, Bonadonna G. High dose chemotherapy for sensitive tumors: is sequential better than current drug delivery? Eur J Cancer Clin Oncol 1989; 25: 1027–30.
16. Peto R, Pike MC, Armitage P et al. Design and analysis of randomized clinical trials requiring prolonged observation of each patient: II. Analysis and examples. Br J Cancer 1977; 35: 1–39.
17. Anderson JR, Canellos GP, Propert KJ et al. MOPP vs ABVD vs MOPP alternating with ABVD as treatment for advanced Hodgkin's disease: results at a median follow-up of 4 years. Ann Oncol 1990 (in press).
18. Day RS. Treatment sequencing, asymmetry, and uncertainty: protocol strategies for combination chemotherapy. Cancer Res 1986; 46: 3876–85.
19. Glick J, Tsiatis A, Chen M et al. A randomized ECOG trial of alternating MOPP-ABVD vs. BCVPP vs. BCVPP plus radiotherapy for advanced Hodgkin's disease. Proc Am Soc Clin Oncol 1988; 7: 223 (abstr).
20. Diehl V, Pfreundschuh M, Löffler M et al. Chemotherapy vs. involved-field radiotherapy for consolidation of remission achieved with three double cycles of cyclophosphamide, vincristine, procarbazine, prednisone (COPP) and doxorubicin, bleomycin, vinblastine, dacarbazine (ABVD) for stages III/IV Hodgkin's disease: a randomized trial of the German Hodgkin Study Group. Proc Am Soc Clin Oncol 1990; 9: 273 (abstr).

Correspondence to:
Gianni Bonadonna, M.D.
Division of Medical Oncology
Istituto Nazionale Tumori
Via Venezian 1
20133 Milano, Italy

Annals of Oncology, Supplement 2 to Volume 2: 63–66, 1991.
© 1991 *Kluwer Academic Publishers*.

Original article —————————————————————————————

Management of relapse and survival in advanced stage Hodgkin's disease: The EORTC experience

J. M. V. Burgers, R. Somers, M. Henry-Amar, M. Tarayre, P. Carde, J. Thomas, A. Hagenbeek, M. Monconduit, B. E. de Pauw, W. P. M. Breed, L. Verdonck, M. Hayat & R. Zittoun
The Netherlands Cancer Institute, Antoni van Leeuwenhoek Huis, Plesmanlaan 121, 1066 CX Amsterdam, The Netherlands

Summary. The EORTC Lymphoma Cooperative Group and the Pierre and Marie Curie Group conducted a multicentre randomised trial on clinical stages IIIB–IV Hodgkin's disease from 1981–1986. Two hundred seven patients were registered and 192 randomised. Actuarial survival at five years for the whole group was 68%. Induction chemotherapy with eight cycles of MOPP resulted in more patients with progressive disease and fewer partial responders than a combination of MOPP and ABVD, for an equal complete remission rate. Half of the partial responders went into complete remission after radiotherapy. At five years there was no significant survival difference between the arms. Progression was recorded in 39 patients of whom only 4 survived. Relapses were most frequent in previously involved unirradiated areas. For 46 relapsed patients, including 21 early relapses within 18 months of start of treatment, the four-year survival rate was 53%. When complete remission was reached, whether early or late with combination chemotherapy or after additional radiotherapy, prognosis was independent of the way in which it was achieved. All efforts should be taken to reach a complete remission for initially progressing patients and for partial responders.

Key words: advanced Hodgkin's disease

Introduction

The EORTC Lymphoma Cooperative Group and the Pierre and Marie Curie Group decided in 1980 to study advanced stage Hodgkin's disease in a cooperative multicentre trial. The investigation compared the effectiveness of chemotherapy using MOPP with that of a combination of MOPP and ABVD. A second aim was to study the prognostic value of early remission. A third set of concerns was survival, disease-free survival, and relapse pattern in this group of clinically staged patients suffering from stage IIIB–IV Hodgkin's disease, after treatment with combination chemotherapy followed by iceberg radiotherapy to bulky or slowly regressing nodal disease only. The present report focuses on the comparison of MOPP with MOPP/ABVD and on the relapse pattern. A more detailed report, also describing the prognostic value of early remission evaluation, is being prepared by the study coordinators, and an earlier presentation was published in 1988 [1].

Materials and methods

Patients were clinically staged, including chest x-ray, lymphangiogram, and liver ultrasound or abdominal CT scan, further bone marrow biopsy and isotopic bone scan, after general and haematologic examination and biopsy of a relevant lymph node. Treatment started with two courses of MOPP (mechlorethamine 6 mg/m^2 on days 1 and 8, Oncovin 1.4 mg/m^2 on days 1 and 8, procarbazine 100 mg/m^2 on days 1–14, and prednisone 25 mg/m^2 on days 1–14). After randomisation, treatment continued with six further courses of MOPP (M arm) or two courses of ABVD, two courses of MOPP, and two further courses of ABVD (doxorubicin [Adriamycin] 25 mg/m^2 on days 1 and 15, vinblastine 6 mg/m^2 on days 1 and 15, bleomycin 10 mg/m^2 on days 1 and 15, and dacarbazine 375 mg/m^2 on days 1 and 15) (M/A arm). Thereafter, radiation treatment was given to nodal areas harbouring disease >5 cm at start of treatment or not in complete remission after four courses of chemotherapy.

Lung, liver, and bone lesions were not irradiated. The radiation dose was 20 Gy; any lymph node area not in complete remission at the time of irradiation received 30 Gy.

From 1981 to 1986, 207 patients between 15 and 70 years of age with Hodgkin's disease clinical stage IIIB and IV were registered by 19 centres. One hundred ninety-two patients were randomised after

Table 1.

	M (96)	M/A (96)
CS III 1–3 nodal areas	18%	15%
> 1–3 nodal areas	32%	34%
CS IV 0–3 nodal areas	21%	19%
> 4 nodal areas	29%	32%
mediast. inv. none	39%	38%
M/T ratio < 1/3	40%	44%
bulky	20%	18%
liver involvement	16%	18%
lung involvement	16%	20%
bone involvement	11%	15%
bone marrow involvement	14%	13%

M = M arm (MOPP only) see text; M/A = M/A arm (MOPP and ABVD) see text; CS = clinical stage; M/T = mediastinum-thorax ratio.

Table 2.

	M (96)	M/A (96)
After CT, 8 cycles		
CR	57%	59%
PR	20%	32%
progression	23%	8% P = 0.014
After CT 8 cycles ± RT		
CR	68%	73%
6 year: RFS	61%	69%
FFP	43%	60% P = 0.025
S	57%	65% P = 0.13

CR = complete remission; PR = partial remission; RFS = relapse free survival; FFP = free from progression; S = overall survival. See also legends Table 1.

two courses of MOPP, while 6 patients refused, 4 showed disease progression, and 5 were not randomised for other reasons. Median age was 34 years, with 29% over 40 years of age; 64% were male; B symptoms were present in 21%. Nodular sclerosing histology was present in 64%, and mixed cellularity in 29%.

Disease extent, in terms of stage, number of involved nodal areas, mediastinal involvement, and organ involvement, is shown in Table 1. The distribution was well balanced between both treatment arms.

All data were stored at the Institut Gustave Roussy, Villejuif, France, using a specific database management program [2]. In 1989 a questionnaire was sent regarding the 85 patients with progression or relapse asking for further information on site of relapse in relation to previous involvement and radiotherapy, and inquiring after further management. Answers were collected for 27 of the 39 patients who had progression before treatment was completed, for 36 of the 46 who later relapsed. For all patients data were updated as of February 1, 1990.

Results

Primary treatment

Among the 96 patients in the M arm, 22 progressions took place, while in the M/A arm only 8 progressions occurred P = 0.014). There was a lesser difference in partial remission, 19 patients in the M arm versus 29 in the M/A arm, half of whom were brought into complete remission by additional irradiation. The complete remission rate after eight cycles was equal, 57 and 55% patients, and the complete remission rate after completion of therapy, with or without additional radiotherapy, was 68% patients and 73% patients, respectively (Table 2). Freedom from progression (FFP) differed significantly, being higher in the M/A arm than in the

EORTC TRIAL ON CS IIIB-IV HD

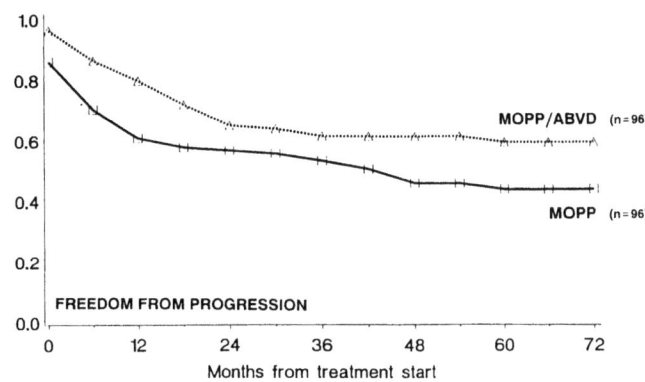

Fig. 1. Freedom from progression for randomised patients, according to treatment arm.

EORTC TRIAL ON CS IIIB-IV HD

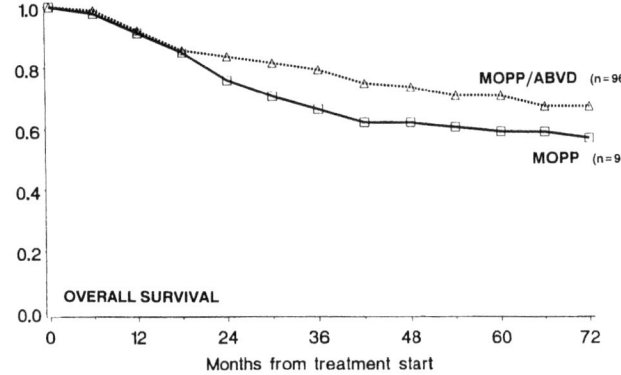

Fig. 2. Actuarial survival for randomised patients according to treatment arm.

M arm, 60 versus 43% at five years, respectively (P = 0.025), while survival was not significantly different (Figs 1 and 2), and relapse-free survival was similar for both arms.

For patients in complete remission, whether reached early, later or only after additional radiotherapy, re-

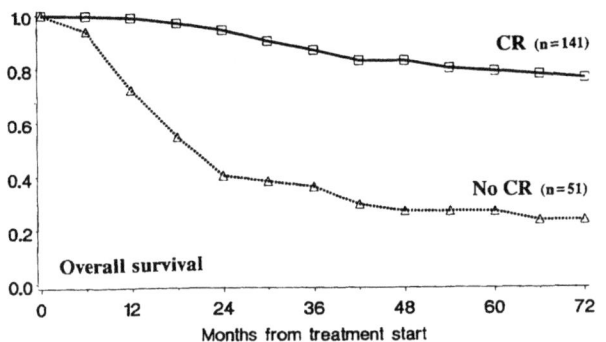

Fig. 3. Complete remission (CR) groups patients in CR after four courses, after eight courses, or after eight courses and radiotherapy. All others combines partial remission (18) and progressions (39). Actuarial survival is plotted from start of treatment.

Table 3.

	196 pt	FFP 6 yr	S 6 yr
CR after 4 cycles	81	64%	72%
CR after 8 cycles	34	71%	77%
CR after 8 cycles + RT	25	48%	75%
Other patients	52	19%	24%
PR	18		
progression	39		
All patients	196	51%	61%

CR = complete remission; PR = partial remission; RFS = relapse free survival; FFP = free from progression; S = overall survival. See also legends Table 1.

lapse-free survival was similar (67% at five years), and survival was 78%. For patients who did not reach complete remission, five-year survival was 28% (Table 3 and Fig. 3). The overall survival for the whole group at five years was 68%.

Progression

During initial treatment, 39 (20%) patients underwent disease progression. Further data are available for 27 of the 39. The site of progression is detailed in Table 4, showing that 16 of 27 patients had progression in sites amenable to radiotherapy. After second-line treatment, a complete remission was reached in 6 patients (treatment included radiotherapy in all); 4 of them survived, 3 now longer than five years. Five patients in partial remission were not irradiated and all died. Fifteen patients had a second progression; their treatment included radiotherapy in 1 and intensive chemotherapy with autologous bone marrow support (ABMT) in 1. These 15 patients all died within two years. Finally, 1 patient died of a non-Hodgkin's lymphoma. The four-year survival rate of this group with progressive disease was 8% (Table 5).

Table 4.

Relapse site:

Progressions	Relapses
11 isolated nodal	22 isolated nodal*
5 lung/bone + nodal	6 lung/bone + nodal
3 bone-marrow	4 isolated organs
8 multiple nodal + extranodal	4 multiple nodal + extranodal
27	36

* 3 in previously involved irradiated areas (20 Gy).
RT = radiotherapy. Answers to questionnaires were collected from 27/39 progressions and 36/46 relapses.

Relapses

After initial complete remission, a relapse was recorded for 46 of 135 patients (34%), in 21 within 18 months of start of treatment (early relapse), and in 25 later than 18 months after start of treatment. For 36 patients more information is available. The site of relapse is detailed in Table 4. Isolated nodal relapse occurred in 22 of 36 patients, and only 3 were within previously irradiated involved areas. Another 6 patients had nodal relapses together with bone or lung lesions. A second complete remission was reached in 23 of these 36 patients through second-line treatment including radiotherapy in 15 and ABMT in 3, and 17 of these 23 remained alive. In these 17 patients, 5 second relapses took place with patients alive at time of reporting. Of the 8 patients who reached partial remission (including 1 who received radiotherapy) and 5 who had further progression (including 2 who received radiotherapy and 1 who received ABMT), 3 patients were alive at time of analysis (Table 5). The four-year survival for all patients with relapse was 53%. Of the 21 patients with early relapse, and the 16 patients with relapse between 18 and 36 months after start of treatment, half of each group remained alive. For the 9 patients who developed a relapse later than 36 months, follow-up thereafter is still too short for meaningful analysis.

Cause of death

Overall, 40 (42%) and 29 (30%) patients died in the M arm and the M/A arm, respectively (Table 6). While

Table 5.

		Progression and relapse (available data)			
		2nd CR	Relapse	Alive	(4 yr)
Progression	27	6 (22%)	1/6	4	8%
Relapse	36	23 (64%)	11/23	20	53%
All patients	88			32	34%

* 3 in previously involved irradiated areas (20 Gy).
RT = radiotherapy. Answers to questionnaires were collected from 27/39 progressions and 36/46 relapses.

66

Table 6.

Causes of death	M (96)	M/A (96)
Died	40	29
HD progression	22	7
After relapse	7	13
Treatment related	3	2
Second malignancy	5	1
Intercurrent	3	6

M = M arm (MOPP only) see text; M/A = M/A arm (MOPP and ABVD) see text; CS = clinical stage; M/T = mediastinum-thorax ratio.

more deaths due to second malignancies occurred in the M arm, more intercurrent deaths occurred in the M/A arm. The main difference between the treatment arms concerns death through progression of Hodgkin's disease, which occurred more often in the MOPP only arm, while death after relapse was more frequent in the M/A arm.

Discussion

The reported trial investigated the value of combination chemotherapy with MOPP/ABVD after initial chemotherapy with MOPP alone (two courses) for clinically stages IIIB–IV Hodgkin's disease patients. In this setting, more progressions occurred in the MOPP alone arm, while in the mixed arm there were partial responders. The complete remission rates were similar for both arms. Half of the patients in partial remission could be brought into complete remission by additional radiotherapy, independent of type of previous chemotherapy, while only a few of the patients with progressive disease could be salvaged.

At progression or relapse, most disease was in previously involved nodal areas as already described by Young [3]. Salvage treatment included chemotherapy and/or radiotherapy, and 5 patients received intensive chemotherapy (with radiotherapy in 2 patients) with autologous bone marrow support. Whether radiotherapy has been used whenever possible cannot be ascertained, especially as only 1 out of 13 patients who achieved again partial remission had radiotherapy and only 1 survived. Nevertheless, half of the relapsed patients have survived both from the early and from the later relapses.

For patients who progressed, the outlook was still grim. An early switch of chemotherapy (M/A arm) seemed able to prevent such progressions and convert them into partial remissions. To reach a complete remission after progression, radiotherapy was essential in the reported patient group. Bloomfield [4] also report-

ed that fewer patients died in the treatment group in which radiotherapy was given early, i.e., in the middle of six courses of CVPP. This was the 'sandwich' arm in the CALGB 7551 study for untreated stage IIIB and IV patients. When studying ABMT data, the best results seem to have been reached by Yahalom [5], who included extensive radiotherapy in his treatment program for progressed or relapsed patients.

Conclusion

The combination of MOPP/ABVD to a total of 8 courses resulted in fewer progressions and more partial responses with a similar complete remission rate, in comparison to 8 courses of MOPP alone. When radiotherapy was used, half of the partial responders were able to achieve a complete remission. In case of complete remission, prognosis was independent of the way in which this was reached. Relapses usually occurred in previously involved unirradiated areas, suggesting that irradiation directly after initial combination chemotherapy could avoid a large proportion of relapses in advanced Hodgkin's disease. Re-treatment of relapse results in a 53% four-year survival rate, whereas almost all patients with progressive disease died within one year of progression. All efforts should be taken to reach a complete remission for initially progressing patients and for partial responders.

References

1. Somers R, Henry-Amar M, Carde P, Najman A. On behalf of the EORTC Lymphoma Cooperative Group and the Group Pierre and Marie Curie: MOPP versus alternating 2 MOPP/2 ABVD in advanced Hodgkin's disease. J Clin Onc 1988; 7: 236.
2. Wartelle M, Kromar A, Jam P, Kruger D. 'PIGAS': an interactive statistical data base management system. In: Hammond R and McCarthy JC (eds). Proceedings of the second international workshop in statistical data base management. Los Altos CA 1983; p 124–32.
3. Young RC, Canellos PG, Chabner BA et al.Patterns of relapse in advanced Hodgkin's disease treated with combination chemotherapy. Cancer 1978; 42: 1001–7.
4. Bloomfield CD, Pajak TF, Glicksman AS et al. Chemotherapy and Combined Modality Therapy for Hodgkin's Disease: A Progress Report on Cancer and Leukemia Group B Studies; Cancer Treat Rep 1982; 66: 835–46.
5. Yahalom J, Gulati S, Shank B et al. Total Lymphoid irradiation, high dose chemotherapy and autologous bone marrow transplantation for chemotherapy-resistant Hodgkin's disease; Int J Rad Onc Biol Phys 1989; 17: 915–922.

Correspondence to:
I. M. V. Burgers
The Netherlands Cancer Institute
Antoni van Leeuwenhoek Huis
Plesmanlaan 121
1066 CX Amsterdam
The Netherlands

Annals of Oncology, Supplement 2 to Volume 2: 67–71, 1991.
© 1991 *Kluwer Academic Publishers*.

Original article

Autologous bone marrow transplantation for refractory or relapsed Hodgkin's disease: The Memorial Sloan-Kettering Cancer Center experience using high-dose chemotherapy with or without hyperfractionated accelerated total lymphoid irradiation

Joachim Yahalom* & Subhash Gulati
Memorial Sloan-Kettering Cancer Center, New York, USA

Summary. Fifty patients with advanced-stage Hodgkin's disease (HD) who relapsed or failed to respond to multiple regimens of combination chemotherapy were entered onto two autologous bone marrow transplantation (AuBMT) protocols. Twenty-eight patients who did not have prior radiation therapy were treated with protocol A. Protocol A consisted of reinduction with conventional doses of combination chemotherapy followed by boost local-field irradiation to areas of residual disease and hyperfractionated accelerated total lymphoid irradiation (TLI). Chemotherapy consisted of high-dose etoposide (VP-16) and cyclophosphamide followed by infusion of cryopreserved, unpurged autologous bone marrow. Twenty-two patients who have had prior radiation therapy were treated with protocol B. Protocol B consisted of reinduction with conventional doses of chemotherapy followed by involved field radiation therapy (when tolerance to residual disease has not been previously reached). High-dose chemotherapy regimen consisted of cyclophosphamide, carmustine (BCNU), and VP-16 (CBV) followed by autologous bone marrow transplantation.

Of the 28 patients in protocol A, 5 patients died during the immediate peritransplant period, 5 patients progressed within six months, and 2 of them died. Two patients relapsed 13 and 39 months post transplant; 1 of them was reinduced into a complete remission (CR). Seventeen patients (61%) are disease free (16 patients in continuous complete remission), 12–54+ months (median 25+ months) following completion of therapy. Of the 22 patients in protocol B, 1 died of cytomegalovirus pneumonitis, and 11 relapsed. Ten patients (45%) are alive and disease free 16–42+ months (median 23+ months) after therapy.

In both protocols, patients who had responded to the reinduction chemotherapy, which was given prior to the transplant regimen, had a significantly better chance of remaining disease free (69 versus 13%, $P < 0.00001$). Treatment with protocol A resulted in a high rate of complete remission and a relative by low relapse rate, but was associated with considerable toxicity. Protocol B was less toxic but carried a higher risk of relapse. Both protocols offer a potential cure for patients with refractory or relapsed Hodgkin's disease who have exhausted conventional modes of therapy.

Key words: autologous bone marrow transplantation, bone marrow transplantation, Hodgkin's disease, salvage therapy, total lymphoid irradiation

Introduction

The choice of salvage therapy in Hodgkin's disease (HD) depends mostly on the history of the prior therapies and length of relapse-free interval [1, 2]. Whereas about 60% of the patients who relapse after radiotherapy alone are cured with standard chemotherapy or combined modality [3], less than 30% of patients who failed chemotherapy will achieve a long-term remission [1]. HD which has been refractory to alternating chemotherapy regimens or to salvage therapy will rarely sustain a response to a third-line chemotherapy regi-

men [1, 4, 5]. Bone marrow transplantation programs using allogeneic [6, 7] or, more commonly, autologous stem cell sources provided a choice of salvage with myeloablative doses of chemotherapy [8]. Wide-field radiotherapy has been successfully used for salvage of chemotherapy failures in a limited number of selected patients [9–11]. However, radiotherapy has not been widely employed in AuBMT programs for HD [8].

In this report we describe our preliminary experience with two AuBMT salvage regimens. One of the regimens incorporated hyperfractionated accelerated total lymphoid irradiation (TLI) with high-dose chemo-

* Dr. Yahalom is a recipient of an American Cancer Society Clinical Oncology Career Development Award.

68

therapy for salvage of previously unirradiated patients who have exhausted standard-dose chemotherapy options.

Patients and methods

Between November 1985 and June 1989, 50 patients with HD were treated with two high-dose therapy regimens and AuBMT at Memorial Sloan-Kettering Cancer Center (MSKCC). Forty-five patients who entered this study had failed at least two alternating or sequential chemotherapy combinations. Five patients who progressed immediately after an adequate course of combination chemotherapy with or without radiation were also enrolled in this program.

Eligibility criteria where as follows: a) pathological diagnosis of HD confirmed at MSKCC, b) bone marrow aspirate and biopsy analysis revealing cellular bone marrow with no involvement by HD, c) absence of other serious organ system diseases and Karnofsky performance status >70, and d) age greater than 15 years and less than 50 years.

Patients who had no history of prior radiation therapy were entered onto protocol A. Patients who had previous radiation therapy were entered onto protocol B. All candidates who met the eligibility requirements and consented to the treatment protocol were entered in this study. The median follow-up for surviving patients is 24 months with a range of 12+ to 54+ months. Patient characteristics in both protocols are summarized in Table 1. In protocol A (TLI, cyclophosphamide, etoposide [VP-16]) patients had a higher rate of extranodal disease (43%) at the time of AuBMT and were less likely (21%) to have achieved a complete response (CR) to therapy prior to salvage as compared to patients in protocol B (cyclophosphamide, VP-16, and carmustine [CBV]) (68%). Upon approval for this study, bone marrow was harvested and cryopreserved without any further treatment (unpurged) using the method of Stiff et al. [12].

In all patients, harvesting yielded adequate quantities of bone marrow. Following satisfactory bone marrow cryopreservation, patients were started on reinduction chemotherapy. Agents chosen for reinduction were those to which the patients were not exposed in the past or those that had shown previous clinical activity in those patients [13]. Most patients received two to three cycles of chemotherapy, and the median interval to bone marrow transplantation was 12 weeks. Patients who were selected to be treated with protocol B were irradiated to areas of residual disease only if the tolerance of the area permitted a meaningful additional dose of radiation. Nine of the 22 patients on protocol B were treated with radiation therapy as part of their conditioning protocol with doses that ranged from 1800 to 4140 cGy.

Upon completion of reinduction, patients on protocol A were treated with the following regimen: Involved field boost radiation therapy to all areas of residual or recurrent disease. This part of the treatment was administered on an outpatient basis over five days, and the total dose was 1500 cGy in 300-cGy daily fractions (14 patients) or 150 cGy per fraction twice daily (13 patients). Only 1 patient, who entered a complete remission following reinduction chemotherapy, was not boosted with radiation. TLI was delivered by a 10-MeV linear accelerator using a beam spoiler for the mantle field. Both mantle and inverted-Y opposed fields were administered at each treatment session. The total TLI dose was 2004 cGy delivered over four days at 167 cGy per fraction three times a day at intervals of five to six hours. Following one day of rest, VP-16 250 mg/m^2/day was administered intravenously for three days followed by IV cyclophosphamide 60 mg/kg/day for two days. After 48 hours, cryopreserved bone marrow was thawed in a water bath at the bedside and rapidly reinfused without any further treatment.

Protocol B consisted of treatment with BCNU 250 mg/m^2 IV on day 1, VP-16 250 mg/m^2 IV on days 2–4, and cyclophosphamide 50 mg/kg on days 5–7 followed by reinfusion of the bone marrow 48 hours later.

Moderate to severe mucositis was managed with frequent mouth care and antifungal medications. Patients were placed on total parenteral nutrition until they were able to eat. All blood products were irradiated to 3 cGy. Post-AuBMT prophylaxis for *Pneumocystis carinii* pneumonia consisted of trimethoprim-sulfamethoxazole orally. All patients with previous herpes simplex virus infection or high viral titers of herpes simplex received prophylactic IV acyclovir.

All patients were evaluated by means of physical examination; blood chemistry profile; peripheral blood count; chest radiography; chest, abdominal, and pelvic computerized tomography; and bilateral bone marrow biopsies. Follow-up was carried out every two to three months after transplantation or as clinically indicated. Complete remission was defined as the complete disappearance of clinical and radiological evidence of HD. Partial remission was defined as reduction of 50%

Table 1. Patient characteristics.

Protocol group	Total	Age (yr) Median (range)	Extranodal disease	Primary TX CR*	Reinduction responsive**
A	28	27 (13–44)	12 (43%) 7-lung 3-liver 2-bone	6 (21%)	17 (61%)
B	22	28 (18–37)	3 (14%)	15 (68%)	18 (82%)
All	50	27	15 (30%)	21 (42%)	35 (70%)

* Patients who achieved a complete response with their original therapy.
** Patients responding to postharvesting reinduction chemotherapy with a complete or partial response.

or more of measurable disease for at least one month. Responders to reinduction are defined as patients who achieved partial or complete remission at the end of reinduction chemotherapy. Relapse-free survival was calculated from the day of marrow transplantation for all patients, and analysis was as of May 20, 1990. The actuarial relapse-free survival curves were plotted according to the method of Kaplan and Meier and were compared by the log-rank test.

Results

Overall response and survival

The results of both protocol groups are summarized in Table 2. In protocol A, 23 patients survived the peritransplant period and are available for evaluation of response (Fig. 1). Patients who died of acute toxicity are scored as nonresponders. Five patients progressed within six months, and two of them died. Two patients relapsed 13 and 39 months after AuBMT. One patient who relapsed after 39 months was the only patient who had not received boost radiotherapy. She had a localized nodal relapse at the site of her initial recurrent disease. This patient achieved a complete response to

additional chemotherapy and was without clinical evidence of disease 15 months post retreatment. Sixteen patients (57%) are alive and free of relapse. Twenty-one patients (75%) are alive, 12–54+ months after AuBMT (median 25+ months).

In protocol B, 15 patients (68%) achieved a CR. Of those, 6 relapsed six to 14 months after AuBMT. Nine patients (41%) are relapse free, and 12 (55%) are alive 16–42+ months (median 23+ months) after AuBMT (Fig. 2).

Response to reinduction

Patients who responded to reinduction chemotherapy with CR or PR were considered responsive. Those progressing or showing only a minimal response to reinduction were labeled resistant. Of the 28 patients in protocol A, 17 (61%) were responsive. In protocol B, 18 of the 22 patients (82%) achieved a response prior to high-dose chemotherapy. In both protocols the relapse-free survival rate for patients who responded to reinduction with CR or PR was significantly higher compared to resistant patients (Protocol A: P < 0.005, Protocol B: P < 0.001). Figure 3 compares the actuarial relapse-free survival according to response to reinduction for all patients in both protocols.

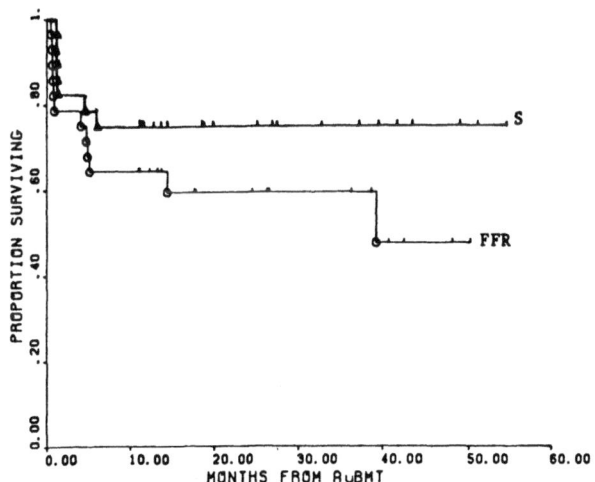
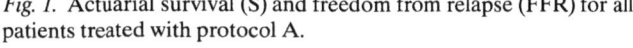

Fig. 1. Actuarial survival (S) and freedom from relapse (FFR) for all patients treated with protocol A.

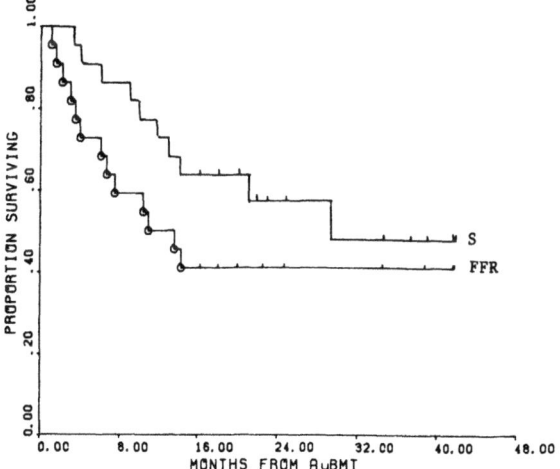

Fig. 2. Actuarial survival (S) and freedom from relapse (FFR) for all patients treated with protocol B.

Table 2. Treatment results.

Protocol	Reinduction response	# of PTS	Toxic death	CR	Relapse	Alive relapse-free
A	Responsive	17 (61%)	2 (12%)	15 (88%)	1	14 (82%)
	Resistant	11 (39%)	3 (27%)	4 (36%)	2	2 (18%)
	Total	28	5 (19%)	19 (68%)	3 (16%)	16 (57%)
B	Responsive	18 (82%)	1	14 (78%)	5	9 (50%)
	Resistant	4 (18%)	0	1	1	0
	Total	22	1 (4.5%)	15 (68%)	6 (40%)	9 (41%)
Both	All	50	6 (12%)	34 (68%)	9 (26%)	25 (50%)

70

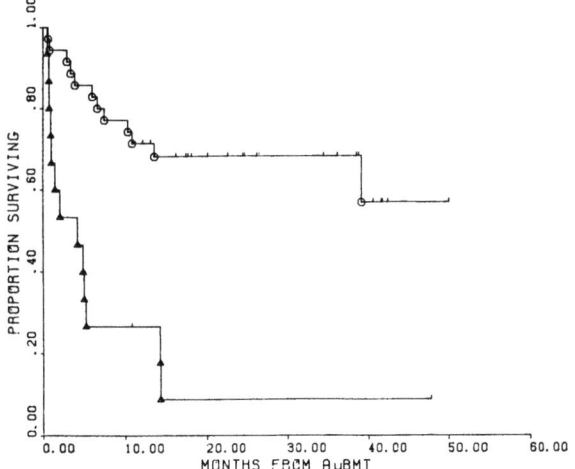

Fig. 3. Actuarial freedom from relapse for responders (○) and non-responders (△) (P < 0.00001). All patients in both protocols.

Toxicity

In protocol A, 5 patients died of treatment-related complications. Two patients died of sepsis during granulocytopenia, one of them also developed pulmonary hemorrhage as a terminal event. Two patients bled from their bronchi and died of pulmonary insufficiency. One patient died with the clinical picture of acute respiratory distress syndrome with chest x-ray findings of diffuse pulmonary infiltrates. In protocol B, 1 patient died at day 117 post AuBMT of cytomegalovirus pneumonia after she had achieved a complete hematological recovery.

Discussion

Programs using high-dose chemotherapy with AuBMT have become available to a growing number of HD patients. The groups of patients that are considered to benefit from AuBMT are (1) patients progressing or not obtaining a CR with conventional chemotherapy, particularly with alternating regimens; (2) patients relapsing within a year after CR; or (3) patients in second relapse [14]. All the patients in this report have met these criteria. Most groups have employed chemotherapy regimens with AuBMT but without radiotherapy [8]. The most commonly used high-dose combination chemotherapy consists of cyclophosphamide, BCNU, and VP-16 (CBV) [16]. Treatment with this regimen has yielded relapse-free survivals of 24–38% with median follow-up periods ranging between two and four years [15–18]. Most centers have elected to escalate the dose of some of these agents, but have not yet shown any response advantage [15, 16]. The only group that has systematically studied dose escalations of this regimen has not been able to demonstrate a benefit, even when considerable toxicity was reached [17]. Our patients treated with CBV (protocol B) have shown relatively little toxicity but a considerable

relapse rate, suggesting that an escalation of doses is warranted.

Radiation therapy has been used in AuBMT programs for HD only in a manner used in conditioning regimens for allogeneic bone marrow transplantation-total body irradiation [7, 19]. This mode of radiation administration was associated with increased pulmonary toxicity in patients previously irradiated to the mediastinum [7, 19]. Most current regimens using AuBMT are confined to chemotherapy alone [15–18]. However, involved-field radiotherapy has been used with favorable results after AuBMT in patients not achieving CR. In one study, 33% of PR patients obtained a CR with post-AuBMT radiotherapy [16]. We were motivated to develop a combined modality regimen with AuBMT for HD [13] by the long-proven efficacy of radiotherapy in early-stage HD, the limited but favorable experience in salvage of chemotherapy failures with wide-field radiation [9–11], and the fact that a considerable number of AuBMT candidates have not been previously irradiated. The observation that recurrences after AuBMT are almost always limited to areas previously involved with HD [7, 19] has prompted us to incorporate boost radiotherapy to areas of residual or recurrent disease in the protocol. Accelerating TLI was designed to shorten the intensive, myelosuppressive part of the therapy prior to AuBMT. Hyperfractionation was employed in order to decrease toxicity, based on our experience with hyperfractionated total body irradiation [20].

The common factor for patients treated with protocol A is that they have not been previously treated with radiation. It is interesting, however, that most of them have never achieved a CR prior to intensive therapy as compared to the previously irradiated patients (protocol B group). There were also more patients in group A with extensive extranodal disease as compared to group B (Table 1). The results of the AuBMT salvage regimen in this group are encouraging, with 57% of the patients free of relapse at a median follow-up of 25+ months. Treatment-related mortality was higher with protocol A (18%) compared to protocol B (4.5%), particularly in patients who had mediastinal disease. Pulmonary complications were the cause of death in 4 patients. We hypothesized that rapid disintegration of a bulky mediastinal tumor after combined-modality treatment may result in pulmonary hemorrhage and respiratory failure. Allowing more recovery time between the boost mediastinal irradiation and TLI may attenuate this process.

Analysis of various patient characteristics and response records has provided prognostic indicators for salvage with AuBMT programs [7, 16, 18]. In a multivariate analysis, Jagannath et al. [16] identified failure of more than two prior chemotherapy treatments and poor performance status to be adverse prognostic factors for survival. Jones et al. [7] showed that the response to standard salvage therapy prior to transplant strongly influenced both the therapy-related mortality rate and the event-free survival following AuBMT. Vose et al. [18] demonstrated that patients transplanted early, after only one or two previous chemotherapy regimens and with no bulky disease, had a lower early death rate and better three-year survival rate compared to patients transplanted late or with bulky disease. Gribben et al. [21] found the tumor mass at AuBMT to affect survival.

We analyzed the response to standard-dose chemotherapy, given as reinduction after harvesting, as an indicator for response to high-dose chemotherapy and radiotherapy in both treatment regimens. For most patients, the time of response to reinduction predicted the outcome of the whole AuBMT program (Fig. 3). We recommend prompt attempt to achieve a response immediately prior to the intensive therapy, since it may significantly affect AuBMT outcome. On the other hand it may not be advisable to offer the aggressive program of AuBMT to patients who have shown complete refractoriness to multiple salvage efforts.

Improved selection criteria and earlier application of AuBMT programs, together with intensification of chemotherapy and appropriate incorporation of radiotherapy, will provide a better chance of survival for patients who have failed the initial treatment attempt.

Acknowledgment

The authors are grateful to Karla Whitmarsh for excellent data management and analysis.

References

1. Buzaid AC, Lippman SC, Miller TP. Salvage therapy of advanced Hodgkin's disease; critical appraisal or curative potential. Am J Med 1987; 83: 523–32.
2. Fisher RI, DeVita VT, Hubbard SP, Simon R, Young RC. Prolonged disease-free survival in Hodgkin's disease with MOPP reinduction after first failure. Ann Intern Med 1979; 90: 761–63.
3. Roach III M, Brophy N, Cox R, Varghese A, Hoppe RT. Prognostic factors for patients relapsing after radiotherapy for early stage Hodgkin's disease. J Clin Oncol 1990; 8: 623–29.
4. Bergasagel DE. Salvage treatment for Hodgkin's disease in relapse (editorial). J Clin Oncol 1987; 5: 525–26.
5. Hagemeister FB, Tannir N, McLaughlin P, Salvador P, Riggs S, Velasquez WS, Cabanillas F. MIME chemotherapy (methyl-GAG, ifosfamide, methotrexate, etoposide) as treatment for recurrent Hodgkin's disease. J Clin Oncol 1987; 5: 556–61.
6. Appelbaum FR, Sullivan KM, Thomas ED, Buckner CD, Clift RA, Deeg HJ, Newman PE, Sanders JE, Stewart P, Storb R. Allogeneic marrow transplantation in the treatment of MOPP-resistant Hodgkin's disease. J Clin Oncol 1985; 3: 1490–4.
7. Jones RJ, Plantadosi S, Mann RB, Ambinder RF, Seifter EJ, Vriesendorp HM, Abeloff MD, Burns WH, May WS, Rowly SD, Vogelsang GB, Wagner JE, Wiley JM, Wingard JR, Yeager AM, Saral R, Santos GW. High dose cytotoxic therapy and bone marrow transplantation for relapsed Hodgkin's disease. J Clin Oncol 1990; 8: 527–37.
8. Armitage JO. Bone marrow transplantation in the treatment of patients with lymphoma. Blood 1989; 73: 1749–58.
9. Roach III M, Kap DS, Rosenberg SA, Hoppe RT. Radiotherapy with curative intent: an option in selected patients relapsing after chemotherapy for advanced Hodgkin's disease. J Clin Oncol 1987; 5: 550–5.
10. Mauch P, Tarbell N, Skarin A, Rosenthal D, Weinstein H. Wide-field radiation therapy alone or with chemotherapy for Hodgkin's disease in relapse from combination chemotherapy. J Clin Oncol 1987; 5: 544–9.
11. Fox KA, Lippman SM, Cassady JR, Heusinkveld RS, Miller TP. Radiation therapy salvage of Hodgkin's disease following chemotherapy failure. J Clin Oncol 1987; 5: 38–45.
12. Stiff PJ, DeRisi MF, Langleben A, Gulati S, Koester A, Lanzotti V, Clarkson BD. Autologous bone marrow transplantation using unfractionated cells without rate-controlled freezing in hydoxyethyl starch and dimethyl sulfoxide. Ann NY Acad Sci 1983; 411: 378–80.
13. Yahalom J, Gulati S, Shank B, Clarkson B, Fuks Z. Total lymphoid irradiation, high-dose chemotherapy and autologous bone marrow transplantation for chemotherapy-resistant Hodgkin's disease. Int J Rad Oncol Biol Phys 1989; 17: 915–22.
14. Armitage JO, Barnett MJ, Carella AM, Dicke KA, Diehl V, Gribben JG, Pfreundschuh M. Bone marrow transplantation in the treatment of Hodgkin's lymphoma: Problems, remaining challenges and future prospects. Recent Results Cancer Res 1989; 117: 246–53.
15. Carella AM, Congiu AM, Gaozza E, Mazza P, Ricci P, Visani G, Meloni G, Cimino G, Mangoni L, Coser P, Cetto GL, Cimino R, Alessandrino EP, Brusamolino E, Santini G, Tura S, Mandelli F, Rizzoli V, Bernasconi C, Marmont AM. High-dose chemotherapy with autologous bone marrow transplantation in 50 advanced resistant Hodgkin's disease patients: an Italian study group report. J Clin Oncol 1988; 6: 1411–6.
16. Jagannath S, Armitage JO, Dicke KA, Tucker SL, Velasquex WS, Smith K, Vaughan WP, Kessinger A, Horowitz LJ, Hagemeister FB, McLaughlin P, Cabanillas F, Spitzer G. Prognostic factors for response and survival after high-dose cyclophosphamide, carmustine and etoposide with autologous bone marrow transplantation for relapsed Hodgkin's disease. J Clin Oncol 1989; 7: 179–85.
17. Wheeler C, Antin JH, Churchill WH, Corne SE, Smith BR, Bubley GJ, Rosenthal DS, Rappaport JM, Ault KA, Schnipper LE, Eder JP. Cyclophosphamide, carmustine, and etoposide with autologous bone marrow transplantation in refractory Hodgkin's disease and non-Hodgkin's lymphoma. A dose-finding study. J Clin Oncol 1990; 8: 648–56.
18. Vose JM, Bierman PJ, Weisenburger DD, Armitage JO. The importance of early autologous bone marrow transplantation in the management of patients with Hodgkin's disease. Proc Amer Soc Clin Oncol 1990; 9: 256.
19. Phillips GL, Wolff SN, Herzig RH, Lazarus HM, Fay JW, Lin HS, Shina DC, Glasgow GP, Griffith RC, Lamb CW, Herzig GP. Treatment of progressive Hodgkin's disease with intensive chemoradiotherapy and autologous bone marrow transplantation. Blood 1989; 73: 2086–92.
20. Shank B, Chu FC, Dinsmore R, Kapoor N, Kirkpatrick D, Teitelbaum H, Reid A, Bonfiglio P, Simpson L, O'Reilly RJ. Hyperfractionated total body irradiation for bone marrow transplantation. Results in seventy leukemia patients with allogeneic transplants. Int J Radiat Oncol Biol Phys Nov 1983; 9: 1607–11.
21. Gribben JG, Linch DC, Singer CRJ, McMillan AK, Jarrett M, Goldstone AH. Successful treatment of refractory Hodgkin's disease by high-dose combination chemotherapy and autologous bone marrow transplantation. Blood 1989; 73: 340–4.

Correspondence to:
Joachim Yahalom, M.D
Department of Radiation Oncology
Memorial Sloan-Kettering Cancer Center
1275 York Avenue
New York, NY 10021, USA

Annals of Oncology, Supplement 2 to Volume 2: 73–76, 1991.
© 1991 Kluwer Academic Publishers.

Original article

Cardiopulmonary toxicity after three courses of ABVD and mediastinal irradiation in favorable Hodgkin's disease

P. Brice, J. Tredaniel, J. J. Monsuez, J. P. Marolleau, C. Ferme, C. Hennequin, J. Frija, C. Gisselbrecht & M. Boiron
Institut d'hématologie, Hôpital Saint-Louis, 1 Avenue Claude Vellefaux, 75010 Paris, France

Summary. The combination of chemotherapy and radiotherapy in Hodgkin's disease has been associated with iatrogenic effects. Forty adult patients were studied to evaluate the early toxicity following three courses of ABVD (cumulative dose of doxorubicin [Adriamycin] 150 mg/m^2, and bleomycin 60 mg) and mediastinal irradiation at 40 Gy. Cardiopulmonary toxicity was assessed from six months to three years after completion of irradiation. Of the 40 patients, all of whom were in complete remission from Hodgkin's disease, 6 experienced dyspnea on exertion. In studies related to Cardiac toxicity, the left ventricular ejection fraction ranged from 50 to 77% (mean 63%); 8 patients had a minor pericardial effusion, 4 had valvular calcification, and 6 had minimal cardiac abnormalities. With regard to pulmonary toxicity, CT scan showed a small pleural effusion with pleural thickening in 19 patients and mediastinal or apical fibrosis in 15 patients. The total pulmonary capacity value was low (<80%), in 19 patients, and decreased carbon monoxide diffusion capacity (<70%) was found in 10 patients. We conclude that early cardiac toxicity was absent despite the use of Adriamycin and mediastinal irradiation. Pulmonary toxicity was present but minor, and it may decrease with the use of smaller fraction sizes for mantle field irradiation.

For many years, Hodgkin's disease (HD) has been the focus of sustained therapeutic interest and extensive investigative research. Modalities available for the treatment of this malignancy included radiation and multiple-drug chemotherapy, which made the disease into one of the first malignancies to be highly curable, with a relapse-free survival rate ranging from 70 to 90% in stages I to IIIA [1]. However, now that the therapeutic effectiveness of this combined therapy has been established, attention has turned to reducing its long-term after effects such as secondary leukemia or male sterility [2].

These adverse effects are related to the most extensively used chemotherapy, a combination known as MOPP (nitrogen mustard, vincristine, procarbazine, and prednisone) [3]. An important issue in current HD therapy is whether another combination, ABVD (doxorubicin [Adriamycin], bleomycin, vinblastine, and dacarbazine [DTIC]) is less leukemogenic than MOPP. A related and equally important issue is whether, and to what extent, ABVD increases cardiac and pulmonary toxicity. We therefore used an ABVD-derived regimen (Table 1) because the ABVD combination resulted in similar cure rates to MOPP in advanced stages of Hodgkin's disease [4]. Mediastinal irradiation has been associated with cardiac and pulmonary toxicity [4–7] which may be potentiated by ABVD [8–9]. This report focuses on the pulmonary and cardiac side effects of a combination of three courses of ABVD chemotherapy and mantle-field irradiation in adult patients treated for favorable HD (stages I to IIIA).

Material and methods

Patients

Between 1985 and 1989, 80 adult patients with newly diagnosed HD (stage I to IIIA) and good prognoses were entered into the H 85 protocol at St Louis Hospital. Among these patients, 40 were followed for cardiopulmonary toxicity. The initial characteristics of the 40 patients are summarized in Table 2. All patients underwent clinical staging at diagnosis with physical examination, routine laboratory studies, postero-anterior chest x-rays, lymphangiography, chest and upper abdominal CT scan, and bone marrow biopsy. They were then staged according to the Ann Arbor staging system [10].

Therapy

Stage IA and IIA patients without bad prognostic factors (mediastinal involvement, histological subtype 3 or

Table 1. The H85 protocol for HD (stages I to III A).

3 courses of ABVD:	Adriamycin 25 mg/m^2 d1 + d8
	Bleomycin 10 mg d1 + d8
	Vindesine 2 mg/m^2 d1 + d8
	Dacarbazine 250 mg/m^2 d1 + d8
	Every 21 days
Mantle field RT	40 Gy with 2.1 or 2.2 Gy per fraction
Splenic and lumboaortic RT	40 and 35 Gy

RT = radiotherapy.

Table 2. Characteristics of the 40 patients.

		No. of patients
Age (mean) mean	16 to 67 years (36 years)	40
Sex	Male	19
	Female	21
Stage	I	6
	II	28
	IIIA	6
B symptoms	yes	11
	no	29
Mediastinal involvement	yes	33
	no	7
RT mediastinal boost	yes	5
	no	35

4, or tumor mass >7 cm) were treated exclusively with radiotherapy; in consequence, they are excluded from this study. The remaining patients with stage I, II and IIIA received combined-modality therapy with three monthly courses of ABVD followed one month later by mantle-field radiotherapy and after one month rest by lumboaortic and splenic radiotherapy (Table 1). Total dose was 150 mg/m^2 for Adriamycin and 60 mg for bleomycin. All radiotherapy was delivered at St Louis Hospital through anterior and posterior fields with an 18-MeV photon accelerator. Radiation doses were at 40 Gy in the mantle-field area (with the option of a boost to the mediastinum of 5 Gy in 5 patients) the fraction size was 2.1 Gy (10 patients) and 2.2 Gy (30 patients). The 40 patients studied were in complete remission after this therapy, although 7 retained a residual mediastinal mass.

Cardiopulmonary toxicity

Cardiopulmonary toxicity was evaluated with thoracic x-ray and CT scan, electrocardiogram, bidimensional echocardiogram (left ventricular ejection fraction was calculated at rest), and pulmonary function tests. All patients were questioned regarding cardiopulmonary symptoms and had a complete physical examination.

This checkup was performed in the outpatient clinic at least six months after completion of mantle-field radiotherapy and up to three years after. The mean time between the end of the treatment and these tests was 13 months. In 10 patients whose initial tests were abnormal, repeat pulmonary function tests were performed six months later.

Table 3. Cardiac function after therapy.

LVEF mean	50 to 75% 61.5%
Pericardial effusion	8 pts
Valvular calcifications	4 pts

Results

Forty patients with normal performance status were studied for cardiopulmonary toxicity.

Cardiac toxicity

All patients had a normal electrocardiogram at rest. The left ventricular ejection fraction (LVEF) ranged from 50 to 77% (mean 63%), and only 2 patients had slightly low LVEF at 50%, the remaining LVEF were above 55% and no patient had clinical symptoms of cardiac failure. A minor asymptomatic pericardial effusion was found in 8 patients. Four patients had valvular calcifications, and 6 patients had minor cardiac abnormalities on echocardiogram (septal hypokinesia in 3 patients, and parietal hypertrophy in 3 patients).

Pulmonary toxicity (Table 4)

Six of 40 patients (15%) experienced dyspnea on exertion, and in 17 (42%) pulmonary function tests showed minor restrictive disease which persisted six months later in 10 patients who were retested. Significantly reduced carbon monoxide diffusing capacity was present in 8 patients (20%). Radiological lesions were frequent (60%) when CT scans were performed; 19 patients had a minor pleural effusion with pleural thickening, and 1 patient with contiguous pleural involvement at diagnosis had a major pleural effusion requiring surgery after therapy. Fifteen patients had mediastinal fibrosis or small pulmonary nodules (<1 cm) in the irradiated field.

Discussion

Now that cure is easily achieved for adults with favorable Hodgkin's disease, it is increasingly important to limit treatment sequelae. The problem is more severe in children, in whom radiotherapy is administered at lower dosage or not used at all [12].

Treatment protocols have moved through the recognition of acute and long-term side effects. Many curative treatment combinations have been used with the

Table 4. Pulmonary function after therapy.

	Percentage of normal values	No. of patients
Total lung capacity	≥80%	23
	<80%	17
Forced expiratory volume/vital capacity	≥80%	31
	<80%	9
DLCO	≥70%	32
	<70%	8
Radiologic lesions	yes	24
	no	16

aim of excellent cure rates and maximal functional outcome. MOPP chemotherapy in combination with radiotherapy is associated with an increased risk of leukemia and secondary cancers [13]. MOPP chemotherapy is also associated with azoospermia in men, with frequent sterility after as few as three courses of chemotherapy. This was not found after three courses of ABVD chemotherapy [14]. Protocols using ABVD were developed to reduce these risks, since ABVD was shown to have the same efficiency in advanced HD [3]. However, bleomycin is known to cause pulmonary injury while Adriamycin has documented cardiac toxicity [9, 15]. These two toxicities may be increased when combined with mediastinal irradiation.

Adriamycin and chest radiotherapy cause cardiac toxicity, and this toxicity is dose related. Cumulative doses Adriamycin of less than 550 mg/m^2 are well tolerated. Chest radiotherapy potentiates the cardiotoxicity of Adriamycin, and lower drug doses are generally recommended in combination with irradiation [16]. In our study the cumulative dose of Adriamycin was 150 mg/m^2. The major early risk of this combination is congestive heart failure, then pericarditis, and later myocardial infarction [4]. These toxicities are usually associated with mediastinal irradiation through a single anterior field, a technique we no longer employ. In our study echocardiography was utilized not only to assess ventricular function, but also to provide specific information about possible pericardial effusion. We did not study LVEF during exercise.

All our patients were asymptomatic for cardiac symptoms, but in 8 we found a minor pericardial effusion and in 6 a minor abnormality. The LVEF was normal in all but 2 patients, but both had high blood pressure.

In this study early cardiac toxicity is absent but longer follow-up is required to evaluate late toxicity such as occlusive coronary artery disease or constrictive pericarditis [5].

Bleomycin has documented adverse effects on pulmonary function in adults. The incidence of this lung toxicity increases with higher dosage and patient age. There are no sensitive clinical tests for the detection of bleomycin-induced lung toxicity, but pulmonary function studies have been correlated with the injury. Serial single-breath carbon monoxide diffusing capacity measurements are the most sensitive indicator of subclinical pulmonary toxicity [16].

Ionizing radiation may also cause pulmonary pathology. Pneumonitis and fibrosis are dose related and associated with decreased total lung capacity on pulmonary function tests.

In our series with a complete reevaluation at least six months after completion of therapy, we found slight pulmonary abnormalities. The reduction of carbon monoxide diffusing capacity was minor and found in only 8 patients (25%). This is explained by the total dose of bleomycin, which was low (60 mg). A recent study observed an increased pulmonary toxicity after

ABVD chemotherapy (compared to MOPP) with mantle-field irradiation, but patients received six courses of ABVD and thus a higher total dose of bleomycin [8].

The most important signs of toxicity were abnormal radiologic findings, and a minor restrictive syndrome (decreased total lung capacity in 17 patients [42%], with dyspnea during exercise in 6 patients [15%]).

This pulmonary toxicity is related to mantle-field irradiation and may be slightly enhanced by combination with bleomycin. Toxicity may be increased if the fraction size employed is larger than 2 Gy. It has already been reported that radiotherapy fraction size larger than 2 Gy can increase functional pulmonary impairment after chemoradiotherapy treatment for HD [9].

In conclusion, administration of three courses of ABVD and radiotherapy is an effective and safe treatment for good prognosis HD. Cardiopulmonary toxicity is minor but needs longer follow-up for optimal evaluation.

References

1. Hagemeister FB. Prognostic factors in decision making in the clinical management of Hodgkin's disease. Hematol oncol 1988; 6: 257–69.
2. Blayney DW, Longo DL, Young RC et al. Decreasing risk of leukemia with prolonged follow up after chemotherapy and radiotherapy for Hodgkin's disease. N Engl J Med 1987; 316: 710–4.
3. Coleman CN, Williams CJ, Flint A, Glatstein EJ, Rosenberg SA, Kaplan HS. Hematologic neoplasia in patients treated for Hodgkin's disease. N Engl J Med 1977; 297: 1249–52.
4. Bonadonna G, Valagussa P, Santoro A. Alternating non cross resistant combination chemotherapy or MOPP in stage IV Hodgkin's disease. Ann Intern Med 1986; 66: 1023–34.
5. Gottdiener JS, Katin MJ, Borer JS, Bacharach SL, Green MV. Late cardiac effect of therapeutic mediastinal irradiation. N Engl J Med 1983; 308: 569–71.
6. Gomez GA, Park JJ, Panahon AM et al. Heart size and function after radiation therapy to the mediastinum in patients with Hodgkin's disease. Cancer Treat Rep 1983; 67: 1099–103.
7. Green DM, Gingell RL, Pearce J, Panahon AH, Ghoorah J. The effect of mediastinal irradiation on cardiac function of patients treated during childhood and adolescence for Hodgkin's disease. J Clin Oncol 1987; 5: 239–45.
8. Dopico GA, Wiley AL, Rao P, Dickie HA. Pulmonary reaction to upper mantle radiation therapy for Hodgkin's disease. Chest 1979; 75: 688–92.
9. Cosset JM, Henry Amar H, Thomas J et al. Increased pulmonary toxicity in the ABVD arm of the EORTC H6 V trial. J Clin Oncol 1989; 8: abst. 985.
10. Lamonte CS, Yeh SDJ, Straus DJ. Long term follow up of cardiac function in patients with Hodgkin's disease treated with mediastinal irradiation and combination chemotherapy including doxorubicin. Cancer Treat Rep 1986; 70: 439–44.
11. Carbone PP, Kaplan HS, Musshoff K, Smithers PW, Tubiana M. Report of committee on Hodgkin's disease staging classification. Cancer Res 1971; 31: 1860–1.
12. Behrewdt H, van Bunningen NF, van Leeuwen EF. Treatment of Hodgkin's disease in children with or without radiotherapy. Cancer 1987; 59: 1870–3.
13. Van Leeuwen FE, Somers R, Taal BG et al. Increased risk of lung cancer, non Hodgkin's lymphoma and leukemia following Hodgkin's disease. J Clin Oncol 1989; 7: 1046–58.

76

14. Viviani S, Santoro A, Ragni G, Boufante V, Besfetti O, Bonadonna G. Gonadal toxicity after combination chemotherapy for Hodgkin's disease. Comparative results of MOPP vs ABVD. Eur J Cancer Clin Oncol 1985; 21: 601–5.
15. Bauer KAA, Skarin AT, Balikian JP, Garnick MB, Rosenthal DS, Canellos GP. Pulmonary complications associated with combination chemotherapy programs containing Bleomycin. Am J Med 1983; 74: 557–63.

Correspondence to:
Dr. P. Brice
HDJ Hematologie
Hôpital Saint-Louis
1 Avenue Claude Vellefaux
75010 Paris, France

Annals of Oncology, Supplement 2 to Volume 2: 77–82, 1991.
© 1991 *Kluwer Academic Publishers.*

Original article ────────────────────

Long-term toxicity of early stages of Hodgkin's disease therapy: The EORTC experience

J. M. Cosset, M. Henry-Amar & J. H. Meerwaldt
for the EORTC Lymphoma Cooperative Group (see the Appendix)

I. Introduction

The ultimate goal of Hodgkin's disease (HD) therapy is no longer merely to achieve the cure of the patients, but to reach the Holy Grail of 'uncomplicated cure.' Actually, a cure associated with a low risk of benign complications might be acceptable in most cases.

In this short and nonexhaustive report, we shall concentrate on the experience gathered by the European Organization for Treatment and Research on Cancer (EORTC) Lymphoma Cooperative Group in two types of long-term toxicity of HD therapy: non-malignant late complications, and second cancers.

This report is based on the analysis of the late effects of treatment which were prospectively recorded in the four trials that the EORTC conducted in early-stage HD: trial H1 (1964–1971), trial H2 (1972–1976), trial H5 (1977–1981), and trial H6 (1981–1988). These trials included 1660 patients (January 1990 update). A basic scheme of each study is presented in Figure 1. The detailed results of these trials were recently published by Tubiana et al. [1].

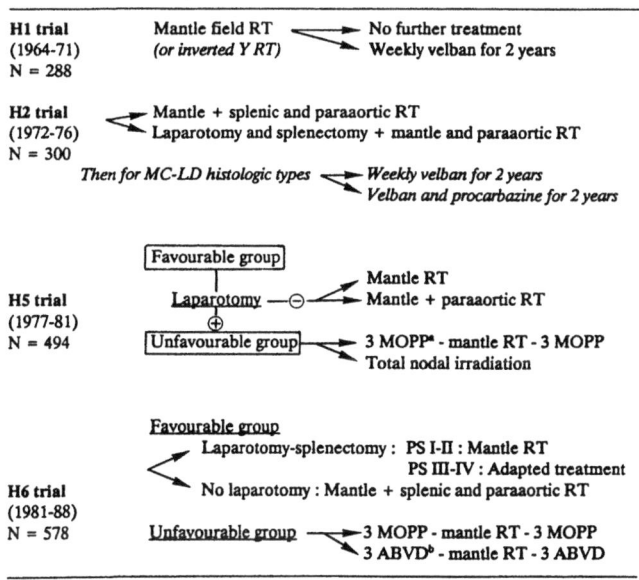

^a MOPP = mechlorethamine hydrochloride, vincristine, procarbazine, prednisone
^b ABVD = doxorubicin, bleomycin, vinblastine, dacarbazine

Fig. 1. Design of the four consecutive EORTC trials H1, H2, H5, and H6 in early stage Hodgkin's disease.

II. Nonmalignant complications

Conflicting data are still being reported in the literature for some types of nonmalignant long-term complications [2]. In the present paper, we shall provide the reader with recent EORTC data on the following complications: late gastrointestinal injuries, late pulmonary function impairment, and cardiac failures.

a. Late injuries of the gastrointestinal tract (GIT)

The late digestive tract problems that the clinicians may have to deal with after HD therapy are essentially ulcers, gastritis, and small bowel injuries (obstruction and perforation). These complications were previously analysed in a series of 775 patients entered in the two consecutive H2 and H5 trials (see Fig. 1), and the results already published [3]. Updated data, with longer follow-up (and thus some additional complication cases) are reported here.

In this series, 41 of 775 patients (5.3%) developed a late GIT injury. As previously reported, these complications were significantly and independently favoured by a previous staging laparotomy and by paraaortic irradiation [3, 4].

Of the 377 patients who underwent a staging laparotomy, 33 (8.8%) experienced a GIT injury, while in the group of 398 patients who were not assigned to laparotomy, only 8 (2%) presented with a GIT complication (P < 0.001).

Of 519 patients who were treated by paraaortic irradiation (RT), 39 (7.5%) experienced a late digestive tract injury, while, in the group of 256 patients who were not given any infradiaphragmatic RT, there were only two cases (0.8%) of digestive tract complications (P < 0.001).

In the radiobiological literature over the last decade, RT fractionation has been shown to be a major determinant of the rate and severity of late RT injuries [5, 6]. This is confirmed by the EORTC experience for late post-RT GIT injuries. In the different European centres, three different fraction sizes were used in the H2 and H5 trials: 2, 2.5 and 3.3 Gy (for the same total dose of 40 Gy to be delivered in four weeks). For patients who did not undergo staging laparotomy, the

Table 1. Late injuries of the gastrointestinal tract in the H2 and H5 EORTC trials.

Previous laparotomy	Paraaortic irradiation	Fraction size (Gy)	Patients at risk	No. of injuries	5-yr cumulative incidence
no	no	–	133	1	<1%
yes	no	–	123	1	1%
no	yes	2.0	183	1	<1%
no	yes	2.5	48	3	8%
no	yes	3.3	34	3	11%
yes	yes	2.0	176	18	8%
yes	yes	2.5	48	5	12%
yes	yes	3.3	30	9	28%

five-year post-RT GIT complication rates significantly increased with the dose per fraction. The rates were <1, 8, and 11% in the three groups, respectively (P < 0.005). For patients who underwent a laparotomy, these rates were 8, 12, and 28% in the same three groups, respectively (P = 0.03). Details are given in Table 1.

Nowadays, laparotomy is no longer part of the staging procedures in most ongoing studies in Europe. It should therefore no longer play a significant role in the incidence of late GIT injuries [1]. On the other hand, paraaortic RT is still being proposed for a significant number of patients. In such a situation, when delivering a standard dose of 36–40 Gy, one of the main parameters of long-term digestive injury appears to be the RT fractionation, and the use of fraction sizes larger than 2 Gy should be firmly discouraged.

b. Late pulmonary function impairment

The evolution of pulmonary function tests after a standard mantle-field irradiation used alone has already been extensively studied [7, 8, 9, 10]. Vital capacity (VC) usually drops to 70–80% of the normal theoretical value 6–12 months after completion of therapy and returns to baseline after 18–24 months in most cases. The addition of MOPP (nitrogen mustard, vincristine, procarbazine, and prednisone) does not appear to significantly alter this evolution in the EORTC experience [11]. In 1982, when introducing the ABVD scheme (doxorubicin [Adriamycin], bleomycin, vinblastine, and dacarbazine) in combination with RT for the first time in a European protocol (H6 unfavourable – see Fig. 1), the EORTC Lymphoma Cooperative Group was aware of the possible increase in lung toxicity which might be associated with the use of (1) an agent with potential toxicity to the lung (bleomycin), and (2) a drug acting in some conditions as an efficient radiosensitizer (Adriamycin) [12].

Therefore, a prospective evaluation of spirometric tests was started in this trial (which compared three cycles of MOPP, followed by mantle-field irradiation, followed by a further three MOPP to three cycles of ABVD, mantle-field irradiation, and a further three

cycles of ABVD). The study included 334 patients. Because spirometric tests could not be systematically performed in some participating centers, only 106 (32%) patients (47 in the MOPP arm and 59 in the ABVD arm) who underwent at least a pre- and a post-therapy examination were included in the analysis. Moreover an additional pulmonary function test was performed one year post-therapy in 69 patients.

Comparisons between the two groups of patients assigned to either combination MOPP-RT or ABVD-RT showed no significant differences in age, sex, clinical presentation, or treatment modalities. Furthermore, there were no significant differences in the results of the pulmonary function tests prior to chemotherapy between the two patient groups. At the end of treatment (after the last course of chemotherapy), the mean VC change, calculated as the ratio of the observed value to the theoretical value in percent, was significantly higher in the ABVD arm (−19%) than in the MOPP arm (−13%) (P = 0.005).

One year after the end of chemotherapy, the mean VC change was −3% in the ABVD arm and −5% in the MOPP arm, a difference that was no longer statistically significant. This was a possible consequence either of the small number of evaluations that were available at that time or of an almost complete recovery of pulmonary function in both treatment arms.

Nevertheless, it should be mentioned that in the ABVD arm, two patients died from lung toxicity while there was no death related to pulmonary complications in the MOPP arm of the study.

This set of data was further analysed using a stepwise logistic regression in which posttreatment pulmonary toxicity (VC <70% of the theoretical value) was considered as the dependent variable, and other parameters as covariables. In this analysis the use of a total radiation dose of more than 37 Gy (relative risk [RR] = 1.90, P = 0.013) and ABVD (RR = 1.67, P = 0.025) were the only significant variables associated with a late functional pulmonary impairment.

The 59 patients included in the ABVD arm, and for whom posttreatment respiratory toxicity data were available, were then further investigated. Neither the cumulative dose of Adriamycin and bleomycin nor the route of administration of bleomycin (intravenous or intramuscular) was found to significantly influence lung function. A logistic regression was used to assess the roles of radiation dose, dose per fraction, bleomycin route of administration, and age on pulmonary toxicity. In this analysis (with 23 patients presenting with posttreatment VC <70%), no parameter was significantly related to lung toxicity.

In conclusion, the use of ABVD may aggravate the late pulmonary function impairment secondary to a standard mantle-field irradiation. However, this still needs to be confirmed after more patients' data are available at one and two years post chemotherapy. Whatever the type of treatment (RT alone or combined modality), RT fraction sizes exceeding 2 Gy should be discarded. Other potential risk factors (e.g., cumulative chemotherapy dose or radiation dose) are currently being prospectively investigated in the ongoing EORTC H7 trial [1].

c. Cardiac failures

Conflicting data have been recently reported in the literature for the incidence of cardiac failure, particularly myocardial infarction (MI), after HD therapy. Some authors claimed that the risk of MI is probably significantly increased after HD treatment [13,14] while others reported an MI rate which is superimposable on that expected in the general population [15, 16].

At the Institut Gustave-Roussy (IGR), cardiac toxicity was studied in two series of clinical stage I–IV HD patients. The first series consisted of 499 patients who were given mantle-field irradiation (with or without chemotherapy, mostly MOPP); the second series consisted of 138 patients who were treated without mediastinal radiotherapy [17]. Thirteen cases of MI (i.e., a 10-year cumulative incidence of 3.9%) were recorded in the first group of patients who were given mediastinal RT, while no cases of MI were registered in the second group of patients (P < 0.05), thus demonstrating that mediastinal irradiation is very likely to play a direct role in coronary and/or myocardial toxicity [18].

Late cardiac toxicity was also considered in the follow-up examination of HD patients treated by the EORTC Lymphoma Group. The incidence of MI was studied among 1048 of the 1082 patients entered in the H1, H2, and H5 trials (including a part of the aforementioned IGR patients), while the cardiac failure mortality was analysed among the overall cohort of patients treated on the four consecutive H1, H2, H5, and H6 protocols.

Morbidity
Twenty-one (2%) cases of MI were recorded among 1048 patients at risk. There were 17 males and 4 females. The MI occurred 3 to 225 months after the treatment was completed. The cumulative incidence rates were 2.4% at 10 years and 4.6% at 15 years.

In this EORTC series, it was impossible to precisely assess the role of mediastinal irradiation, since all patients were previously given mantle-field RT. No effect of RT dose fractionation could be shown, possibly because of the relatively small number of events.

Mortality
Twenty-four (1.5%) deaths due to cardiac failure were observed among 1650 patients at risk [19]. They occurred in males, 3 to 237 months after the treatment was completed. The 20-year cumulative death rate was 6.7%. All but 3 patients were in first complete remission. All patients were initially irradiated on the mediastinum. In addition, combination chemotherapy

was administered to a total of 5 patients, either as part of initial treatment (2 patients) or when a relapse occurred (3 patients). Compared to the general population, the standardized mortality ratio (SMR) was 10.17 (P < 0.001). It was higher in patients younger than 40 years (SMR = 15.38, P < 0.001) than in older (SMR = 8.24, P < 0.001). The analysis showed that SMR increased with time, with a peak between 3–11 years post treatment.

In conclusion, these data strongly suggest that mediastinal irradiation has been responsible for an increase in the risk of myocardial infarction that led to an increased risk of dying from cardiac failure in patients cured of HD. No EORTC data concerning cardiac function evaluation are available concerning long-term toxicity, and the importance of chemotherapy-associated toxicity (particularly with Adriamycin) is still to be investigated. Furthermore, it remains an open question whether or not the present way of delivering mantle irradiation (high-energy photons, two equally weighted beams being used at each session, fraction size of 1.8–2 Gy, and dose reduced to 30–36 Gy to the inferior mediastinum by using a subcarinal block when possible) is now able to partly, or totally, overcome the cardiac toxicity inherent in the older techniques.

III. Second cancers

Second cancers (SC) were diagnosed in 63 (3.8%) of the 1650 patients entered in the four consecutive EORTC trials. Ten patients with basal cell carcinoma of the skin, 2 patients with in situ carcinoma of the uterine cervix, and 4 patients with unspecified histological diagnosis were excluded from the study. While sex ratio (M/F) was 1.3 in the overall EORTC HD population, it was 1.9 among SC patients. A similar sex ratio was observed regardless of the type of SC.

a. Acute nonlymphocytic leukemias (ANLL)

In the EORTC series, 17 cases of ANLL, or myelodysplastic syndrome, were registered. Their cumulative incidence from the time of initial treatment is plotted in Figure 2. The probability for developing ANLL was 1.2% at 10 years, and 2.3% at 15 years. The risk seemed to reach a plateau level after 12–14 years. The standardized incidence ratio (SIR), that is, the ratio of observed number of ANLL to expected number, was 36.6 (95% confidence limits [CL] 21.3–58.5; P < 0.001).

By Cox regression analysis, the only factor found to be associated with an increase in risk of ANLL was the combination of radiation and MOPP chemotherapy (RR = 13.6; P < 0.001), thus confirming previously published data [20, 21, 22, 23]. In this series, splenectomy was not found to play any role in secondary ANLL risk, in contrast with some previously reported data [23, 24, 25, 26].

CUMULATIVE INCIDENCE OF SECOND CANCER

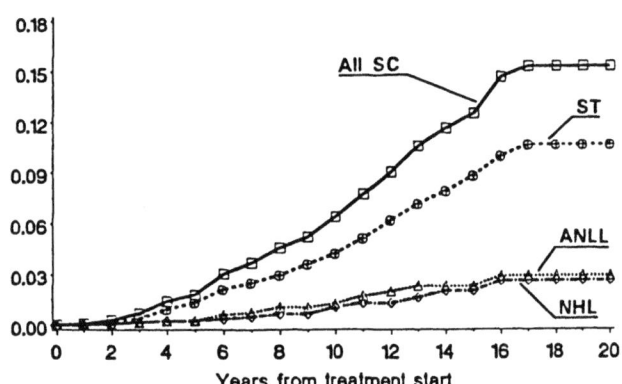

Fig. 2. Cumulative incidence of all second cancer (SC), solid tumor (ST), ANLL, and NHL for the entire EORTC cohort (N = 1650).

b. Non-Hodgkin's Lymphomas (NHL)

In the EORTC series, 13 cases of NHL were diagnosed. Their cumulative incidence is plotted in Figure 2. The NHL curve closely parallels that of ANLL, also exhibiting a plateau after 12–14 years. The probability of developing NHL was 1% at 10 years and 1.9% at 15 years. The SIR was 33.3 (95% CL 17.8–57; P < 0.001).

By Cox regression analysis, two factors were found to be significantly associated with an increased risk of developing NHL: age at HD diagnosis greater than 40 years (RR = 6.6, P < 0.01), and a combination of radiation and MOPP chemotherapy (RR = 6.0, P < 0.01) [20].

c. Solid tumors (ST)

Thirty-three (2%) cases of secondary solid tumors were registered. The cumulative incidence rate (Fig. 2) increases to 4.2% at 10 years and to 8.8% at 15 years. In contrast to ANLL and NHL evolution, the annual risk of ST appears to increase continuously (the apparent plateau after 16 years should be considered with caution because of the small number of patients still at risk

after 15 years of follow-up). An increased incidence was observed for some specific ST types: salivary glands (parotid) in males and females (SIR > 50, P < 0.001), gastric carcinoma in males (SIR = 7.1, P < 0.001), and bronchial carcinoma in males (SIR = 3.3, P = 0.001). In addition, twenty-three solid tumors were located within previously irradiated volumes (SIR = 3.2, P < 0.001). Overall, the SIR for ST was 1.7 (95% CL 1.2–2.4, P < 0.005).

By Cox regression analysis, two factors were found to be significantly associated with an increased risk of developing a secondary ST: age at HD diagnosis greater than 40 years (RR = 3.6, P < 0.001) and extended-field radiotherapy (total or subtotal nodal irradiation) (RR = 2.0, P = 0.05) [20].

IV. Treatment-related long-term toxicity and mortality

In the entire EORTC cohort, 320 deaths were recorded. Of these 169 (53%) were due to HD progression or relapse [19].

Treatment-related (toxic) deaths (Table 2) accounted for 26 demises. In addition, 24 fatal cardiac failures were registered. Second cancers were responsible for 46 deaths; 13 from ANLL (or myelodysplasia), 9 from NHL, and 24 from solid tumors. Intercurrent deaths occurred in 32 cases. For 23 patients, the cause of death could not be specified (Table 2).

The proportion of deaths related to long-term treatment toxicity can be estimated as the excess mortality calculated as the total number of toxic deaths (n = 26) plus cardiac failure deaths (n = 24) plus second cancer deaths (n = 46) minus the total number of expected deaths from a normal matched population (i.e., 3 cardiac failures plus 12 second cancers) (Table 2). This led to an overall number of 81 deaths most probably related to some adverse effects of treatment, i.e., as much as one quarter of the deaths recorded in the entire cohort. This proportion is certainly underestimated, since an unknown percentage of the deaths due to intercurrent and unspecified causes (total 55 cases) could actually be related to an unrecognized long-term toxicity of therapy.

V. Discussion and conclusion

It is now well established that the risk of death from HD is constantly decreasing with time. This is clearly shown by the analysis of the EORTC data [19] as well as by the analysis of the International Database on Hodgkin's Disease (IDHD) [27, 28]. For example, in the latter series, only 75 (0.6%) of 12 301 patients relapsed 10 years or more after initial therapy [27].

However, the annual death rate of the HD population does not significantly decrease with time. This is explained by a 'balance' between a progressive decrease in mortality from HD and an increasing death

Table 2. Observed (O) and expected (E) deaths for the entire EORTC cohort (N = 1650 patients).

	O	E	O/E*	95% CL
All deaths	320	40.14	7.97	7.02–8.90
Deaths from Hodgkin's disease	169			
Treatment-related deaths	26			
Cardiac failures	24	2.78	8.63	5.53–12.83
Second cancers	46	11.98	3.84	2.81–5.12
Intercurrent deaths	32			
Unspecified cause	23			

* All differ significantly from 1; P < 0.001 (two-sided test).
95% CL: 95% confidence limit assuming a Poisson distribution for O.
From Henry-Amar [19].

rate related to other causes. In the EORTC cohort, there was a steadily increasing mortality due to second cancers, intercurrent diseases, and cardiac failure [19]. After 20 years, data showed that the main causes of death were second cancers (with a cumulative incidence of 9.3%), intercurrent diseases (cumulative incidence 7.6%) and cardiac failures (cumulative incidence 5.7%) [19].

This increasing rate of deaths unrelated to HD, which has been observed in both the European and the international series [19, 27], explains why the survival curve of the patients previously treated for HD never parallels that of the general population. These patients, even when cured of their disease, remain at a higher risk of death than the general population 10 years and more post therapy. There is now evidence that this fact is partly related to long-term treatment toxicity.

As a consequence, our efforts should now be devoted to decreasing the incidence of these late complications, and the search for (1) less leukemogenic chemotherapy schemes, (2) safer ways of delivering HD radiotherapy, and (3) less toxic schedules of CT-RT combinations should become the highest priority for HD studies in the 1990s.

Appendix

Chairmen of the EORTC Lymphoma Cooperative group: M. Tubiana (1964–1967), K. Breur (1967–1969), B. van der Werf-Messing (1969–1972), J. Henry (1973–1975), J. Abbatucci (1975–1977), J. M. V. Burgers (1977–1980), M. Hayat (1980–1982), R. Somers (1983–1987), and J. H. Meerwaldt (1987–present). *Statistician*: M. Henry-Amar. *Data manager*: N. Dupouy. *Scientific secretaries*: A. Laugier (1964–1972), M. Hayat (1972–1975), M. Urbajtel (1975–1977), E. van der Schueren (1977–1980), P. Carde (1980–1985), J. H. Meerwaldt (1985–1987), and J. Thomas (1987–present). *Committee of pathologists*: M. J. J. T. Bogman, J. Bosq, B. Caillou, N. Duplay, R. Gérard-Marchant, E. Halkin, P. van Heerde, R. Heiman, P. M. Kluin, A. M. Mandard, R. Menon, M. F. Prins, J. A. M. van Unnik, L. Vrints, and C. de Wolf-Peeters. *Committee of radiologists*: C. Bergiron, J. L. Chassard, W. Feremans, R. W. Kropholler, J. Masselot, and P. Markovits.

Cooperating centres in The Netherlands: Antoni van Leeuwenhoek Ziekenhuis, Amsterdam *(J. M. V. Burgers and R. Somers)*; University Hospital, Leiden *(E. M. Noordijk)*; St. Radboud Academic Hospital, Nijmegen *(C. Haanen, B. E. de Pauw, and D. Wagener)*; Rotterdamsch-Radiotherapeutisch Instituut, Rotterdam *(J. H. Meerwaldt, M. Qasim, W. Sizoo, and B. van der Werf-Messing)*; Ziekenhuis Leyenburg, The Hague *(H. Kerkhofs)*; University Hospital, Utrecht *(J. G. Nyssen, H. van Peperzeel, and L. Verdonck)*; Stichting Ignatius-Ziekenhuis, Breda *(A. C. J. M. Holdrinet)*; Catharina Ziekenhuis, Eindhoven *(W. P. M. Breed)*; and Acad. Ziekenhuis, Rotterdam *(J. Michiels)*.

Cooperating centres in Belgium: Institut Jules Bordet, Brussels *(D. Bron, J. Henry, J. Lustmann-Maréchal, R. Reinier)*; Centre René Goffin, La Louvière *(J. C. Goffin)*; Hôpital de Bavière, Liège *(R. Lemaire)*; Acad. Ziekenhuis St. Rafaël, Leuven *(J. Thomas and E. van der Schueren)*; and Ziekenhuis St Jan, Brugge *(A. Van Hoof and A. Louwagie)*.

Cooperating centres in Italy: Istituto di Radiologia, Università di Firenze *(L. Cionini and G. De Giuli)*; and Ospedale San Giovanni, Torino *(R. Musella)*.

Cooperating centres in France: Fondation Bergonié, Bordeaux *(B. Hoerni and C. Lagarde)*; Centre François-Baclesse, Caen *(J. S.*

Abbatucci and A. Tanguy); Centre G. F. Leclerc, Dijon *(P. Fargeot and J. C. Horiot)*; Centre Léon-Bérard, Lyon *(J. Papillon and L. Revol)*; Centre Antoine-Lacassagne, Nice *(C. Lalanne, M. Schneider, and A. Thyss)*; Hôtel-Dieu, Paris *(M. C. Blanc and R. Zittoun)*; Institut Jean-Godinot, Reims *(A. Cattan)*; Centre Henri-Becquerel, Rouen *(R. Le Fur, M. Monconduit, and H. Piguet)*; Centre Cl. Regaud, Toulouse *(F. Rigal-Huguet)*; Institut Gustave-Roussy, Villejuif *(J. L. Amiel, P. Carde, J. M. Cosset, M. Hayat, and M. Tubiana)*; and Institut de Cancérologie et d'Immunogénétique, Hôpital Paul Brousse, Villejuif *(G. Mathé and J. L. Misset)*.
Cooperating centre in Germany: Universität zu Köln *(H. Sack)*.

References

1. Tubiana M, Henry-Amar M, Carde P et al. Towards comprehensive management tailored to prognostic factors of patients with clinical stage I and II in Hodgkin's disease. The EORTC lymphoma group controlled clinical trials 1964–1987. Blood 1989; 73: 47–56.
2. Hohl RJ, Schlilsky RL. Non malignant complications of therapy for Hodgkin's disease. Hematology/Oncology Clinics of North America 1989; 3: 331–43.
3. Cosset JM, Henry-Amar M, Burgers JMV et al. Late radiation injuries of the gastro-intestinal tract in the H2 and H5 EORTC Hodgkin's disease trials: Emphasis on the role of exploratory laparotomy and fractionation. Radiother Oncol 1988; 13: 61–8.
4. Gallez-Marchal D, Fayolle M, Henry-Amar M et al. Radiation injuries of the gastro-intestinal tract in Hodgkin's disease: The role of exploratory laparotomy and fractionation. Radiother Oncol 1984; 2: 93–9.
5. Thames HD, Hendry JH. Fractionation in radiotherapy. London: Taylor and Francis, 1987.
6. Cosset JM, Henry-Amar M, Girinsky T et al. Late toxicity of radiotherapy in Hodgkin's disease: The role of fraction size. Acta Oncologica 1988; 27: 113–29.
7. Host H, Vale JR. Lung function after mantle field irradiation in Hodgkin's disease. Cancer 1973; 32: 328–32.
8. Evans RF, Sagerman RH, Ringrose TL et al. Pulmonary function following mantle field irradiation for Hodgkin's disease. Radiology 1974; 111: 729–31.
9. Watchie J, Coleman CN, Raffin TA et al. Minimal long term cardiopulmonary dysfunction following treatment for Hodgkin's disease. Int J Radiat Oncol Biol Phys 1989; 16: 79–84.
10. Smith LM, Mendenhall NP, Cicale MJ et al. Results of a prospective study evaluating the effects of mantle irradition on pulmonary function. Int J Radiat Oncol Biol Phys 1989; 16: 79–84.
11. Cosset JM, Henry-Amar M, Thomas J et al. Increased pulmonary toxicity in the ABVD arm of the EORTC H6-U trial. Proc Am Soc Clin Oncol 1989; 8: 253.
12. Zucali R, Pagnoni AM, Zanini M et al. Radiobiological and spirometric evaluation of mediastinal and pulmonary late effects after radiotherapy and chemotherapy for Hodgkin's disease. J Eur Radiother 1981; 2: 169–76.
13. Boivin JF, Hutchison GB. Coronary heart disease mortality after irradiation of Hodgkin's disease. Cancer 1982; 49: 2470–5.
14. Pohjola-Sintonen S, Totterman KJ, Salmo M et al. Late cardiac effects of mediastinal radiotherapy in patients with Hodgkin's disease. Cancer 1987; 60: 31–7.
15. Hancock SL, Hoppe RT, Horning SJ et al. Intercurrent death after Hodgkin's disease therapy in radiotherapy and adjuvant MOPP trials. Ann Int Med 1988; 109: 183–9.
16. Van Rijswijk REN, Verbeek J, Haanen C et al. Major complications and causes of death in patients treated for Hodgkin's disease. J Clin Oncol 1987; 5: 1624–33.
17. Cosset JM, Henry-Amar M, Pellae Cosset B et al. Pericarditis and myocardial infarctions after Hodgkin's disease therapy at

82

the Institut Gustave-Roussy. Int J Radiat Oncol Biol Phys 1990 (in press).

18. Corn BW, Trock BJ, Goodman RL. Irradiation-related ischaemic heart disease. J Clin Oncol 1990; 8: 741–50.
19. Henry-Amar M, Somers R. Long-term survival in early stages Hodgkin's disease: The EORTC experience. In: Treatment Strategy in Hodgkin's disease, Somers R, Henry-Amar M, Meerwaldt JH, Carde P (eds). Colloque INSERM no 196. London, Paris: INSERM/John Libbey Eurotext, 1990; 151–66.
20. Henry-Amar M. Risk of second cancer after therapy for early stage Hodgkin's disease: The EORTC experience. Int J Radiat Oncol Biol Phys 1990 (in press).
21. Henry-Amar M, Pellae-Cosset B, Bayle-Weisgerber C et al. Risk of secondary acute leukemia and preleukemia after Hodgkin's disease. The Institut Gustave-Roussy experience. In: New aspects in the diagnosis and treatment of Hodgkin's disease. Diehl V, Pfreundschuh M, Loeffler M (eds). Recent results in Cancer Res 1989; 117: 270–83.
22. Pedersen-Bjergaard J, Specht L, Larsen SO et al. Risk of therapy-related leukemia and preleukemia after Hodgkin's disease. Relation to age, cumulative dose of alkylating agents, and time from chemotherapy. Lancet 1987; ii: 83–88.
23. Kaldor JM, Day NE, Clarke EA et al. Leukemia following Hodgkin's disease. N Engl J Med 1990; 322: 7–13.
24. Van Leeuwen FE, Somers R, Hart AAM. Splenectomy in Hodgkin's disease and second leukemia. Lancet 1987; ii: 210–1.
25. Van Leeuwen FE, Somers R, Tall BG et al. Increased risk of lung cancer, non-Hodgkin's lymphoma, and leukemia following Hodgkin's disease. J Clin Oncol 1989; 7: 1046–58.
26. Van der Velden JW, van Putten WL, Gurnee VF et al. Subsequent development of acute non-lymphocytic leukemias in patients treated for Hodgkin's disease. Int J Cancer 1988; 42: 252–5.
27. Henry-Amar M, Somers R. Survival outcome after Hodgkin disease. A report from the International Database on Hodgkin disease (IDHD). Seminars in Oncology 1990 (in press).
28. Somers R, Henry-Amar M, Meerwaldt JH, Carde P (eds). Treatment Strategy in Hodgkin's disease. Statistical report, part X. Colloque INSERM no 196. London, Paris: INSERM/John Libbey Eurotext, 1990; 381–418.

Correspondence to:
J. M. Cosset
Radiotherapy Department and INSERM U247
Institut Gustave-Roussy
94805 Villejuif Cedex – France

Annals of Oncology, Supplement 2 to Volume 2: 83–92, 1991.
© 1991 *Kluwer Academic Publishers*.

Original article _____

Non-Hodgkin's lymphoma arising in patients treated for Hodgkin's disease in the BNLI: A 20-year experience

M. H. Bennett,[1] K. A. MacLennan,[2] G. Vaughan Hudson[3] & B. Vaughan Hudson[3]
from the British National Lymphoma Investigation
[1]*Mount Vernon Hospital,* [2]*the Royal Marsden Hospital, Fulham Road and* [3]*UCMSM, Middlesex Hospital, London, United Kingdom*

Summary. Twenty-two of 3033 patients with Hodgkin's disease (HD) randomised into the clinical trials of the BNLI have developed non-Hodgkin's lymphomas (NHLs) at periods up to 16 years after presentation (1 simultaneous and 1 composite), giving an incidence of 0.7%. The frequency of NHL varied from 3.8% in lymphocyte-predominant HD to 0.3% in nodular sclerosing HD. In this series, 16 patients developed high-grade NHL (12 B cell; 4 peripheral T cell) and 6 developed low-grade NHL (all B cell). The histological subtype of NHL did not appear to be related to initial histological subtype of HD or the treatment received. In histological subtypes other than lymphocyte predominant, there was commonly evidence of immunosuppression in the form of low presentation lymphocyte counts, advanced stage and systemic (B) symptoms. The results suggest that these patients have a propensity for lymphoproliferative disorders, possibly associated with some immune deficiency and the subsequent development of NHL is not treatment related. The findings also emphasise how important it is to biopsy recurrent disease.

Key words: Hodgkin's disease, secondary non-Hodgkin's lymphoma, second malignancies in HD, composite lymphoma, non-Hodgkin's lymphoma in Hodgkin's disease

Introduction

The development of non-Hodgkin's lymphoma (NHL) in patients with Hodgkin's disease (HD) is a well-recognised though infrequent event [1–6a] and may occur subsequent to or simultaneously with the diagnosis of HD [7–8a] when the term composite lymphoma has been used.

The incidence of NHL following HD ranges from 0–5.9% [5] with a disproportionate relative frequency in patients whose original HD was of the lymphocyte-predominant histological type. The majority of NHLs occurring after HD are high-grade B-cell tumours; some T-cell tumours have also been described [2, 9–12].

In the British National Lymphoma Investigation (BNLI) [13], we have encountered similar cases, most of the NHLs being of B-cell type but 4 having been peripheral T-cell lymphomas. We wish to report our 20-year experience.

Materials and methods

Between January 1970 and April 1989, 3033 patients have been registered as HD and randomised into the clinical trials of the BNLI. Up to January 1990, 22 of these patients have subsequently developed an immunophenotypically confirmed NHL and an additional 2 patients had synchronous presentation of HD and NHL.

In all cases the original sections upon which the diagnosis was made have been reviewed and immunocytochemistry performed in the majority (18 of 24) where additional paraffin sections were available. An avidin-biotin complex immunoperoxidase technique was used [14] with primary antisera directed against CD20 (L26; Dako, [15]), CD45 Ro (UCHL 1; Dako, [16]), and CD15 (Dako M1 [17]).

Clinical data were obtained from the files of the BNLI.

In two patients the original diagnosis of HD was changed to one of T-cell-rich B-cell lymphoma [18]. These were composed of large B-cells (L26-positive), some of which were pleomorphic, resembling lacunar, Hodgkin, or Reed-Sternberg cells, scattered in a background of UCHL1-positive small T-cells (large B-cell lymphoma with a high content of reactive T-cells) [19]. In both cases the new lymphoma was of diffuse large B-cell type. For the remaining 22 cases the diagnosis of HD was confirmed on review; 7 were classified as lymphocyte predominant (LP), 8 as nodular scerosis (NS), and 6 as mixed cellularity (MC).

Results

Lymphocyte predominant HD

The seven patients were all males with an age range of 36 to 55 years and all had the nodular subtype of LP

Table 1. Lymphocyte predominant nodular.

LI	Age/sex	Site	Stage	Therapy	NHL	T/B	Site	Interval	A/D months
224	M36	Groin	IIA	PRT	DLL	B	Thigh	18 yr	D6
227	M38	Axilla	IVA	MOPP	D Mix	T	Liver	6 yr	D9
1886	M38	Abdo	IVA	MOPP	DLL	B	Neck	9 yr	D1
3750	M36	Groin	IIA	LRT	DLL	B	Abdo	7 yr	D25
3876	M46	SM	IA	PRT	DLL	B	Caecum Liver	10 yr	A8
5585	M51	SM	IA	LRT (LOPP)	D Mix	T	Skin	4 yr	A48
8056	M55	SCF	IIA	PRT	DLL	T	Spleen Liver	1 yr	D1

LRT – local radiotherapy, PRT – prophylactic radiotherapy. D Mix – diffuse mixed small and large cell cytology, DLL – diffuse large lymphoid cell cytology. SM – Submandibular, SCF – supraclavicular fossa, Med. – mediastinum.

(Table 1). Five were stage I or II at presentation but two cases were classified as having stage IV disease; one (Case 227) by reason of a lung lesion seen on chest x-ray and the other (Case 1886) because of a clinically enlarged liver though two biopsy specimens taken at staging laparotomy were histologically negative. None of the patients had B symptoms.

Four patients developed a high-grade B-cell lymphoma of diffuse large-cell type at 7, 9, 10 and 18 years after the diagnosis of HD, two being in extranodal sites (Case 24 in thigh and Case 3876 in caecum). Three of the patients had been treated with radiotherapy only, achieving complete remission (CR) with no relapse until the development of NHL. One patient (Case 1886) was clinically stage IV at presentation but with disease confined to the abdomen. This patient was treated with combination chemotherapy, achieving CR, but was given two further courses of chemotherapy at five and

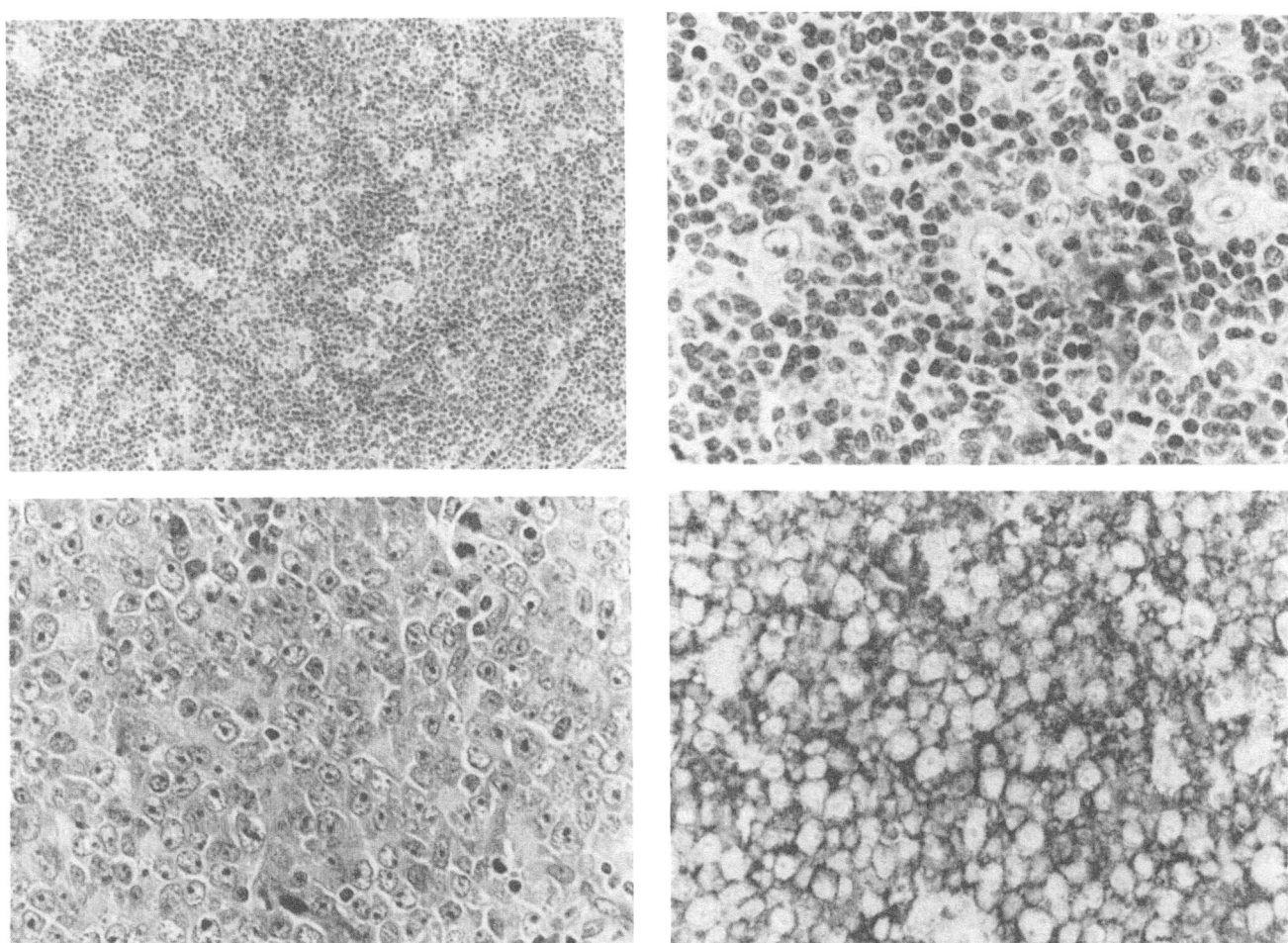

Fig. 1. Case 1886 (A; top left) presentation paraaortic lymph node biopsy showing LP nodular HD (H & E × 125). (B; top right) same biopsy showing typical L & H Hodgkin cells (H & E × 400). (C; bottom left) Secondary large B-cell NHL which developed nine years later. Biopsy of lymph node in the neck (H & E × 310). (D; bottom right) same biopsy immunostained for CD20 (L 26) (ABC × 310).

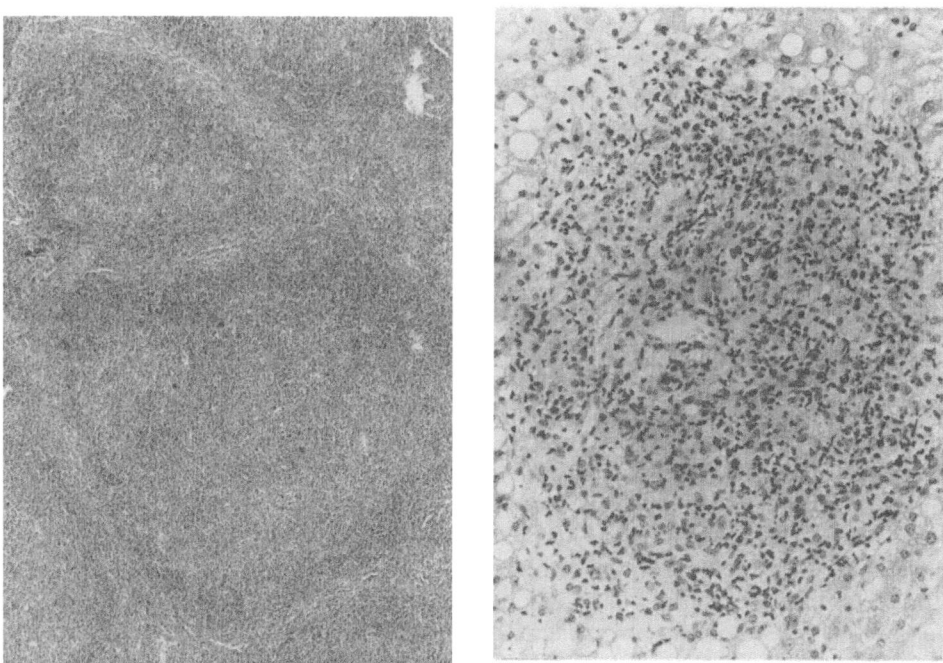

Fig. 2. Case 227 (A; left) Biopsy of axillary lymph node showing LP nodular HD (H & E × 30). (B; right) needle biopsy of liver six years later showing a polymorphous mixed small and large cell infiltrate in the portal tract (H & E × 125).

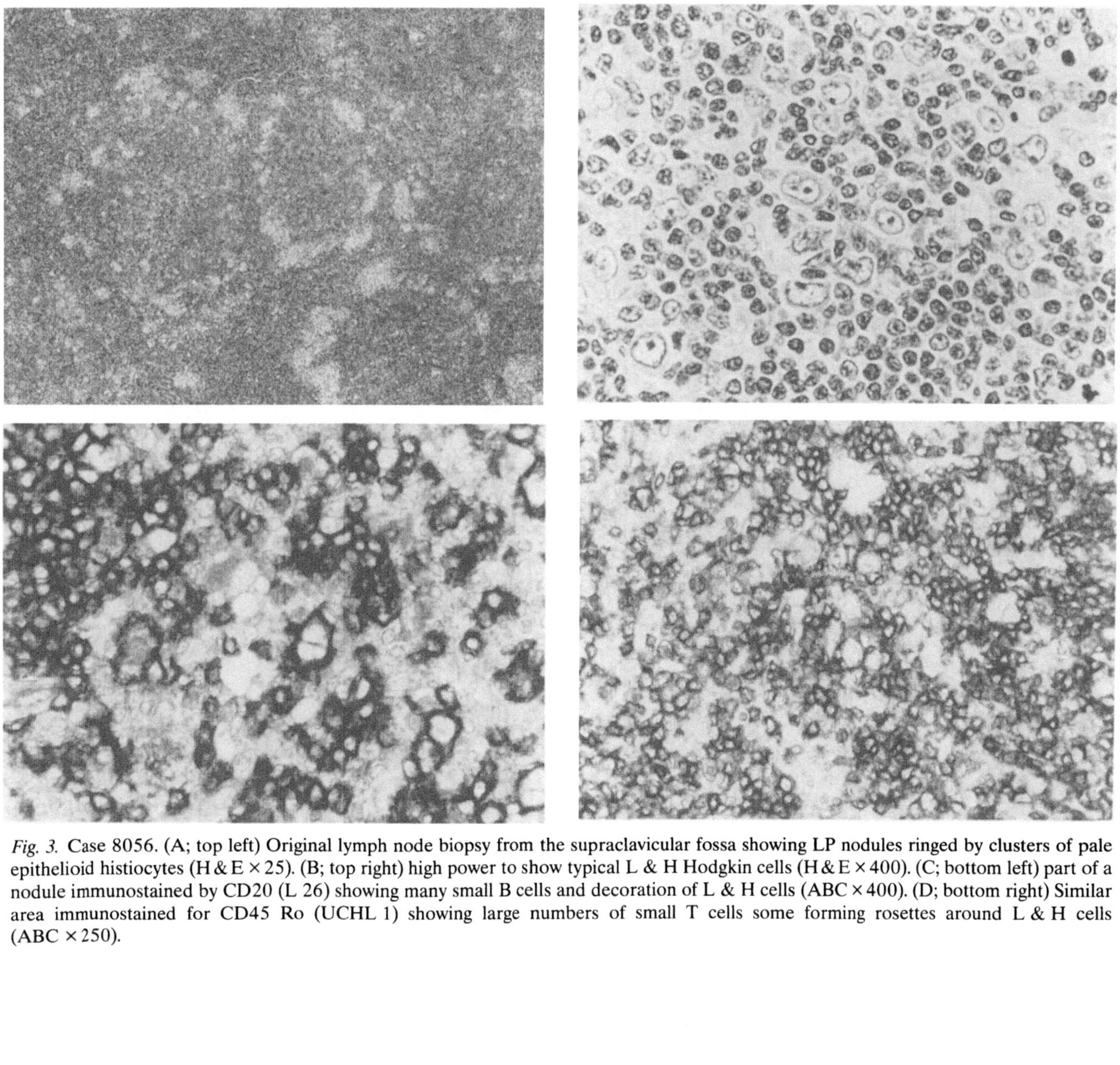

Fig. 3. Case 8056. (A; top left) Original lymph node biopsy from the supraclavicular fossa showing LP nodules ringed by clusters of pale epithelioid histiocytes (H & E × 25). (B; top right) high power to show typical L & H Hodgkin cells (H & E × 400). (C; bottom left) part of a nodule immunostained by CD20 (L 26) showing many small B cells and decoration of L & H cells (ABC × 400). (D; bottom right) Similar area immunostained for CD45 Ro (UCHL 1) showing large numbers of small T cells some forming rosettes around L & H cells (ABC × 250).

seven years for relapse in the abdomen, for which no biopsy was performed. He developed further disease in the neck at nine years, which on biopsy was a diffuse large B-cell NHL (Fig. 1).

In three patients the NHL was of T-cell type, developing in extranodal sites one, four, and six years after the diagnosis of HD. Case 227 was treated with chemotherapy, achieved CR, and did not relapse until he presented with malaise and a large liver six years later. Needle biopsy showed dense portal tract infiltration by a mixture of small and large T-lymphoid cells (positive with UCHL1) and devoid of any L26- or Leu M1-positive large cells (Fig. 2).

Case 5585 was treated originally with local radiotherapy for disease confined to the submandibular region. He relapsed at two years in the neck; biopsy confirmed recurrent Hodgkin's disease of LP nodular type and he was treated with combination chemotherapy. At four years he developed multiple skin lesions with on biopsy showed a dense infiltrate of small and large UCHL1-positive lymphocytes consistent with a cutaneous T-cell lymphoma. He was given further chemotherapy with regression of the lesions, but four years later had recurrent skin lesions and enlarged cervical lymph nodes. Further biopsies have been requested.

Case 8056 is of particular interest, presenting initially with a three-year history of a slowly enlarging node in the supraclavicular. A biopsy specimen showed HD of LP nodular subtype but with large numbers of T-cells infiltrating the nodules (Fig. 3). The patient was treated with mantle radiotherapy and achieved CR but at one year was unwell with a palpable spleen and liver. Chemotherapy was started but as response was poor and there was evidence of hypersplenism, a splenectomy and liver biopsy were performed. Macroscopically the spleen was enlarged by ill-defined, large, swollen, dark red areas which on histological examination were composed of large T-cells with sinusoidal infiltration (Fig. 4). The liver showed extensive portal tract infiltration.

Nodular sclerosing HD

Of the 8 patients, 4 were male and 4 female with ages ranging from 44 to 71 years at presentation with HD (Table 2). Four patients presented with stage III or IV disease and 5 had B symptoms. Four were treated with chemotherapy alone and 3 with radiotherapy alone, all achieving CR and remaining disease free until the development of NHL. One patient (Case 469) presented

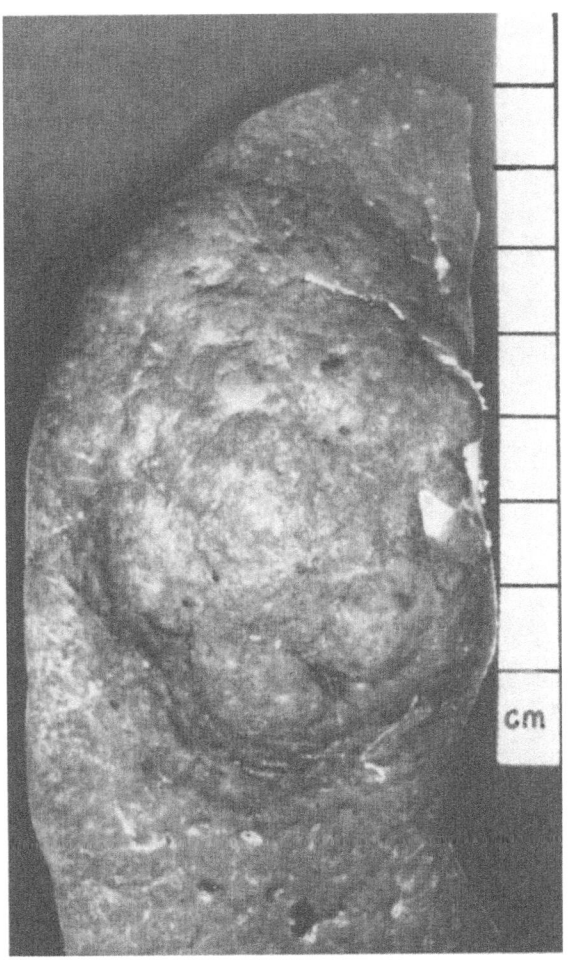
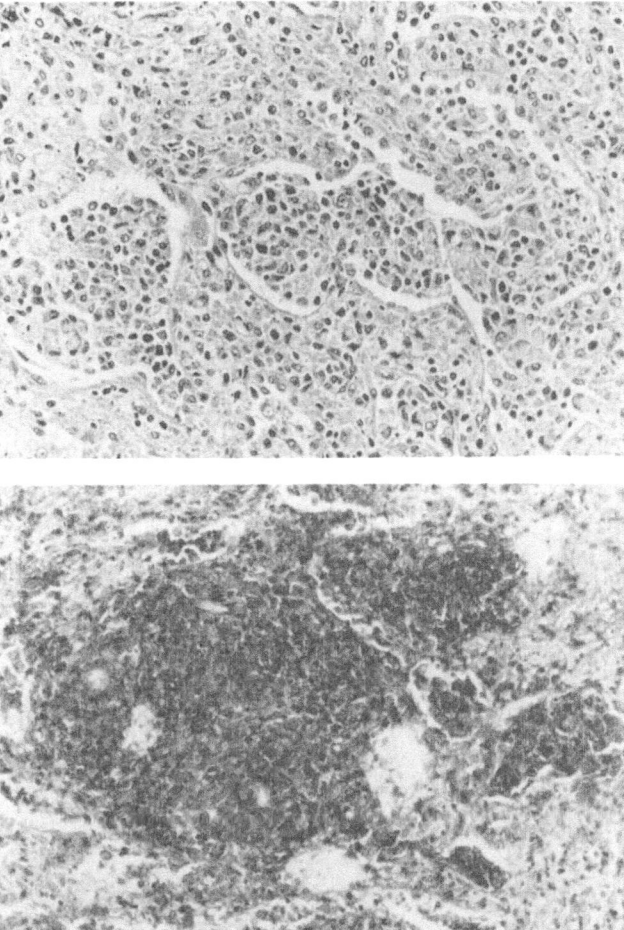

Fig. 4. Case 8056 (A; left) Spleen removed one year after presentation showing swollen, nodular areas. (B; top right) Section of spleen showing large-cell lymphoma with sinusoidal infiltration (H & E × 150). (C; bottom right) section immunostained for CD45 Ro (UCHL 1) showing positive staining of tumour cells in parenchyma and sinuses (ABC × 100).

Table 2. Nodular sclerosis.

LI	Age/sex	Site	Stage	Therapy	NHL	T/B	Site	Interval	A/D months
180	F60	Neck	IIB	LRT	DLL	B	Groin	6 yr	D7
360	M48	Groin	IIIB	MOPP	DLL	B	Axilla	12 yr	D30
469	M44	SCF	IA	PRT (LOPP)	DLL	B	Neck	16 yr	A23
666	F57	Axilla	IVB	MOPP	FL mx	B	Spleen	3 yr	D96
2729	M64	Neck	IIIB	MOPP	DLL	B	Neck	5 yr	D24
5466	F70	E.T.	IA	LRT	DLL	B	Skin	6 yr	A27
6328	M61	Groin	IA	LRT	FL mx	B	Neck	2 yr	A?
6619	F71	Axilla	IIIB	LOPP	DLL	B	Caecum	5 yr	D12

LRT – local radiotherapy, PRT – prophylactic radiotherapy. LOPP – substitution of Chlorambucil for Mustine in MOPP. FL mx – follicular lymphoma, mixed small and large cell type, D Mix – diffuse mixed small and large cell cytology, DLL – diffuse large lymphoid cell cytology. E.T. – epitrochlear, SCF – supraclavicular fossa.

with disease limited to one supraclavicular fossa; staging laparotomy was negative and he was treated with mantle radiotherapy but relapsed in the abdomen at 19 months. Following chemotherapy he remained disease free until developing a large B-cell NHL in the neck at 16 years (Fig. 5).

All 8 patients developed B-cell NHLs; 6 were high-grade large cell lymphomas occurring from 5 to 16 years after presentation with HD. Of these, 4 were

nodal disease and 2 extranodal, 1 in the caecum and 1 in the subcutaneous tissue of the eyebrow. Three had received chemotherapy alone, 2 radiotherapy and 1 (Case 469) radiotherapy followed by chemotherapy for early relapse. Two patients developed low-grade follicular lymphoma of mixed small and large cell type (Fig. 6) two and three years after the diagnosis of HD. One of these patients originally received chemotherapy and the other radiotherapy alone.

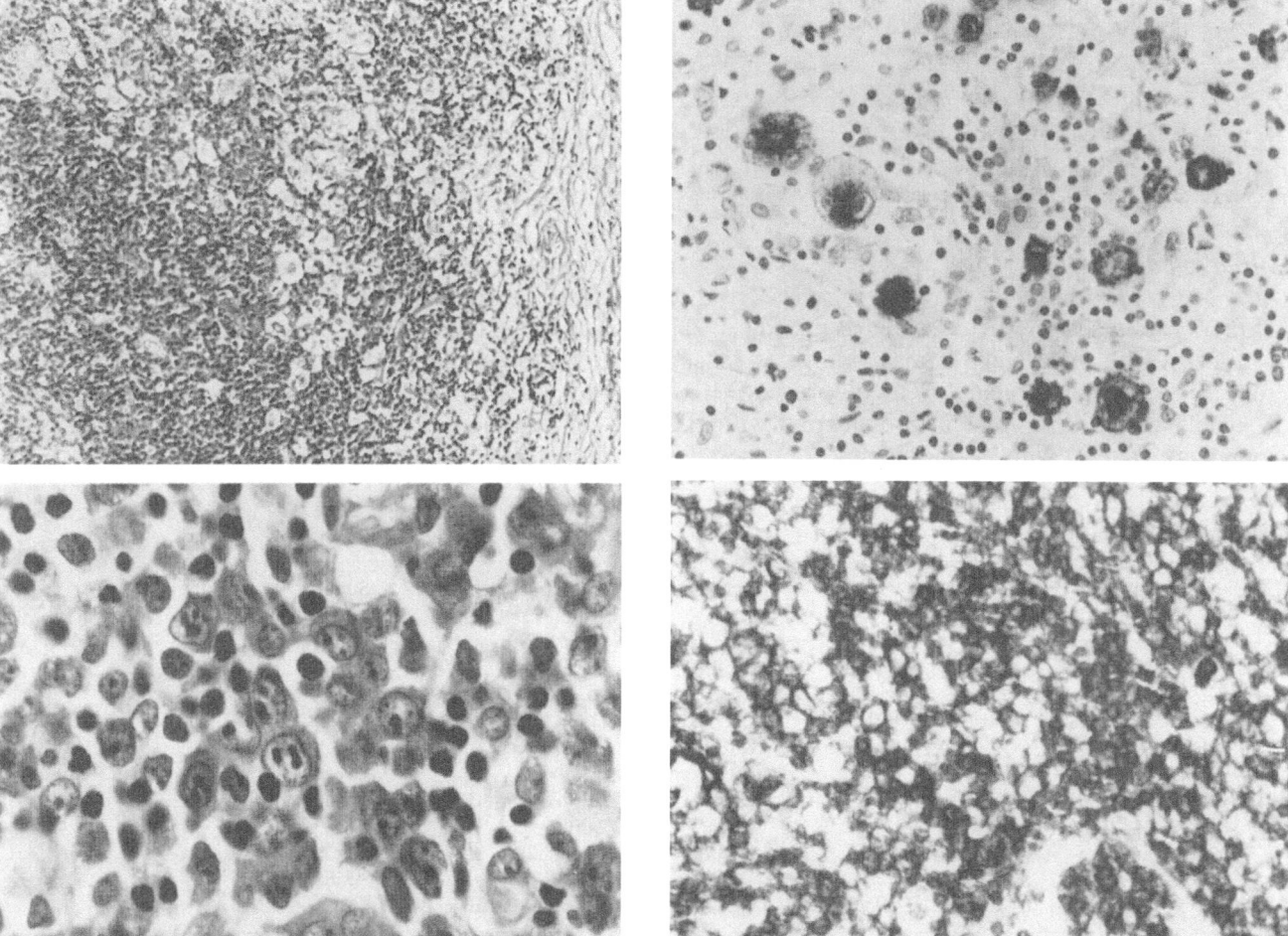

Fig. 5. Case 469 (A; top left) presentation supraclavicular lymph node biopsy showing NS HD (H & E × 100). (B; top right) Immunostaining of same biopsy with CD15 (Dako M1) showing strong golgi and cytoplasmic staining of R-S cells (ABC × 250). (C; bottom left) Biopsy of neck node at 16 years showing large cell lymphoma with centroblastic morphology (H & E × 500). (D; bottom right) Same biopsy immunostained for CD20 (L 26) (ABC × 310).

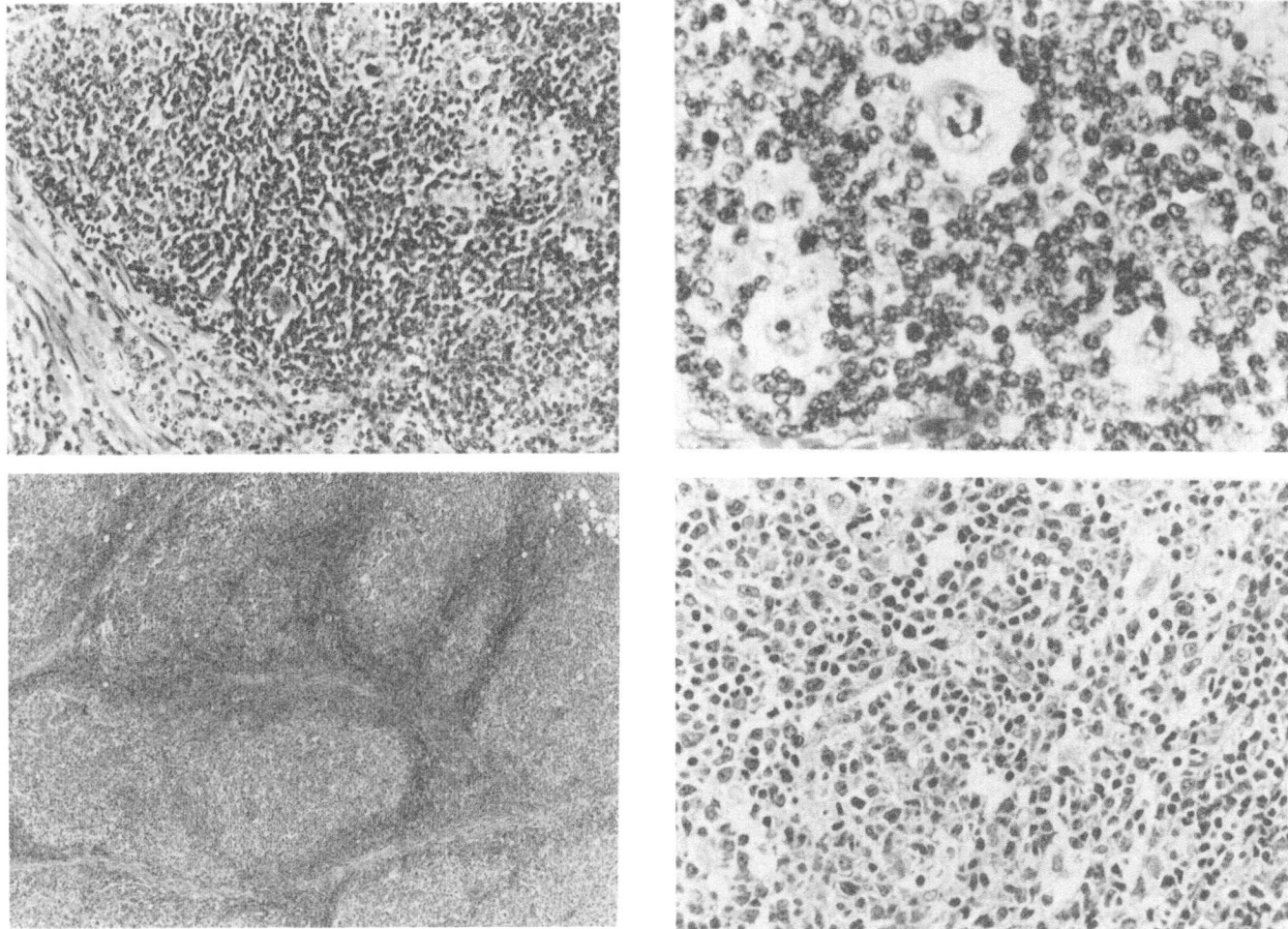

Fig. 6. Case 6328. (A; top left) Presentation biopsy of groin lymph node showing NS HD with scanty lacunar cells (H & E × 150). (B; upper right) same biopsy showing lacunar cells (H & E × 400). (C; bottom left) biopsy of neck lymph node 2 years later showing follicular lymphoma (H & E × 30). (D; bottom right) same lymph node showing cytology of neoplastic follicle (H & E × 250).

Mixed cellularity HD

Of the 7 patients who were classified as mixed cellularity HD, 6 were male and 1 female with ages ranging from 27 to 63 years (Table 3). Three were stage III or IV and 5 had B symptoms at presentation with HD. Four were treated with chemotherapy, 2 with radio-

therapy and one with radiotherapy and chemotherapy for relapse at three years. Two patients developed high-grade B-cell lymphomas of large-cell type (Case 152 in the small bowel at 8 years and Case 224 in an inguinal node at 16 years). Two patients developed low-grade B-cell lymphomas two years after presenting with HD (Case 5414 follicular lymphoma in an axillary node

Table 3. Mixed cellularity.

LI	Age/sex	Site	Stage	Therapy	NHL	T/B	Site	Interval	A/D months
152	M58	Axilla	IVB	MOPP	DLL	B	Small Bowel	8 yr	D5
224	M27	Neck	IIB	LRT (MOPP)	DLL	B	Groin	16 yr	A35
3399	M32	Neck	IA	PRT	D Mix	T	Groin	8 yr	A45
5414	M61	Groin	IA	LRT	FL mx	B	Axilla	2 yr	A63
7375	M47	Med.	IIIB	LOPP	LPIC	B	BM	2 yr	A20
9175	F63	Neck Axilla	IIB	LOPP	FL small	B	Neck Axilla	0 yr	A22
9531	M50	PA	IVB	CHOP	FL small	B	Mes.	0 yr	A12

LRT – local radiotherapy, PRT – prophylactic radiotherapy. LOPP – substitution of Chlorambucil for Mustine in MOPP. FL small – follicular lymphoma, predominantly small cell type, FL mx – follicular lymphoma, mixed small and large cell type, D Mix – diffuse mixed small and large cell cytology, DLL – diffuse large lymphoid cell cytology, LPIC – lymphoplasmacytic immunocytoma. Med. – mediastinum, PA – para-aortic, Mes. – mesenteric.

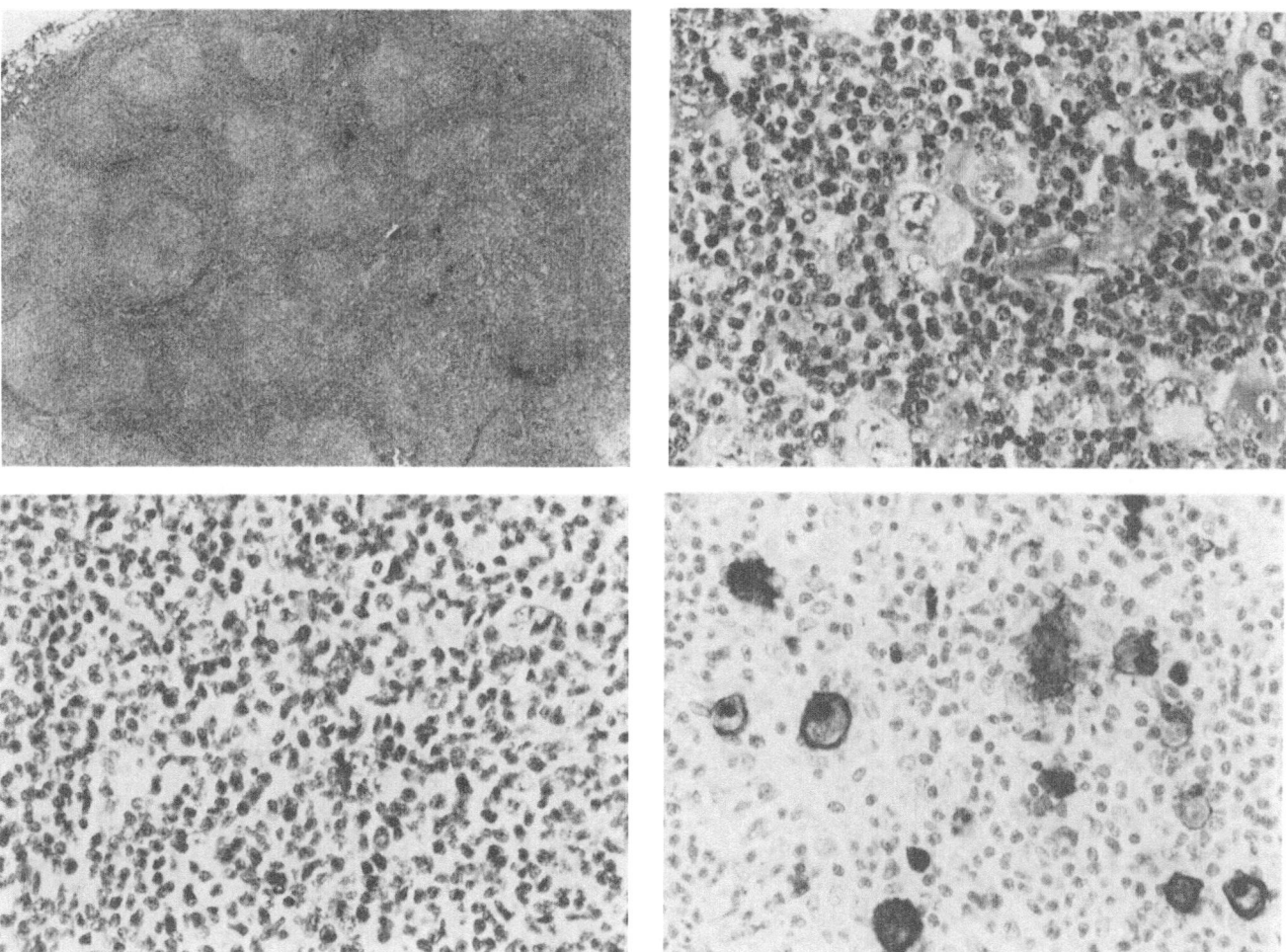

Fig. 7. Case 9175. (A; top left) Composite lymphoma showing follicular and diffuse areas (H & E × 15). (B; upper right) Detail from diffuse area showing R-S cells (H & E × 350). (C; bottom left) cytological detail from follicular area typical of CB/CC NHL (H & E × 310). (D; bottom right) diffuse area immunostained for CD15 (Dako M1) showing positive R-S cells (ABC × 310).

and Case 7375 a lymphoplasmacytoid lymphoma in the bone marrow with Waldenström's macroglobulinaemia).

Two patients had simultaneous presentation of HD and follicular lymphoma small cleaved-cell type. Case 9531 showed HD in paraortic nodes and follicular lymphoma in mesenteric nodes. Case 9175 was a true composite lymphoma with HD and NHL in different parts of both cervical and axillary nodes (Fig. 7), a pattern which was maintained in two recurrences at one and two years. One patient, Case 3399, developed a peripheral T-cell lymphoma of mixed small and large cell type in an inguinal node (Fig. 8).

Discussion

Twenty-two of 3033 patients with HD in the BNLI have developed NHL, giving an overall incidence of 0.7% which is lower than reported by other workers [1, 2, 5, 11] but is very similar to recent results from the EORTC international workshop on treatment strategy in HD where 106 of 12, 128 (0.87%) evaluable patients developed NHL [20].

Krikorian et al. [1] suggest that combined-modality

therapy for HD may be a causative factor for subsequent development of NHL as appears to be the case for acute leukaemia [21]. All their patients had presented 4–10 years previously with NS HD. However, most other reports [4, 6, 8] refer to patients with LP HD and either simultaneous or subsequent development of large-cell NHL.

The incidence in this series differs considerably with the different histological subtypes of HD. LP constitutes only 6% (182 patients) of HD in the BNLI but 7 cases of NHL arose in this group giving an incidence of secondary NHL of 3.8% in patients presenting with LP HD, or expressed in a different way, 31% of patients developing secondary NHL in this study presented with the LP histological subtype. Similar results were reported by Kim et al. [11]. Four of our patients developed large B-cell lymphoma at periods from 7 to 18 years later; this represents an incidence of B-cell lymphoma of 2% which is similar to the observations of Hansmann et al. [6] (14 of 537; 2.6%) but much lower than the series reported by Miettinen et al. [4] (5 of 51; 9.8%). The development of high-grade B-cell NHL in LP nodular HD is regarded by some as tumour progression (because of the germinal centre origin of this subtype of HD [22]) and not as a second neoplastic

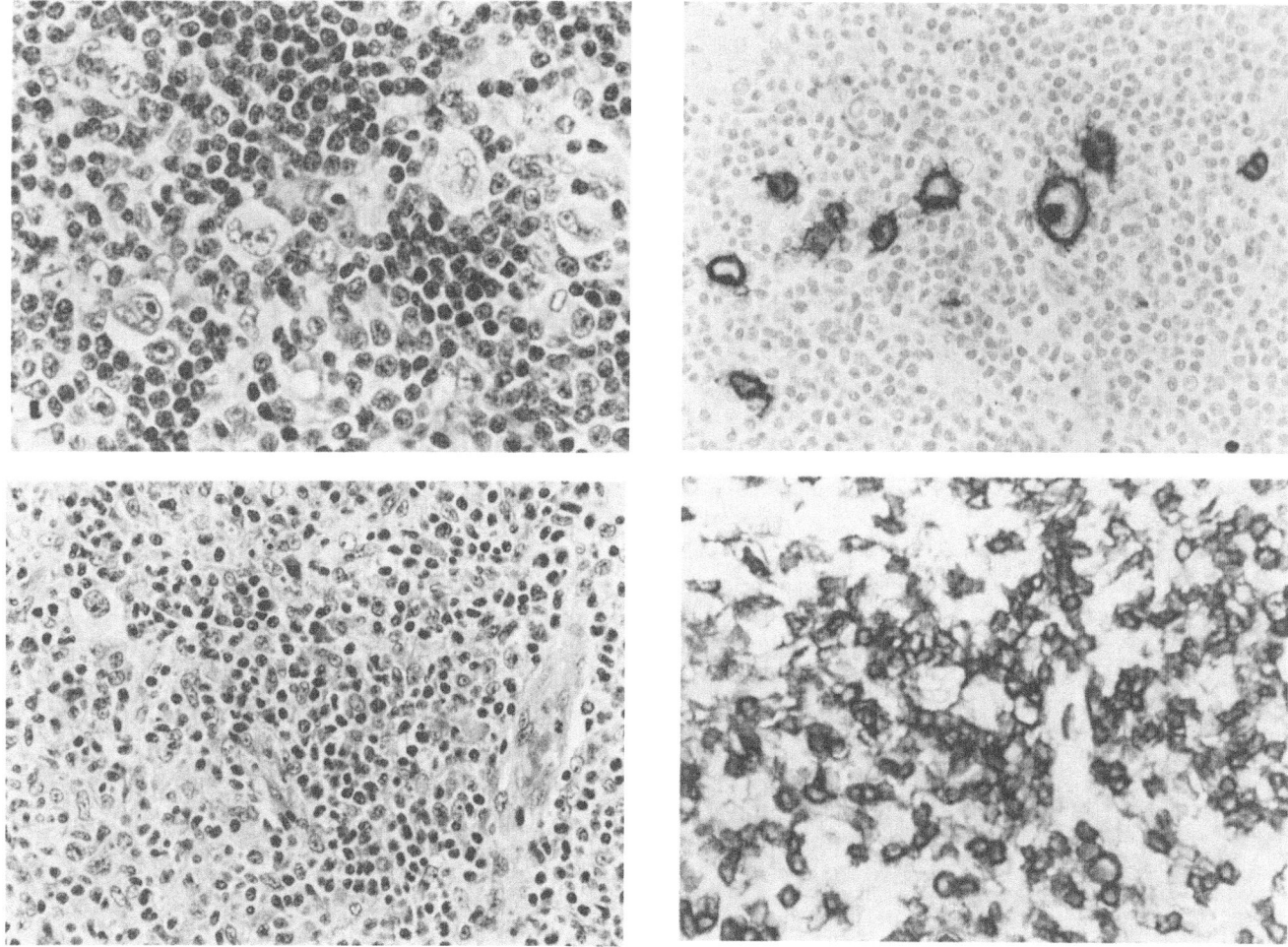

Fig. 8. Case 3399. (A; top left) biopsy of neck node showing MÇ HD with typical R-S cell (H & E × 400). (B; top right) same biopsy immunostained for CD15 (Dako M1) showing typical positive staining pattern of R-S cells (ABC × 310). (C; bottom left) biopsy of groin node eight years later showing a peripheral T-cell lymphoma of mixed small and large cell type (H & E × 250). (D; bottom right) Same biopsy immunostained for CD45 Ro (UCHL 1) showing positive staining of small, medium, and large cells (ABC × 310).

event [6]. This intriguing concept is supported by the observation of transitional states between LP nodular and large-cell NHL where the nodules of HD gradually become replaced by a predominantly large-cell population [8, 23]. It is more difficult to explain the emergence of peripheral T-cell NHL from LP nodular HD, which to our knowledge has not been previously described. Of the 3 patients subsequently developing T-cell lymphomas, 1 had received radiotherapy alone, 1 chemotherapy, and 1 RT followed by chemotherapy for early relapse. However, the NHL developed one, four, and six years after initial therapy. This is probably a rather short interval for the new disease to be therapy-induced and these may represent coincidental or composite disease. None of the 7 LP patients had B symptoms or a raised erythrocyte sedimentation rate (ESR) at presentation and in the 5 patients in whom the data were recorded, none had a low lymphocyte count.

The commonest subtype is NS which constitutes 74% of patients (2244) in the BNLI series and has the lowest incidence of subsequent NHL, 0.3% (8 patients). It is interesting to note that no patient with NS developing secondary NHL was younger than 40,

whereas the majority of patients with NS HD are between 10 and 30 years of age. Similar findings were observed by Henry-Amar in the EORTC workshop data where the relative risk of secondary NHL following HD increased in patients in their fourth and subsequent decades [20]. In the patients with NHL originally presenting with NS HD, all developed B-cell NHL. Six were high-grade large-cell type arising between 5 and 16 years after the diagnosis of HD. Of these patients, 3 had received RT alone, 2 chemotherapy alone and only one both modalities. For this one patient whose NHL developed 16 years later and who was stage IA with a normal ESR and lymphocyte count at presentation, the NHL may have been therapy related. Of the other 5 patients with high-grade NHL, 4 had B symptoms with high ESR and 3 had low presentation lymphocyte counts, perhaps indicating an impaired immune state.

Mixed cellularity forms 19% of HD cases in the BNLI (576 cases) and 7 of these patients (1.2%) developed NHL. Only 2 developed high-grade large B-cell lymphomas; one at 8 years after chemotherapy alone and one at 16 years after receiving radiotherapy following by chemotherapy for a relapse at 3 years. In this latter case the emergent NHL could be therapy related but both patients presented with B symptoms and low lymphocyte counts. One patient developed a peripheral T-cell lymphoma in the groin at eight years having presented with stage IA HD in the neck with a normal ESR and lymphocyte count. The remaining 4 patients had low-grade B-cell lymphomas, 2 being diagnosed at two years after presenting with HD and 2 being synchronous diagnoses, one having HD in paraortic nodes and follicular lymphoma in mesenteric nodes and the other being a true composite lymphoma with both HD and follicular lymphoma in different parts of the same node. These low-grade NHLs must therefore represent coincidental or composite disease and cannot be treatment related.

The majority of the secondary NHLs reported in this study were high-grade (77%; 17 of 22) and many presented at extranodal sites (9 of 22). These features are also seen in patients with immunodefficiency states [24] and in many of the patients who have developed secondary NHL in this series there was evidence of systemic disturbance [25] and immunodefficiency at the time of their presentation with HD. Notable exceptions to this were patients with LP nodular HD, none of whom showed systemic disturbance.

There appears to be little correlation between the original histological subtype of HD and the subsequent NHL save that no low-grade NHLs developed in the LP subgroup. B-cell lymphoma was the commonest (12 high-grade and 6-low grade), but 4 high-grade immunohistochemically proven T-cell lymphomas were also found (3 in LP and 1 in MC).

Conclusions

Patients with LP HD have the highest risk of developing NHL. This supports previous suggestions that the large B-cell lymphomas arising in patients with LP HD represent histological progression of disease and are not treatment related.

Combined-modality therapy for HD is known to be associated with an increased risk of subsequent acute leukaemia, but in this series only 3 patients of 24 received both RT and chemotherapy and this cannot therefore have been a major causative factor for the subsequent NHL.

All of the low-grade B-cell lymphomas occurred within three years of the onset of HD and the T-cell lymphomas at one, four, and six years, and it is therefore most unlikely that the treatment for HD played a part in their causation.

The results therefore suggest that these patients have a propensity to develop lymphoproliferative disease. This could possibly be related to the prolonged immunodeficiency associated with HD, and in support of this it is interesting to note that 10 patients had B symptoms and 7 had low lymphocyte counts at presentation. However, none of the LP HD cases had B symptoms or

low presentation lymphocyte counts, yet they developed similar secondary NHL at similar time intervals to the other types of HD. It could in some cases merely be the chance occurrence of two different lymphoproliferative diseases.

Whatever the relationship, if any, between treatment and development of NHL in HD patients, we would stress how important it is to perform biopsies in recurrent disease whenever possible, since the treatment required will be different if NHL is diagnosed. Furthermore if biopsy of recurrent disease were routine, more cases of NHL arising in patients treated for HD might come to light.

Acknowledgements

We would like to acknowledge the enthusiastic support of the many clinicians who collaborate in the studies of the BNLI and enter patients into the clinical trials. We are also grateful to the many pathologists who have generously provided pathological material. Financial support for the BNLI is provided by the Cancer Research Campaign, Cooperative Clinical Cancer Therapy Trust Fund, the Isle of Man Anti-Cancer Association, the Lisa Lear fund, the Jean Shanks Foundation and many friends and well-wishers. We are grateful to Miss Sonia Noble, Mrs Angela O'Halloran and Mrs Frances Daley for expert technical assistance.

References

1. Krikorian JG, Burke JS, Rosenberg SA, Kaplan HS. Occurrence of non-Hodgkin's lymphoma after therapy for Hodgkin's disease. N Engl J Med 1979; 300: 452–8.
2. Armitage JO, Dick FR, Goeken JA, Foucar K, Gingrich RD. Second lymphoid malignant neoplasms occurring in patients treated for Hodgkin's disease. Arch Internal Med 1983; 143: 445–50.
3. Jacquillat C, Khayat D, Desprey-Curely JP et al. Non-Hodgkin's lymphoma occurring after Hodgkin's disease. Cancer 1984; 53: 459–62.
4. Miettinen M, Franssila KO, Saxen E. Hodgkin's disease, lymphocytic predominance nodular increased risk for subsequent non-Hodgkin's lymphoma.Cancer 1983; 51: 2293–300.
5. Zarrabi MH, Rosner F. Second neoplasms in Hodgkin's disease: Current controversies. Haematol./Oncol. Clinics of North America 1989; 3: 303–18.
6. Hansmann M-L, Stein H, Fellbaum C et al. Nodular paragranuloma can transform into high-grade malignant lymphoma of B type. Hum Pathol 1989; 20: 1169–75.
6a. Karp SJ, Bennett MH. Non-Hodgkin's lymphoma following radiotherapy for Hodgkin's disease. Clinical Radiology 1986; 37: 479–481.
7. Kim H, Hendrickson MR, Dorfman RF. Composite Lymphoma. Cancer 1977; 40: 959–76.
8. Sundeen JT, Cossman J, Jaffe ES. Lymphocyte predominant Hodgkin's disease with coexistent 'large cell lymphoma': Histological progression or composite malignancy? Am J Surg Pathol 1988; 12: 599–606.
8a. Hansmann ML, Fellbaum CM, Hui PK, Lennert K. Morphological and immunohistochemical investigation of non-Hodgkin's lymphoma combined with Hodgkin's disease. Histopathology 1989; 15: 35–48.

9. Lowenthal RM, Harlow RWH, Mead AE, Tuck D, Challis DR. T-cell non-Hodgkin's lymphoma after radiotherapy and chemotherapy for Hodgkin's disease. Cancer 1981; 48: 1586–9.

10. Bouchiex C, Zittoun R, Reynes M, Diebold J, Bernadou A, Bilski-Pasquier G. A typical T-cell leukaemia terminating Hodgkin's disease. Cancer 1979; 44: 1403–7.

11. Kim H, Zelman RJ, Fox MA et al. Pathology panel for lymphoma clinical studies: A comprehensive analysis of cases accumulated since its inception. JNCI 1982; 68: 43–67.

12. Caya JG, Choi H, Tieu TM, Wollenberg NJ, Almagro UA. Hodgkin's disease followed by mycosis fungoides in the same patient. Cancer 1984; 53: 463–7.

13. Jelliffe AM, Vaughan Hudson G. The evolution of the British National Lymphoma Investigation. Clinical Radiology 1981; 32: 483–90.

14. Hsu SM, Raine L, Fanger H. Use of avidin-biotin-peroxidase complex (ABC) in immunoperoxidase techniques: a comparison between ABC and unlabeled antibody (PAP) procedures. J Histochem Cytochem 1981; 29: 577–80.

15. Ishii Y, Takami T, Yuasa H, Takei T, Kikuchi K. Two distinct antigen systems in human B lymphocytes: identification of cell surface and intracellular antigens using monoclonal antibodies. Clin Exp Immunol 1984; 58: 183–92.

16. Norton AJ, Ramsay AD, Smith SH, Beverly PCL, Isaacson PG. Monoclonal antibody (UCHL1) that recognises normal and neoplastic T cells in routinely fixed tissues. J Clin Path 1986; 39: 399–405.

17. Hall PA, D'Ardenne AJ. Value of CD 15 immunostaining in diagnosing Hodgkin's disease: a review of published literature. J Clin Pathol 1987; 40: 1298–304.

18. Ramsey AD, Smith WJ, Isaacson PG. T-cell-rich-Bcell lymphoma. Am J Surg Pathol 1988; 12: 433–43.

19. Ng CS, Chan JKC, Hui PK, Lau WH. Large B-cell lymphomas with a high content of reactive T cells. Hum Pathol 1989; 20: 1145–54.

20. Henry-Amar M. Second Malignancies in Hodgkin's disease. In: Treatment strategy in Hodgkin's disease, EORTC symposium. Sommers R, Henry-Amar M, Meerwaldt JH, Carde P (eds), 1990; John Libbey, London, Paris.

21. Colman M, Selby P. Second malignancies and Hodgkin's disease. In: Hodgkin's Disease. Selby P, Mcelwain TJ 1987; Blackwell Scientific Publications, Oxford. Chapter 14: 361–77.

22. Tiemens W, Visser L, Poppema S (1986): Nodular lymphocyte predominance type of Hodgkin's disease is a germinal centre lymphoma. Lab Invest 1989; 54: 457–61.

23. Banks PM, Lust JA, Thibodeau SN. Nodular lymphocyte predominance Hodgkin's disease (NLPHD) and its transition to large cell lymphoma (LCL): Immunophenotypic and genetic probe analysis. Lab Invest 1989; 60: 5A (28).

24. Riggs S, Hagemeister FB. Immunodeficiency states: A predisposition to lymphoma. In Hodgkin's disease and Non-Hodgkin's lymphoma in adults and children. LM Fuller et al. (eds); Raven Press, New York, pp 451–78.

25. Vaughan Hudson B, MacLennan KA, Bennett MH, Easterling MJ, Vaughan Hudson G, Jelliffe AM. Systemic disturbance in Hodgkin's disease and its relation to histopathology and prognosis. Clinical Radiology 1987; 38: 257–261.

Correspondence to:
Dr. K. A. MacLennan
Dept of Histopathology
The Royal Marsden Hospital
Fulham Rd, London SW 3 6 JJ, UK

Annals of Oncology, Supplement 2 to Volume 2: 93–97, 1991.
© 1991 *Kluwer Academic Publishers*.

Original article _____

Direct sequence analysis of 14_{q+} and 18_{q-} chromosome junctions at the MBR and MCR revealing clustering within the MBR in follicular lymphoma

F. E. Cotter,[1] C. Price,[1] J. Meerabux, E. Zucca[2] & B. D. Young[1]

[1] *ICRF Department of Medical Oncology, St Bartholomew's Hospital, London EC1A 7BE, England;* [2] *Division of Oncology, Ospedale San Giovanni, 6500 Bellinzona, Switzerland*

Summary. The t(14;18) translocation is a highly consistent feature of follicular lymphoma although the underlying mechanism generating this fusion remains uncertain. The breakpoints on chromosome 18 are at one of two sites, designated mbr and mcr, in the *bcl-2* gene. A polymerase chain reaction strategy has been developed for amplification and direct sequencing of the resultant 14_{q+} and 18_{q-} reciprocal junctions. Sequence analysis of the amplified 14_{q+} junction established that 21 tumours contained a *bcl-2* (mbr) sequence to an immunoglobulin J_H region, the majority being J_5 or J_6. A nonrandom pattern of breakpoints within the mbr region was found. Clustering of the breakpoint occurred with over 60% of the translocations clustering within 10 bases. There was a second cluster within the mbr 50 bases 3′ of the first cluster. One of these junctions had an unusual configuration with the *bcl-2* and J_H sequences separated by a recognisable D_H region. This suggests that at least some of the junctional sequences, previously thought of as N insertions, may be fragments of unrecognised D_H regions. In one of these tumours it was possible to sequence the reciprocal 18_{q-} junction, showing it to consist of a D_H/*bcl-2* (mbr) fusion. Analysis of both reciprocal junctions for a translocation in the mcr region of *bcl-2*, showed that this 18_{q-} junction also consisted of D_H fused to a *bcl-2* sequence. In contrast to previous analyses, which demonstrated either loss or duplication of *bcl-2* sequences at the breakpoints, the *bcl-2* sequence was conserved during the mbr and mcr translocations in this study. Although the precise mechanism of the t(14;18) translocation remains unclear, these data demonstrate that breakpoints are nonrandomly distributed within the mbr.

Introduction

Approximately 85% of follicular lymphomas and 30% of diffuse large-cell lymphomas carry the t(14;18)(q32.3;q21.3) chromosomal translocation by cytogenetic and molecular techniques [1, 2]. The breakpoints on chromosome 18 occur within or near a transcriptional unit called the *bcl-2* gene [2–6] with approximately 60% of the breakpoints clustering over 150 base pairs in a 3′ untranslated region of the *bcl-2* gene [2, 7], known as the 'major breakpoint region' (mbr). A further 25% have breakpoints at a site 20 kb 3′ to the mbr sequence in a region called the 'minor cluster region' (mcr) [2]. All the mcr breakpoints occur within 500 base pairs of each other, and some tighter clustering to within 3 base pairs has been reported [8]. On chromosome 14, the breakpoints occur in the joining (J_H) region of the immunoglobulin heavy chain gene [4, 5, 6]. The translocation is postulated to result from an error during VDJ joining [7, 8, 9]. The 14_{q+} derivative chromosome at the breakpoint junction has short segments of unidentifiable nucleotides thought to represent 'N' insertions normally found at the VD and DJ junctions following IgH rearrangement [7, 9]. Fewer 18_{q-} derivative chromosome breakpoints have been studied [7, 10], but predominantly immunoglobulin heavy chain diversity regions (D_H) are joined to the *bcl-2* gene with loss of the 5′ J_H region suggesting a de-

letion between D_H and J_H in t(14;18) translocation in lymphomas [7]. The translocation results in a hybrid *bcl-2*/IgH transcript but a normal *bcl-2* protein due to the structurally unaltered coding region. There is a deregulation of *bcl-2* protein production resulting in its increased expression within the cells containing the t(14;18) translocation [11, 12].

The clustering of the majority of breakpoints on *bcl-2* facilitates the use of the polymerase chain reaction (PCR) for amplification and analysis of the t(14;18) breakpoints. *Bcl-2* oligonucleotide primers (either mbr [13] or mcr [8]) flanking the translocation have been used, with a consensus J_H sequence found at the 3′ end of each J_H exon, to amplify the 14_{q+} junctions. This approach has been extended to the 18_{q-} junctions using a primer based on part of the recombination signal sequences known to flank germ line D_H sequences. It was possible to sequence junctions produced by translocations in either the mbr or mcr regions in a series of follicular lymphomas and to determine if further subclustering occurs with the mbr.

Methods

Enzymatic amplification

DNA was extracted as previously described [14] from

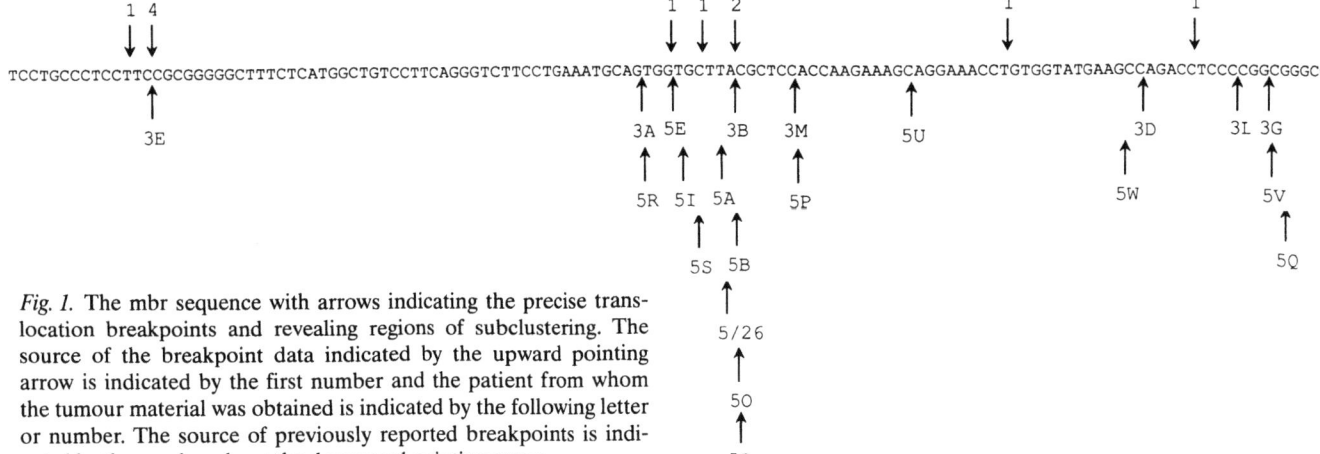

Fig. 1. The mbr sequence with arrows indicating the precise translocation breakpoints and revealing regions of subclustering. The source of the breakpoint data indicated by the upward pointing arrow is indicated by the first number and the patient from whom the tumour material was obtained is indicated by the following letter or number. The source of previously reported breakpoints is indicated by the number above the downward pointing arrow.

patients with histologically proven centroblastic/centrocytic follicular lymphoma. Enzymatic amplification was carried out by the PCR [15] using an automated Perkin-Elmer DNA Thermal Cycler. The final reaction volume included 1 μg of tumour DNA, oligonucleotide primers (1 mM), 1.5 units of Taq DNA polymerase (Amplitaq-Cetus), gelatin (0.01% w/v) in 100 μL of Taq buffer (50 mM KC1, 10 μM tris-C1 pH8.3, 1.5 mM MgCl$_2$). Amplification of the mbr-J$_H$ and mcr-J$_H$ junctions on chromosome 14$_{q+}$ was performed with primers previously described [8, 16]. The D$_H$-mbr and D$_H$-mcr junctions on chromosome 18$_{q-}$ were amplified with primers DH1 (5'-GTGAGGTCTGTGT*CACTGTG*-3')-BC2 (5'-ATATTCCATATTCATCACTTTGAG-3') and DH1-BC6 (5'-TTATTGAGTGGTCCTTCCTTTC-3') respectively. Thirty cycles of amplification were performed as previously described and analysed by electrophoresis in a 2% agarose gel stained with ethidium bromide.

Direct sequence analysis

Direct nucleotide sequence analysis by the dideoxy chain termination method [17] was carried out on PCR products. DNA from the reaction mixture was purified using a Sephadex G50 column followed by ethanol precipitation, freeze-drying and resuspension in distilled water. Sequencing was carried out using *bcl-2* internal oligonucleotides as sequencing primers with the modified T7 DNA polymerase (Sequenase), a five-minute labelling reaction at 15 °C and a five-minute termination reaction at 37 °C. The mbr-J$_H$ junctions were sequenced with kinase-labelled aliquots of primer BC3 (5'-CACAGACCCACCCAGAGCCC-3') and the D$_H$-mbr junctions with primer BC4 (5'-GTCTGATCA TTCTGTTCCCTG-3'), the mcr-J$_H$ junctions with BC7 (5'-TCAGTCTCTGGGGAGGAGTGG-3'), and the D$_H$-mcr junctions with BC8 (5'-TCATTTCAGTTGAGTG CTGTG-3').

Results

Analysis of mbr junctions in bcl-2

Enzymatic amplification using primers for the mbr-J$_H$ junction was performed on each DNA sample and electrophoresis revealed specific products from 21 samples (data not shown). Under the conditions of amplification, normal human DNA yielded no fragments. Direct sequence analysis using primer BC3 revealed the structure of these products and the precise breakpoint on *bcl-2* at the mbr is summarised in Figure 1. The most striking feature of the mbr breakpoint sequence analysis is the subclustering within the mbr region, over 60% of the breakpoints occurring on or within 10 bases of base 70 and possibly a further subclusters 50 bases 3' of the first cluster. The full sequence across the translocation breakpoint for seven cases is shown in Figure 2 demonstrating a fusion between a *bcl-2* sequence and members of the immunoglobulin heavy chain joining region exons (J$_H$), confirming the presence of the t(14;18) translocation in these tumours. The breakpoint on *bcl-2* fell within the range of previously determined [7] breaks in the mbr region. There was a clear preponderance (5 of 7) for the J$_6$ member of the J$_H$ family. Most of the J$_H$ sequences had some single base differences when compared with their germ line equivalents. This could be due to either polymorphic variation or somatic mutation which is known to occur during D-J recombination. In contrast the *bcl-2* sequence showed no evidence of mutation. In every junction there was an intervening sequence between *bcl-2* and J$_H$, although in Patient D this consisted of only a single base. In Patient E there was a particularly large intervening sequence which, on further analysis, was found to contain a recognisable D$_H$ region (Fig. 2). The D$_H$ (diversity) regions recombine with J$_H$ in normal Ig gene rearrangement and thus this junction (*bcl-2*-D$_H$-J$_H$) could result from translocation after D$_H$-J$_H$ recombination. Thus this junction consisted of *bcl-2* fused to D$_H$ which in

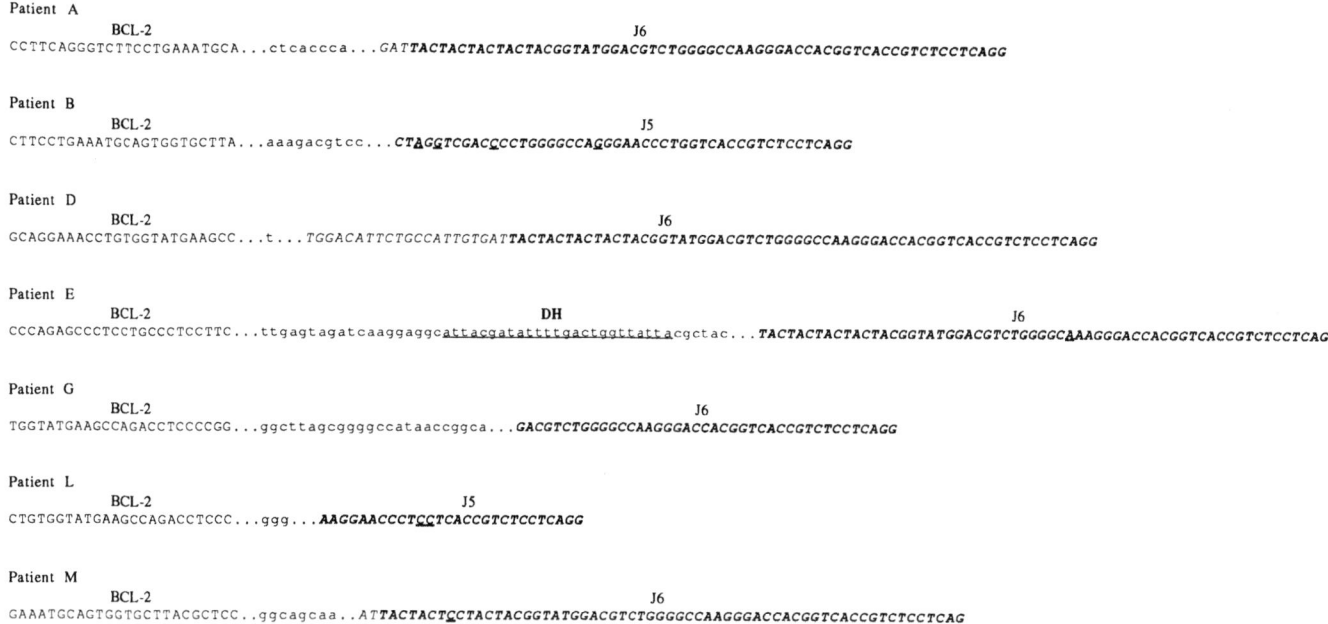

Patient A
```
        BCL-2                                                    J6
CCTTCAGGGTCTTCCTGAAATGCA...ctcaccca...GATTACTACTACTACTACGGTATGGACGTCTGGGGCCAAGGGACCACGGTCACCGTCTCCTCAGG
```

Patient B
```
        BCL-2                                                    J5
CTTCCTGAAATGCAGTGGTGCTTA...aaagacgtcc...CTAGGTCGACCCCTGGGGCCAGGGAACCCTGGTCACCGTCTCCTCAGG
```

Patient D
```
        BCL-2                                                    J6
GCAGGAAACCTGTGGTATGAAGCC...t...TGGACATTCTGCCATTGTGATTACTACTACTACTACGGTATGGACGTCTGGGGCCAAGGGACCACGGTCACCGTCTCCTCAGG
```

Patient E
```
        BCL-2                              DH                                            J6
CCCAGAGCCCTCCTGCCCTCCTTC...ttgagtagatcaaggaggcattacgatattttgactggttattacgctac...TACTACTACTACTACGGTATGGACGTCTGGGGCAAAGGGACCACGGTCACCGTCTCCTCAGG
```

Patient G
```
        BCL-2                                                    J6
TGGTATGAAGCCAGACCTCCCCGG...ggcttagcggggccataaccggca...GACGTCTGGGGCCAAGGGACCACGGTCACCGTCTCCTCAGG
```

Patient L
```
        BCL-2                         J5
CTGTGGTATGAAGCCAGACCTCCC...ggg...AAGGAACCCTCCTCACCGTCTCCTCAGG
```

Patient M
```
        BCL-2                                                    J6
GAAATGCAGTGGTGCTTACGCTCC..ggcagcaa..ATTACTACTCCTACTACGGTATGGACGTCTGGGGCCAAGGGACCACGGTCACCGTCTCCTCAG
```

Fig. 2. Sequences of the chromosome 14q+ junctions in 7 follicular lymphomas. *Bcl*-2 sequence is shown in upper case and joining region sequence is in upper case italics with the coding exons in bold type. Differences between the J_H sequences and their germ-line equivalents are underlined. The intervening sequences between *bcl*-2 and J_H are indicated in lower case. The part of the intervening sequence which is identical to a previously identified D_H region is underlined (Patient E).

turn was fused to J_6. None of the other intervening sequences had significant homology to each other or to any other known D_H or putative N insertion sequences.

The primer DH1 in combination with the *bcl*-2 primer BC2, was used for amplification of the reciprocal junctions on chromosome 18q-. In Patient B, direct sequencing revealed the structure of the 18q- junction in which a putative D_H region is fused to the mbr region of *bcl*-2, and has been compared with the 14q+ and normal chromosome 18 sequence in the same tumour in Figure 3a. It is clear that, during breakage and rejoining, the *bcl*-2 gene has been conserved without any of the short duplications or deletions noted by others [7, 10].

Analysis of mcr junctions in bcl-2

A similar analysis was performed using oligonucleotide primers for the mcr region of *bcl*-2. It was possible to sequence both 14q+ and 18q- junction and the results for one of the patients are shown in Figure 3b. The 14q+ junction is similar to those reported by others [8] with mcr sequence fused to a member of the J_H family. There is very little sequence which could be called an N-insertion and the breakpoint in mcr is precisely at a position which has been broken in two previously analysed tumours [8]. The sequence of the reciprocal 18q- junction is also shown in Figure 3b and as in Figure 3a there has been no net loss or gain of *bcl*-2 sequence.

3(a)

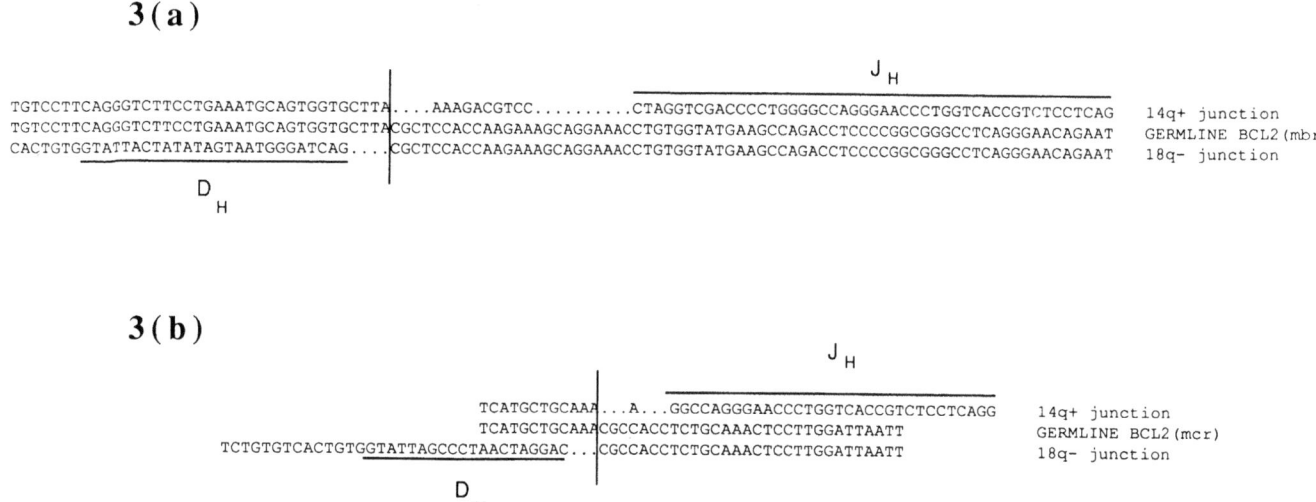

```
                                                                    J H
TGTCCTTCAGGGTCTTCCTGAAATGCAGTGGTGCTTA....AAAGACGTCC.........CTAGGTCGACCCCTGGGGCCAGGGAACCCTGGTCACCGTCTCCTCAG   14q+ junction
TGTCCTTCAGGGTCTTCCTGAAATGCAGTGGTGCTTACGCTCCACCAAGAAAGCAGGAAACCTGTGGTATGAAGCCAGACCTCCCCGGCGGGCCTCAGGGAACAGAAT   GERMLINE BCL2(mbr)
CACTGTGGTATTACTATATAGTAATGGGATCAG....CGCTCCACCAAGAAAGCAGGAAACCTGTGGTATGAAGCCAGACCTCCCCGGCGGGCCTCAGGGAACAGAAT   18q- junction
                    D
                     H
```

3(b)

```
                                        J H
                        TCATGCTGCAAA...A...GGCCAGGGAACCCTGGTCACCGTCTCCTCAGG   14q+ junction
                        TCATGCTGCAAACGCCACCTCTGCAAACTCCTTGGATTAATT               GERMLINE BCL2(mcr)
            TCTGTGTCACTGTGGTATTAGCCCTAACTAGGAC..CGCCACCTCTGCAAACTCCTTGGATTAATT  18q- junction
                    D
                     H
```

Fig. 3. The sequences of the reciprocal 14q+ and 18q- junctions for breakpoints at the mbr (a), patient B, and the mcr (b) [16].

96

Furthermore, as with mbr translocations, this function is composed of a D_H sequence fused to *bcl-2*.

Discussion

The use of the D_H-based primer (DH1) offers a means to amplify and analyse rapidly a proportion of the 18_{q-} junctions. As a means of detecting the presence of the $t(14;18)$ it appears to be less efficient than the equivalent strategy for the 14_{q+} junctions [16]. Although the proportion of tumours in which the 18_{q-} junctions can be successfully amplified are fewer, it is possible that other strategies, such as the use of a V_H consensus primer [18], might be successful.

Previous studies have shown that the 14_{q+} junctions are often characterised by short stretches of unrecognisable sequences, which because of their position adjacent to a joining region, have been thought of as N-insertions. There are, however, several features of these sequences which question this interpretation. Firstly, these translocation N-regions tend to be longer than normal N-region sequences, which rarely exceed 10 bases and are usually shorter [19]. Secondly, the normal N-regions are GC-rich whereas translocation N-regions are less so [19]. Finally, Ngan et al. [8] noted that two different tumours had an identical stretch of 11 bases in their putative N-regions and speculated that such regions could be derived instead from previously unrecognised D_H sequences. The tumour from patient E (Fig. 2) has been shown to contain a complete D_H sequence within its putative N-region. This finding supports the idea that at least some of the putative N-regions could contain fragments of D_H regions. Interestingly, this D_H sequence is identical to one previously shown to be located 150 bases 5' to a D_H involved in a follicular lymphoma translocation [7]. Comparison with this sequence indicates that the germ line recombination signals are missing from the 5' end of the D_H sequence (Fig. 2), suggesting that either the translocation has occurred as a mistake in VD joining with a subsequent N-insertion or that VDJ recombination had taken place prior to translocation. The former explanation has been invoked to explain a translocation in the Daudi Burkitt lymphoma cell line as a mistake in VD joining with the DJ already rearranged [20]. The latter course of events has been proposed [21] to account for a $t(8;22)$ translocation in Burkitt's lymphoma in which the Ig lambda light chain complex was thought to be rearranged before translocation.

The underlying mechanism which generates the $t(14;18)$ translocation has been the subject of some debate. It has been suggested that the translocation occurs as a result of mistakes in VDJ recombination. This is based on the presence of sequences on chromosome 18, close to some breakpoints, which bear a similarity to the heptamer-nonamer signal sequences mediating VDJ recombination [9]. The homology, however, is weak and breakpoints are not always associated with such sequences. Also if this mechanism were operative the reciprocal set of recognition signals with a 23-base pair spacer would be expected within mbr and these have not been found [7]. An alternative explanation for the breakage of *bcl-2* has been proposed which does not depend on the presence of heptamer-nonamer signal sequences. Bakhshi et al. [7] analysed the reciprocal junctions of a follicular lymphoma and noted a 3-base pair duplication at the junction. It was proposed that this could be the result of a staggered double-stranded break of the type known to result in direct repeats flanking the insertion of foreign DNA. However, subsequent analysis of two tumours [10] has revealed small deletions, rather than duplications, of *bcl-2* sequence at junctions. Moreover, in our study both tumours analysed showed conservation of *bcl-2* sequence and therefore the duplication of junctional *bcl-2* sequence is not a general feature of the $t(14;18)$ translocation.

Interestingly, the breakpoint in mbr on chromosome 18 for Patient B is at a location identical to that found in a tumour analysed by Tsujimoto et al. [10] in which a deletion of 2 base pairs had occurred. This effectively rules out the possibility that the gain or loss of *bcl-2* sequence is, in some way, dependent on the position of the breakpoint. The analysis of the reciprocal junctions for the translocation in mcr (Fig. 3b) revealed a similar structure to that found in mbr breakpoints. In particular, the fusion of a D_H to mcr sequence forming the 18_{q-} junction has the same configuration as that found in mbr translocations. This suggests that similar mechanisms are involved in mcr translocations. This breakpoint lies at exactly the position of two previously analysed breaks in mcr [8] which themselves were part of a tight cluster of 5 breaks within 4 bases of each other. An interesting feature of this cluster is that it is bounded by two direct repeats [CTGCAAAC] 7 bases apart. It is of considerable interest that two similar tight clusterings of breakpoints are revealed at the mbr in the translocations analysed. Although the underlying mechanism for the $t(14;18)$ translocation in follicular lymphoma remains unclear, similar factors appear to operate for breaks in both the mbr and mcr regions, and the breakpoints appear to take place at definite sites within these regions in a nonrandom manner. This suggests that the sequence of the *bcl-2* gene may have an important role in the mechanism of the $t(14;18)$ translocation. In addition our sequence data suggest that, at least in some cases, it is possible that translocation has taken place after DJ rearrangement.

Acknowledgements

The authors gratefully acknowledge the synthesis of oligonucleotides by I. Goldsmith and the clinical support of T. A. Lister and A. Z. Rohatiner. Some of the data have been previously published.

References

1. Yunis JJ, Oken MM, Kaplan ME, Ensrud KM, Howe RR, Theologides A. Distinctive chromosomal abnormalities in histologic subtypes of non-Hodgkin's lymphomas. N Engl J Med 1982; 307: 1231–3.

2. Weiss LM, Warnke RA, Sklar J, Cleary ML. Molecular analysis of the t(14;18) chromosomal translocation in malignant lymphomas. N Engl J Med 1987; 317: 1185–9.

3. Cleary ML, Sklar J. Nucleotide sequence of a t(14;18) chromosomal translocation breakpoint in follicular lymphoma and demonstration of a breakpoint cluster region near a transcriptionally active locus on chromosome 18. Proc Natl Acad Sci USA 1985; 82: 7439–43.

4. Cleary ML, Galili N, Sklar J. Detection of a second t(14;18) breakpoint cluster region in follicular lymphomas. J Exp Med 1986; 164: 315–20.

5. Bakhshi A, Jensen JP, Goldman P, Wright JJ, McBride OW, Epstein AL, Korsmeyer SJ. Cloning the chromosome breakpoint of t(14;18) human lymphomas: Clustering around J_H on chromosome 14 and near a transcriptional unit on 18. Cell 1985; 41: 899–904.

6. Tsujimoto Y, Cossman J, Jaffe E, Croce CM. Involvement of the *bcl*-2 gene in human follicular lymphomas. Science 1985; 228: 1449–3.

7. Bakhshi A, Wright JJ, Graninger W, Seto M, Owens J, Cossman J, Jensen JP, Goldman P, Korsmeyer SJ. Mechanism of the t(14;18) chromosomal translocation: Structural analysis of both derivative 14 and 18 reciprocal partners. Proc Natl Acad Sci USA 1987; 84: 2396–400.

8. Ngan B-Y, Nourse J, Cleary ML. Detection of chromosomal translocation t(14;18) within the minor cluster region of *bcl*-2 by polymerase chain reaction and direct genomic sequencing of the enzymatically amplified DNA in follicular lymphomas. Blood 1989; 73: 1759–62.

9. Tsujimoto Y, Gorham J, Cossman J, Jaffe E, Croce CM. The t(14;18) chromosome translocations involved in B-cell neoplasms result from mistakes in VDJ joining. Science 1985; 229: 1390–3.

10. Tsujimoto Y, Louie E, Bashir MM, Croce CM. The reciprocal partners of both the t(14;18) and t(11;14) translocations involved in B-cell neoplasms are rearranged by the same mechanism. Oncogene 1988; 2: 347–51.

11. Cleary ML, Smith SD, Sklar J. Cloning and structural analysis of cDNAs for *bcl*-2 and a hybrid *bcl*-2/immunoglobulin transcript resulting from the t(14;18) translocation. Cell 1986; 47: 19–28.

12. Ngan BY, Chen-Levy Z, Weiss LM, Warnke RA, Cleary ML. Expression in non-Hodgkin's lymphoma of the *bcl*-2 protein associated with the t(14;18) chromosomal translocation. N. Engl J Med 1988; 318: 1638–44.

13. Lee M-A, Chang K-S, Cabanillas F, Freireich EJ, Trujillo JM, Stass SA. Detection of minimal residual cells carrying the t(14;18) by DNA sequence amplification. Science 1987; 237: 175–8.

14. Cotter FE, Hall PA, Young BD. Extraction of DNA from small sections of frozen tissue with simultaneous histological examination. J Clin Pathol 1988; 41: 1125–7.

15. Saiki RK, Gelfand DH, Stoffel S, Scharf SJ, Higuchi R, Horn G, Mullis KB and Erlich HA. Primer-directed enzymatic amplification of DNA with a thermostable DNA polymerase. Science 1988; 239: 487–91.

16. Cotter FE, Price C, Zucca E and Young BD. Direct sequence analysis of the 14_{q+} and 18_{q-} chromosome junctions in follicular lymphoma. Blood 1990; 76: 131–35.

17. Sanger F, Nicklen S, Coulson AR. DNA sequencing with chain-terminating inhibitors. Proc Natl Acad Sci USA 1977; 74: 5463–6.

18. Ward ES, Gussow D, Griffiths AD, Jones PT, Winter G. Binding activities of a repertoire of single immunoglobulin variable domains secreted from E Coli. Nature 1989; 341: 544–6.

19. Roth DB, Chang X-B, Wilson JH. Comparison of filter DNA at immune, nonimmune and oncogenic rearrangements suggests multiple mechanisms of formation. Mol Cell Biol 1989; 9: 3049–57.

20. Haluska FG, Tsujimoto Y, Croce CM. The t(14;18) chromosome translocation of the Burkitt lymphoma cell line Daudi occurred during immunoglobulin gene rearrangement and involved the heavy chain diversity region. Proc Natl Acad Sci USA 1987; 84: 6835–9.

21. Showe LC, Moore RCA, Erikson J, Croce CM. MYC oncogene involved in a t(8;22) chromosome translocation is not altered in its putative regulatory regions. Proc Natl Acad Sci USA 1987; 84: 2824–8.

Correspondence to:
Finbarr E Cotter
ICRF Dept. of Medical Oncology
St. Bartholomew's Hospital
London EC1A 7BE
England

Annals of Oncology, Supplement 2 to Volume 2: 99–105, 1991.
© 1991 Kluwer Academic Publishers.

Original article ————————————————————

The significance of B-clonal excess in peripheral blood in patients with non-Hodgkin's lymphoma in remission

Anna Johnson,[1] Eva Cavallin-Ståhl[1] & Måns Åkerman[2]
Departments of [1]Oncology and [2]Pathology & Cytology, University Hospital of Lund, Sweden

Summary. By taking advantage of the monoclonal nature of non-Hodgkin's lymphoma (NHL) it has been possible to detect small numbers of lymphoma cells which are not evident by routine morphological methods. These new methods are based on the detection of either a restricted light chain expression – clonal excess analysis (CE) or a monoclonal rearrangement of the Ig or T-cell receptor genes. We have studied the impact on relapse and survival of CE in peripheral blood in 202 patients in remission. The patients were sampled repeatedly during follow-up in remission. Median follow-up was 55 months (range 1–180). CE was found more frequently during remission in patients with low-grade NHL 18% as compared to 8% in high-grade NHL. There was no correlation with initial stage and the occurrence of CE in remission. Survival and time to relapse did not differ in those with CE and those with a normal light chain distribution. The conclusion is that CE in remission does not herald a poor prognosis and that an isolated finding of CE in remission is not an indication to start therapy.

Introduction

With increasingly more sensitive methods to detect malignant cells in non-Hodgkin's lymphoma (NHL) it has become evident that tumour spread is much more extensive than was previously understood. These novel methods take advantage of the monoclonal nature of NHLs. By analysing either the genotypic or phenotypic expression of the immunoglobulin (Ig) or T-cell receptor genes concerning monoclonality, it is possible to detect minimal numbers of lymphoma cells in admixtures of normal lymphocytes. The monoclonal B-cell phenotype is defined by Ig light chain restriction. By studying $\kappa:\lambda$ ratio or more sophisticated $\kappa:\lambda$ distribution with flow cytometric methods, it is possible to detect a clonal excess (CE) constituting around 1–10% of the cell population [1–7]. The B-phenotypic CE method has its limitations. Varying proportions of lymphomas express too little Ig on the cell surface to be detected by this method [8], and a few are of T-cell lineage. If instead genotypic analyses of monoclonal rearrangements of Ig- and T-cell receptor genes are studied with Southern blot analyses, these problems are overcome. The sensitivity of gene rearrangement analysis is probably superior to that of CE analysis, and approximately 1–5% of lymphoma cells can be identified [9–10]. Even more powerful tools of molecular genetics such as the polymerase chain reaction (PCR) are now becoming available. Using specific translocations as markers of monoclonality, it is possible to detect one lymphoma cell among 100 000 normal ones [11–12].

A prerequisite for cure in cancer therapy is the ability of a treatment to induce complete remission. If tumour cells remain after treatment it seems logical to assume that a clinical relapse will be evident sooner or later.

In the present study we have investigated the impact of CE in peripheral blood on survival and time to relapse in NHL patients in first remission.

Patients

Two hundred two patients treated for NHL, equal numbers of males and females, were included. They were all studied after termination of therapy in first complete remission (CR). Median age at diagnosis was 63 years (range 21–91). The patients were diagnosed in 1974–1989. All patients were treated and followed in our department. After variable times the patients were referred to their local hospitals.

Diagnosis was based on a surgical specimen in all but 5 patients, where only cytologic material was available. All lymphomas were examined by one pathologist (MÅ). Histological classification was performed according to the Kiel classification from 1981 onward. Older biopsy specimens were reclassified according to Kiel. The NHLs were grouped into low-grade NHL, 46%, and high-grade NHL, 54%. Immunohistochemical analysis was used as an adjunct to routine histologic examination from 1985 onward. In the lymphomas classified as high-grade malignant, a panel of monoclonal antibodies was used either on fresh, frozen, or formalin-fixed, paraffin-embedded tissue to ascertain lymphocyte origin. Positive staining with CD45 (Dako-LC, Dakopatts, Copenhagen) confirmed the lymphoma diagnosis in 70 of 110 high-grade NHL patients, and the analysis was not performed for various reasons in the other 40 patients in this group. In the lymphomas classified as low-grade malignant, immunohistochemistry was performed only occasionally. In addition, surface Ig expression was analysed when fresh material was available for preparation of cell suspensions. A light chain restricted population was identified by flow cytometry in 33 of 48 biopsy specimens.

Staging according to the Ann Arbor system was performed using physical examination, fine-needle biopsy of suspicious sites, chest x-ray, CT scan of the abdomen, scintigraphy of the liver and spleen, bone marrow aspiration, and trephine biopsy. Biopsies from Waldeyer's ring were performed in patients with gastric lymphomas. Cerebrospinal fluid was examined in patients with high-grade NHL and bone marrow infiltration. Routine biochemical tests, haematology and a differential white blood cell count were also performed. Forty-six percent (93) of the patients presented with stage I disease, 52% (106) with stage II–IV, and 2% were not completely staged (Table 1). In stage I disease treatment consisted of involved-field irradiation to a target absorbed dose of 40–44 Gy over four to five weeks.

Table 1. Clonal excess (CE) in peripheral blood in relation to histologic grade (Kiel) and stage.

Stage Histology	I CE/n	%	II–IV CE/n	%	n.d. CE/n	All pat. CE/n	%
Low-grade NHL	8/44	18	9/48	19	–	17/92	18
High-grade NHL	3/49	6	5/58	9	1/3	9/110	8
Total	11/93	12	14/106	13	1/3	26/202	13

Abbreviations:
CE = clonal excess.
n.d. = not done.

In stage II–IV, treatment for low-grade NHL generally consisted of prednimustine or CVP (cyclophosphamide, vincristine, and prednisone) and in high-grade NHL either CHOP (cyclophosphamide, doxorubicin, vincristine, and prednisone), CHOP + methotrexate, MEV (methotrexate, cyclophosphamide, and vincristine) or, in the last three years, MACOP-B (methotrexate, doxorubicin, cyclophosphamide, vincristine, prednisone, and bleomycin). In some patients with high-grade NHL and bulky disease (>7 cm) or bone destruction, radiation therapy was added after chemotherapy.

Complete remission (CR) was determined by reevaluating initially involved sites using the staging methods described above. Survival and time to relapse were calculated from termination of therapy in CR. Survival curves were constructed according to the lifetable technique, and differences in survival between groups were tested using the generalized Wilcoxon test.

Methods

Sampling

At regular follow-up visits of NHL patients in first remission, analysis of CE in peripheral blood was performed together with routine haematology and clinical examination. A differential white blood cell count was performed routinely from 1986 onward. The majority of the patients were examined several times. The median was 4 (range 1–10) in the group with normal peripheral blood analysis, and the median was 5 (range 1–9) in the group with CE. Median time from CR to the first CE analysis was 13 months (range 1–140) in the group with normal peripheral blood analysis and 10 months (range 1–89) in the group with CE. The overall median was 12 months (range 1–140). The result of the CE analysis was not available to the responsible physician. Median follow-up was 55 months (range 1–180).

Immunofluorescence staining

Mononuclear cells were isolated from 10 ml of heparinised blood by standard gradient centrifugation and washed in Dulbecco buffer solution (Oxoid Ltd.) supplemented with 0.2% bovine serum albumin and 0.1% NaN_3 (DBA). The cells were frozen overnight in RPMI (Flow Laboratories) with 10% DMSO and 10% fetal calf serum at −70 °C and stored in liquid nitrogen until analysed. In the first five years of the study, analyses were performed fresh in a slightly modified way [7]. The cells were thawed and $0.5–1 \times 10^6$ cells per well were spun down on a microtitre plate. The pellets were incubated with FITC-conjugated polyclonal F(ab')₂ fragments of rabbit anti-human κ and λ (Kallestad Lab Inc 1981–86, Dakopatt 1986–) and FITC-conjugated mouse monoclonal antibodies directed against CD3 and CD19 (Dakopatt). The incubation was performed at saturating conditions at room temperature for 5–15 minutes, and the cells were then washed three times in DBA before the CE analysis.

CE analysis

The fluorescence analysis was performed as described previously [7]. Briefly, a flow cytometer (Ortho System 50-H) was used, and the signals were processed by a data handling system (2140, Data General MP 200). Excitation was performed with an Argonion laser at 488 nm (200 mW), and the emission was measured in a 515–555 nm filter combination. The lymphocyte population was identified by axial light extinction and right-angle scatter. The relative amount of κ and λ per cell was measured in approximately 20×10^3 cells. The κ and λ distributions were visually compared. An unequivocal incongruence between the two distributions was interpreted as a clonal excess (CE) denoting either clonal κ- or λ-bearing cells, i.e. lymphoma cells [1, 2].

was considered to have circulating lymphoma cells if at least one CE analysis in follow-up was distinctly abnormal.

Results

Correlation with pretreatment characteristics

Histology
During a median observation time in remission of 55 months (range 1–180), CE was observed in 13% (26 of 202) of the patients. In low-grade NHL the figures were 18% (17 of 92) and in high-grade NHL 8% (9 of 110) (Table 1). The difference is significant (P = 0.049).

Lymphocytic/immunocytic (lc/ic) lymphomas showed the highest incidence of CE, 32% (6/19) in CR. In the follicular center cell (FCC) lymphomas of centroblastic-centrocytic (cb-cc) type, the incidence of CE was 18% (11/61) and in the high-grade equivalent, centroblastic (cb) lymphoma, CE was found in 8% (6/73) (Table 2).

In cb-cc lymphoma the incidence of CE was 10% (4/40) in those with follicular or follicular and diffuse growth pattern as compared to 43% (3/7) in entirely diffuse cb-cc, resulting in an overall percentage of 15 (7/47) in nodal cb-cc lymphomas. In extranodal cb-cc lymphoma the frequency of CE was 29% (4/14).

In the high-grade NHLs there was no difference between the various histologic subgroups with regard to CE, with 8% in centroblastic (6/73) and immunoblastic (1/12) and 9% (2/23) in high-grade NOS (Table 2). Only two patients with B-lymphoblastic lymphoma were included in the study, and both showed a normal CE analysis.

Stage
There was no difference in occurrence of CE in CR when comparing stage I with stage II–IV irrespective of histologic grade (Table 1). In stage I low-grade NHL, CE was present in 18% (8/44) compared to 6% (3/49) in high-grade NHL. In stage I extranodal lymphoma CE was present in 15% (8/52), and the corresponding figure for stage I nodal disease was 7% (3/41), data not shown. Neither difference was significant.

Haematological parameters
In patients with suspicious or definite bone marrow involvement at diagnosis, CE was found in remission in 35% (6/17). In those with a morphologically normal bone marrow at diagnosis, the corresponding figure was 11% (19/179). The difference is significant (P = 0.01). There was a slight difference in lymphocyte count during initial staging in those who had circulating monoclonal cells in CR compared to those who had not, median 1.5×10^9 L^{-1} (range 0.7–9.2) versus 1.3×10^9 L^{-1} (range 0.1–5.6), (P = 0.03, Wilcoxon Rank Sum Test). Only five patients presented with lymphocyte counts just above the normal upper limit

($>4 \times 10^9$ L^{-1}) at diagnosis, and two of these showed CE at follow-up in CR despite normalized lymphocyte counts.

A monoclonal serum Ig component was found in routine protein electrophoresis in 7 of 188 (4%) patients at primary staging. In none of these patients was there any sign of CE in CR.

Table 2. Clonal excess (CE) in peripheral blood in different histologies.

Kiel groups		n	CE	
Low grade malignant				
m.l. lymphocytic		4	2	
m.l. immunocytic		15	4	
m.l. centrocytic		3	–	
m.l. centroblastic/	F, F + D	40	4	
centrocytic	D	7	3	
	X	14	4	
m.l. low grade NOS		9	–	
Total		92	17	(18%)
High grade malignant				
m.l. centroblastic		73	6	
m.l. immunoblastic		12	1	
m.l. lymphoblastic		2	–	
m.l. high grade NOS		23	2	
Total		110	9	(8%)

m.l. = malignant lymphoma.
X = extra nodal.
F = follicular.
D = diffuse.
NOS = not otherwise specified.

Data in remission

Haematological parameters
The number of B cells and T cells in peripheral blood mononuclear cell fraction was quantitated in parallel with CE. In patients with CE, the mean percentage of B cells (CD19-positive) in CR was 19% (range 0–85) as compared to 18% (range 0–61) in those without CE. The corresponding mean percentages for T cells (CD3) were 48% (range 10–89) for those with CE and 54% (range 12–90) for those without CE in remission.

The median total lymphocyte count in remission was 1.5×10^9 L^{-1} (range 0.4–4.0) in the group with CE and 1.5×10^9 L^{-1} (range 0.1–5.9) in the group without CE.

Relapse and survival analyses
Time to relapse did not differ between those with and those without CE in remission (P = 0.23) (Fig. 1). There was a slight, but insignificant difference (P = 0.07), in high-grade NHL (Fig. 2). In low-grade NHL there was no such difference (P = 0.74) (Fig. 2). Survival did not differ between those with and those without CE in remission (P = 0.72) (Fig. 3). Nor was there any difference in survival when looking separately at high (P = 0.73) and low grade NHL (P = 0.82) with regard to the occurrence of CE (Fig. 4).

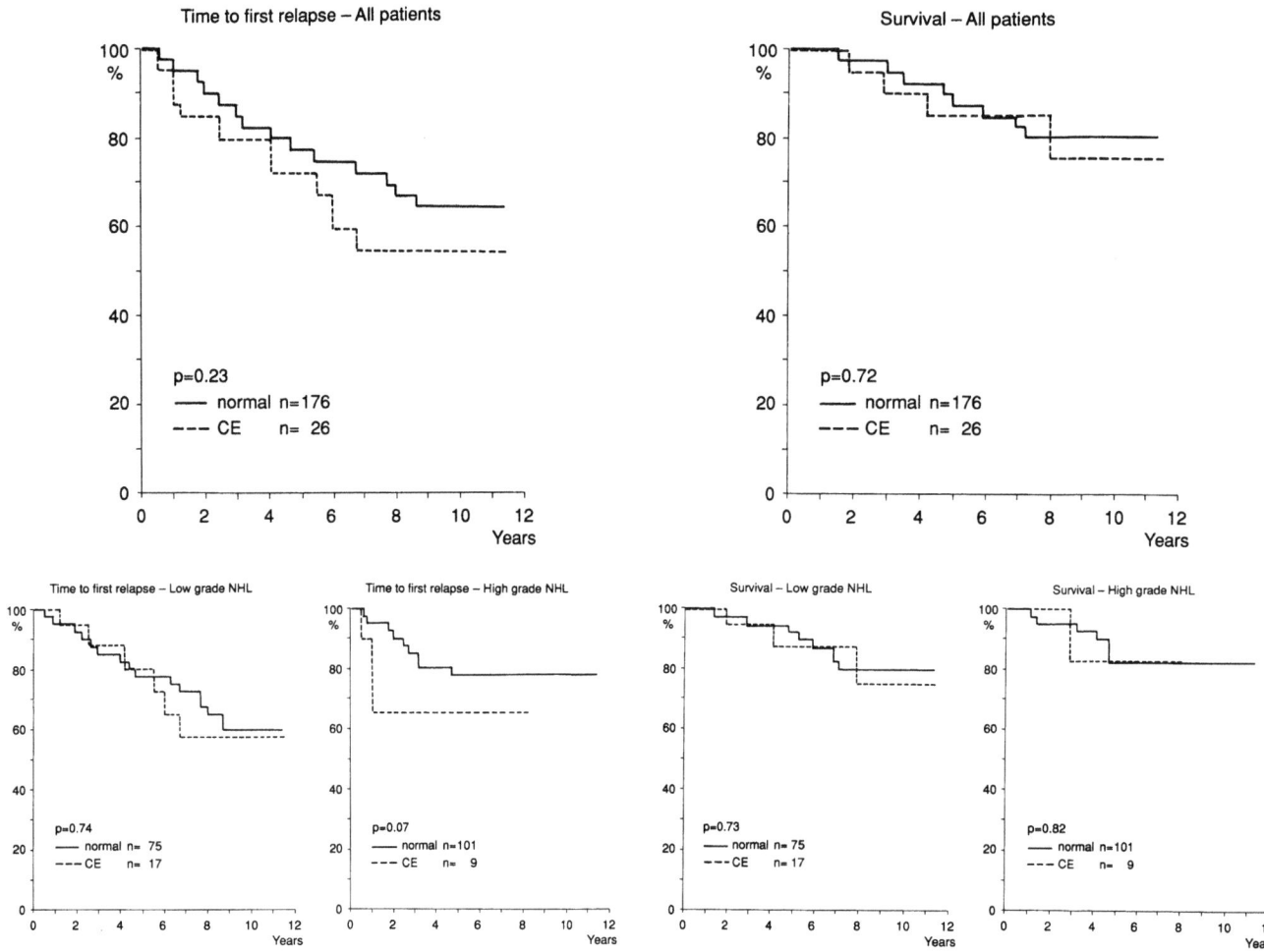

Case reports

Table 3 presents data for patients with high-grade NHL who had CE during remission. Three of these are presented more in detail below and referred to in the discussion.

Patient 1 presented with cb lymphoma stage IVA with generalized lymphadenopathy and tonsillar and bone marrow infiltration but a normal blood lymphocyte count. After eight cycles of CHOP the lymph nodes and bone marrow were cleared, but remaining

Table 3. Clonal excess (CE) in peripheral blood in 9 patients with high grade NHL in remission.

Pat	Data at staging					Data at relapse				FU
	Hist	Stage	X-site	BM	Ly	TTR	Hist	BM	Ly	
1	cb	IVA		+	3.6	11	n.d.	+	5.7	84+
2	cb	II_EA	gastric	–	2.1	–				12+
3	high NOS	n.d.	epiglottis	n.d.	3.6	–				25+
4	high NOS	I_EA	ear canal	–	1.6	–				48+
5	cb	IA		–	0.7	–				75+
6	ib	I_EA	sinus	–	2.1	–				53+
7	cb	III_EA	tonsil	–	n.d.	9	cb	–	n.d.	34
8	cb	IV_EB	ovaries	–	1.0	–				34+
9	cb	IVB		+	7.4	4	cb	–	2.2	4+

Abbreviations:
Hist = histology.
X-site = extranodal.
BM = bone marrow morphology.
Ly = lymphocyte count ($\times 10^9$ L^{-1}).
TTR = time to relapse (months).
FU = follow up (months).
n.d. = not done.

disease was found in the tonsillar region. CR was established after radiotherapy, and CE was found at first analysis eight months after completion of therapy. The patient remained well, but eleven months later the lymphocyte count was above the normal limit and repeated CE analysis showed an expanding CE. Lymphocytes continued to increase slowly, and therapy was instituted six years later when anaemia and thrombocytopaenia developed. The lymphocyte count was then $364 \times 10^9 L^{-1}$ and the blood microscopy showed small indented lymphocytes but no blasts. CE analysis confirmed a 100% monoclonal lymphocyte population in the peripheral blood.

Patient 4 presented with an infiltrating mass in the right external auditory canal. Biopsy confirmed high-grade NHL NOS. No other lymphoma manifestations were present. Bone marrow biopsy showed a slight lymphocyte increase, which was assessed as not malignant. The aspiration was normal and the peripheral blood lymphocyte count was $1.6 \times 10^9 L^{-1}$ with a distinct CE. After radiotherapy she has remained in clinical remission with a normal lymphocyte count for four years and repeated analyses have shown a stable CE.

Patient 9 presented with a very fast-growing cervical mass. Biopsy verified cb lymphoma and immunotyping on cell suspension showed G : κ, CD10-positive phenotype. Enlarged retroperitoneal nodes and a slightly enlarged spleen were identified by CT scan, and bone marrow biopsy showed discrete infiltration, mostly of small lymphocytes. In the marrow aspiration a blastic lymphocyte infiltration was identified and in peripheral blood there was a slight elevation of the lymphocyte count, $7.4 \times 10^9 L^{-1}$, but no blasts were found in the blood smear.

Immunological analysis of blood and bone marrow confirmed κ-positive CE. After MACOP-B therapy for 12 weeks and intrathecal methotrexate, CR was established with normalization of all involved sites but with persistent CE in blood and bone marrow. Four months later she relapsed at the initial site in the neck with cb lymphoma. Peripheral blood and bone marrow was morphologically normal but lymphoma cells were identified by immunoanalysis with a stable CE.

Discussion

It was evident early that assessments of clonal excess using different types of analyses of light chain restriction are more sensitive methods of detecting clonal expansions than are routine haematological analyses including differential white blood cell count [1–2]. Definite proof that these clones represent circulating B-lymphoma cells was provided by Southern blot analysis of Ig-gene rearrangements showing identical rearrangements in tumour material and peripheral blood [13].

The clinical significance of increasingly sensitive methods of detecting tumour spread has remained un-

certain. It has been proposed that the occurrence of CE in peripheral blood at diagnosis is an adverse prognostic sign [14, 15]. Evidence of remaining tumour cells in remission might therefore be even more distressing information. Although the presence of CE in patients in presumed remission has been reported [2, 4], clinical data on the relevance of circulating lymphoma cells have been lacking.

The present study was focused on the prognostic value of CE in the peripheral blood of patients with no other signs of disease. A clinician might instinctively feel inclined to reinstitute treatment when tumour cells are identified, at least in patients with high-grade malignant NHL.

There was no correlation between initial stage and the occurrence of CE in remission with 12% CE in stage I and 13% CE in stage II–IV. Despite this, there was a correlation between initial bone marrow involvement and CE in remission, 35 versus 11% CE for those with normal bone marrow. The association between CE in peripheral blood and morphological bone marrow involvement in active disease has been reported by others [5, 14].

No patient with overt leukaemic dissemination at diagnosis was included, but five presented with slightly elevated lymphocyte counts, two of whom showed CE in remission. There was a slight tendency toward higher lymphocyte counts at primary staging in the group with CE, median $1.5 \times 10^9 L^{-1}$, compared to those without, median $1.3 \times 10^9 L^{-1}$. In remission there was no such difference in median lymphocyte count between the two groups. Nor was there any obvious difference in the two populations with regard to relative numbers of T and B cells in follow-up. These findings suggest that the circulating clones are generally small. In low-grade NHL, overt leukaemic dissemination and bone marrow involvement are more common findings than in high-grade NHL, lymphoblastic lymphoma excluded [16]. In B-CLL, circulation in the peripheral blood is an inherent feature of the malignant cell. It is therefore not surprising that the incidence of occult circulating lymphoma cells was highest in the low-grade histologies, occurring in 18%, and was especially common in the lc/ic subgroups with 32% CE.

In the nodal cb-cc lymphomas there seemed to be a difference in occurrence of CE when comparing those with a follicular growth pattern and those with a purely diffuse pattern, 10 and 43% respectively. The number of patients is, however, too small to allow any definite conclusion (P = 0.056, Fisher's exact test).

The characteristic chronic relapsing pattern of low-grade NHL is compatible with the finding of remaining tumour cells in remission. One might have expected an even higher incidence of CE. Inherent limitations in the CE analysis due to undetectable or absent Ig expression on the surface of the NHL cell might be one explanation. Gene rearrangement studies would overcome this obstacle, and even more sensitive methods, such as detection of bcl-2 translocations or the use of idiotypic probes combined with PCR, will make it possible to detect extremely small numbers of lymphoma cells [17–19].

In high-grade NHL there was no difference between the various subcategories with an incidence of CE around 8%. In high-grade nonlymphoblastic NHL, leukaemic dissemination is rare and usually associated with final progressive disease. Knowing the generally aggressive and rapidly proliferative nature of these diseases, it seems unlikely that the circulating cells during remission represent the blastic population. The present results indicate that a subset of patients with high-grade lymphomas are apparently healthy despite the presence of circulating lymphoma cells following therapy. An explanation might be the occult occurrence of discordant lymphoma or transformed lymphoma, where the aggressive disease has been eradicated by treatment but the indolent low-grade malignant population persists. At least three of our patients, as described in the case reports, may illustrate this hypothesis. Furthermore, one patient with stage I high-grade NHL and repeatedly normal CE analysis developed a slight lymphocyte increase, $5.0 \times 10^9 \, L^{-1}$, three months post therapy. He has remained well with stable blood lymphocyte counts for three years. Since repeated CE analyses and T- and B-cell quantitations were normal, Southern blot analysis was performed. This confirmed our suspicion by revealing an unequivocally monocolonal J_H rearrangement. In this case, Southern blot analysis was able to demonstrate a small clonal excess on the genetic level that was not detectable by flow cytometry, presumably because of very low surface Ig expression. Thus it might well be that there are a number of patients with circulating lymphoma cells in the group without CE, which might be a confounding factor in the analysis of the prognostic information. The magnitude of this problem has not yet been determined, but in studies comparing CE with gene rearrangements there is generally a higher sensitivity in the gene rearrangement analyses [13, 20].

The relapse rate did not differ significantly between those with and those without CE. This was also apparent when low- and high-grade NHL were analysed separately. Nor did survival differ between those with and those without CE despite follow-up for a median of 55 months (range 1–180). However, since there were rather few patients in the CE group, the survival data should be interpreted with some caution. In addition, the same patients were subject to many CE analyses, suggesting a possibility of selection bias towards longevity in the CE group. This objection does not seem to be important, however, since the observation time and the number of samples per patient are equal in both groups.

Many of our findings are in agreement with a recent study by Horning and colleagues of gene rearrangement in peripheral blood of patients with NHL [21]. The incidence of genetically identified circulating lymphoma cells in remission was 10%, a figure much lower than was expected on the basis of previous studies and of estimates of the sensitivity of flow cytometric CE analysis versus genetic probing. It compares fairly well, however, with our figures of CE, which are slightly higher, probably as a consequence of repeat analyses. Horning and colleagues reported that the occurrence of clonal gene rearrangements in peripheral blood did not correlate with clinical relapse, that is, the results were in agreement with our observations.

In conclusion the present results confirm that CE-analysis is a more sensitive method of detecting circulating lymphoma cells than routine haematology and blood microscopy. The occurrence of CE in peripheral blood in remission is a rather unusual phenomenon and does not seem to herald relapse or a worse prognosis. A future goal must be to find out if CE analysis combined with other sensitive molecular genetic methods will better identify those patients who will achieve a clinical relapse. The clinical implication is that an isolated finding of CE in remission is not an indication to start therapy in either low-grade or high-grade NHL.

Acknowledgements

This work was supported from The John and Augusta Persson Fund for Medical Scientific Research at the University of Lund, The Medical Faculty of the University of Lund, The Funds for Medical Research at the University Hospital of Lund, The Bertha Kamprad Foundation for Research in Cancer, and The Swedish Medical Research Council (B87-12X-05946-07A). The authors thank Marie Billgren and Ann Brun for skillful technical assistance.

References

1. Ault K. Detection of small numbers of monoclonal B lymphocytes in the blood of patients with lymphoma. N Engl J Med 1979; 300: 1401–5.
2. Ligler F, Vitetta E, Smith G et al. An immunological approach for the detection of tumor cells in the peripheral blood of patients with malignant lymphoma; implications for the diagnosis of minimal disease. J Immunol 1979; 123: 1123–6.
3. Ligler F, Smith G, Kettman J et al. Detection of tumor cells in the peripheral blood of nonleukemic patients with B-cell lymphoma: Analysis of 'Clonal excess.' Blood 1980; 55: 792–800.
4. Smith B, Weinberg S, Robert N et al. Circulating monoclonal B lymphocytes in non-Hodgkin's lymphoma. N Engl J Med 1984; 311: 1476–81.
5. Sobol R, Dillman R, Collins H et al. Applications and limitations of peripheral blood lymphocyte immunoglobulin light chain analysis in the evaluation of non-Hodgkin's lymphoma. Cancer 1985; 56: 2005–10.
6. Nakano M, Kuge S, Kuwabara S et al. The basic study on κ λ imaging by δ-curve for the detection of a monoclonal B-cell population in the peripheral blood. Blood 1988; 72: 1461–6.
7. Johnson A, Cavallin-Ståhl E, Åkerman M. Flow cytometric light chain analysis of peripheral blood lymphocytes in patients with non-Hodgkin's lymphoma. Br J Cancer 1985; 52: 159–65.
8. Ostberg-Landaas T, Godal T, Marton P et al. Cell-associated immunoglobulins in human non-Hodgkin's lymphoma. A com-

parative study of surface immunoglobulins on cells in suspensions and cytoplasmatic immunoglobulin by immunohistochemistry. Acta path microbiol scand Sect A 1981; 89: 91–101.

9. Cleary M, Chao J, Warnke R et al. Immunoglobulin gene rearrangement as a diagnostic criterion of B-cell lymphoma. Proc Natl Acad Sci USA 1984; 81: 593–7.

10. Cleary M, Trela M, Weiss L et al. Most null large cell lymphomas are B lineage neoplasms. Lab Invest 1985; 53: 521–5.

11. Lee M-S, Chang K-S, Cabanillas F et al. Detection of minimal residual cells carrying the t(14;18) by DNA sequence amplification. Science 1987; 2: 175–9.

12. Crescenzi M, Seto M, Herzige GP et al. Thermostable DNA polymerase chain amplification of t(14;18) chromosomal breakpoints and detection of minimal residual disease. Proc Natl Acad Sci USA 1988; 85: 4869–72.

13. Berliner N, Ault K, Martin P et al. Detection of clonal excess in lymphoproliferative disease by κ/λ analysis: Correlation with immunoglobulin gene DNA rearrangement. Blood 1986; 67: 80–5.

14. Lindh J, Johansson H, Lenner P et al. Monoclonal B-cells in blood in non-Hodgkin lymphoma. Correlation with clinical features and prognoses. Acta Oncol 1989; 28: 641–6.

15. Lindemalm C, Mellstedt H, Biberfeld P et al. Clonal blood B-cell excess in relation to prognosis in untreated non-leukemic patients with non-Hodgkin's lymphoma (NHL). In Malignant Lymphomas and Hodgkin's Disease: Experimental and Therapeutic Advances. Cavalli F, Bonadonna G, Rozencweig M (ed.). Martinus Nijhoff Publishing, 1985; 225–32.

16. Lennert K. Malignant lymphomas other than Hodgkin's disease. In: Handbuch der speziellen pathologischen Anatomie und Histologie. Volume I/3 Lymph Nodes Part B. Berlin, Springer Verlag, 1978.

17. Tycko B, Palmer JD, Link MP et al. Polymerase chain reaction amplification of rearranged antigen receptor genes using junction-specific oligonucleotides: Possible application for detection of minimal residual disease in acute lymphoblastic leukemia. In: Cancer Cells 7/ Molecular Diagnostics of Human Cancer, Cold Spring Harbor Laboratory, 1989; 47–52.

18. Hansen-Hagge T, Yokota S, Bartram C. Detection of minimal residual disease in acute lymphoblastic leukemia by in vitro amplification of rearranged T-cell receptor delta chain sequences. Blood 1989; 74: 1762–7.

19. Deane M, Norton J. Detection of immunoglobulin gene rearrangement in B lymphoid malignancies by polymerase chain reaction gene amplification. Br J Haematol 1990; 74: 251–6.

20. Lindh J, Lindström A, Lenner P et al. Immunoglobulin heavy-chain gene rearrangement in peripheral blood mononuclear cells in non-Hodgkin's lymphoma – Correlation with kappa:lambda analysis and clinical features. Eur J Haematol 1989; 42: 134–42.

21. Horning S, Galili N, Cleary M et al. Detection of non-Hodgkin's lymphoma in the peripheral blood by analysis of antigen receptor gene rearrangements: Results of a prospective study. Blood 1990; 75: 1139–45.

Correspondence to:
Dr. Anna Johnson
Dept of Oncology
University Hospital of Lund
S-221 85, Lund, Sweden

Annals of Oncology, Supplement 2 to Volume 2: 107–113, 1991.
© 1991 *Kluwer Academic Publishers.*

Original article

Expression of myelomonocytic antigens is associated with unfavourable clinicoprognostic factors in B-cell chronic lymphocytic leukaemia

A. Pinto,[1,2] L. Del Vecchio,[3] A. Carbone,[1,4] M. Roncadin,[5] R. Volpe,[4] D. Serraino,[6]
S. Monfardini,[1,7] A. Colombatti[1,2] & V. Zagonel[1,7]

[1] *The Leukaemia Unit and Divisions of* [2] *Experimental Oncology 2,* [4] *Pathology,* [5] *Radiotherapy,* [6] *Epidemiology,* [7] *Medical Oncology, Centro di Riferimento Oncologico, Aviano I-33081, Italy;* [3] *Blood Transfusion Service, Cardarelli General Hospital, Naples, Italy*

Summary. The cross-lineage expression of five myelomonocytic antigens (CD11b, CD11c, CD13, CD14, and CD15) was analysed in neoplastic lymphocytes from 100 consecutive B-cell chronic lymphocytic leukaemia (B-CLL) patients. CD14 antigen was detected on lymphocytes from more than 50% of patients whilst smaller percentages of samples were positive for CD11b (21%), CD11c (26%), CD13 (22%), and CD15 (7%). The presence of the CD13 antigen on neoplastic lymphocytes showed a statistically significant association with the two most important unfavourable clinicoprognostic factors in B-CLL: advanced clinical stage (CD13, $P < 0.01$ by the Rai staging system; $P < 0.05$ by the Binet staging system) and the diffuse pattern of bone marrow infiltration (CD13, $P < 0.001$). A multiple logistic regression analysis showed that the increased risk for CD13-positive patients (13.7-fold higher than CD13-negative cases; $P = 0.001$) of presenting a diffuse pattern of bone marrow infiltration is independent of all other prognostic factors analysed including sex, age, lymphocyte counts, and clinical stage. A statistically significant association of CD11c ($P = 0.002$) and CD11b ($P = 0.032$) expression with the pattern of bone marrow infiltration was also found.

Our results indicate for the first time a statistically significant association of CD13, CD11c, and CD11b antigens with unfavourable prognostic factors in B-CLL. They suggest that the cross-lineage expression of myeloid-associated surface peptidase (CD13-aminopeptidase N) and/or cell adhesion molecules (CD11c-LeuCAMc, CD11b-LeuCAMb) may influence the biological and clinical behaviour of chronic lymphoproliferative disorders of B cells.

Key words: B cell chronic lymphocytic leukaemia, bone marrow infiltration, cell adhesion molecules, cell surface peptidases, myelomonocytic antigens, prognostic factors

Introduction

B-cell chronic lymphocytic leukaemia (B-CLL) is a haematological neoplasm characterized by the clonal proliferation and accumulation of small morphologically mature B lymphocytes [1]. B-CLL cells express monoclonal (light chain-restricted) surface immunoglobulins (SIg) along with a number of B cell-associated antigens such as CD19, CD20, CD21, and CD24, receptors for mouse erythrocytes (MRBC), and, typically, the 67-kd T cell-associated glycoprotein (CD5) [2]. This peculiar membrane phenotype and the absence of markers related to late stages of B-cell differentiation, led to the hypothesis that B-CLL arises from the proliferation of a unique subset of immature B lymphocytes [2, 3]. B-CLL cells are in fact phenotypically arrested at an intermediate stage of differentiation between late pre-B and intermediate/mature B cells [2, 3]. Minor normal B-cell subpopulations showing a B-CLL-like phenotype (CD5+, MRBC+) have been detected in the peripheral edge of the germinal centre

in tonsillar and lymph node tissues of normal adults [4], in fetal lymphoid tissues, and during the early phases of B-cell reconstitution following allogeneic bone marrow transplantation [2, 5].

Despite the apparent uniformity of the cytomorphological and pathological picture [1], the clinical course and the prognosis of B-CLL are highly variable [5, 6]. Some patients display a very aggressive form, while others have an indolent disease course and may survive for more than 10 years [6, 7]. Clinical diversity is also reflected in the great heterogeneity of leukaemic B lymphocytes as recognized by immunological phenotyping using cell surface markers and monoclonal antibodies directed against B cell-associated membrane antigens [2, 3]. Phenotypic heterogeneity of B-CLL is evidenced by the broad range in the proportion of leukaemic cells stained with pan-B specific antibodies among different cases, by the variable intensity of B-cell antigen expression on malignant lymphocytes, and by the failure to express an anticipated antigen [3, 5]. Immunological heterogeneity led to the idea that various B-CLL phenotypes might encompass a relatively broad spectrum of B lymphocyte ontogeny and/or reflect membrane phenotypes of different minor subpopulations of normal B cells [2, 3].

B-CLL staging systems [8, 9], however, do not take into account intrinsic biological features of leukaemic cells such as the membrane phenotype, even though the correlations between a given cell surface antigenic pattern and the clinical outcome have been increasingly reported for several other haematological malignancies. For example, in acute leukaemias of both lymphoid and myeloid lineage (ALL, AML), and multiple myeloma (MM), immunological phenotyping has provided a further tool to allocate patients to prognostic subgroups not identifiable on conventional cytomorphological grounds [10]. In particular the 'cross-lineage' expression of myelomonocytic antigens on ALL cells giving rise to 'mixed-lineage' or 'hybrid' leukaemias is now a well-recognized phenomenon with important biological and clinical implications [11, 12]. Adult patients with myeloid antigen-positive ALL (expressing CD13, CD33 and CD11b determinants) show a low remission rate and a very short survival when treated with conventional chemotherapy regimens [13]. Similar findings have been reported for pediatric ALL and AML [14]. More recently a subset of MM patients whose malignant cells expressed several myelomonocytic antigens (CD11b, CD11c, CD13, CD14, and CD15) has been identified [15, 16]. Even in this case, myelomonocytic antigen-positive myeloma patients displayed an advanced clinical stage at presentation and a poorer clinical outcome as compared to negative ones [15]. Following these reports, many investigators have suggested that 'mixed lineage' leukaemias represent distinct biological and clinical entities so that specific therapeutic strategies should be devised for such forms [11, 12].

Recently we identified a subset of B-CLL characterized by the expression of several myelomonocytic antigens (CD11b, CD11c, CD13, and CD33) and high levels of c-fos oncogene mRNA [17]. Similar results were independently reported by another group of investigators which correlated myeloid antigen expression on a B-CLL subset with interleukin-1 (IL-1) secretion by leukaemic cells [18]. No conclusions were drawn, however, as to the clinicoprognostic implications of those findings. In addition, we showed that myelomonocytic-associated antigens can be induced on B-CLL cells upon in vitro activation/differentiation by several agents such as TPA, vitamin D3, or LPS [19]. Since such 'aberrant' antigen expression seems to correlate with important functional characteristics of leukaemic B cells (IL-1 secretion and c-fos expression), it may provide an additional tool to dissect B-CLL heterogeneity and possibly identify patients with a different clinical outcome.

In order to determine the frequency and the possible clinical relevance of myelomonocytic antigen expression in this lymphoproliferative B cell disorder, we prospectively investigated a large series of B-CLL patients. The correlations between the presence of each myeloid antigen on leukaemic cells and the most important clinicoprognostic factors of B-CLL (including clinical stage and the pattern of bone marrow infiltration) have been analysed.

Materials and methods

Patients

Leukaemic cells were obtained from the peripheral blood of 100 consecutive patients with a clinical, morphological, and immunological diagnosis of B-CLL. Diagnostic criteria for B-CLL were those usually recommended, and recently revised by the NCI-sponsored CLL working group [20], along with the immunological demonstration of B-cell origin (SIg$^+$, CD19$^+$, CD20$^+$, or CD24$^+$ and of kappa or lambda light chain restriction. Patients with a clinically and immunologically proven diagnosis of prolymphocytic leukaemia (PLL), hairy cell leukaemia (HCL), or non-Hodgkin's lymphoma (NHL) were excluded. More than 80% of patients had never been treated, while the rest had received no therapy (chlorambucil and/or corticosteroids) for at least six months. Patients were staged according to the Rai [8] and Binet [9] systems.

Leukaemic-cell isolation and immunophenotyping

Peripheral blood mononuclear cells were obtained by Ficoll-Hypaque (Pharmacia, Sweden) centrifugation of citrate-dextrose anticoagulated whole blood.

Table 1. Monoclonal antibody panel used for immunophenotyping of B-CLL cases.

Cluster designation*	Antibody	Source	Recognized membrane component*	Main Cellular distribution*
CD19	B4	Coulter-Corp.	gp95	B
CD20	B1	Coulter	p37-32	B
CD21	B2	Coulter	p140	B sub, DRC
CD23	B3	Coulter	gp45-50	B sub, DRC, (act M) §
CD5	Leu 1	Becton-Dickinson	gp67	T, B sub
CD11b	MO1	Coulter	gp155-95	M, G, NK
CD11c	Leu M5	Becton-Dickinson	gp150-95	M, G, NK, B sub, act T
CD13	MY7	Coulter	gp150	M, G
CD14	MY4	Coulter	gp55	M, Macro sub, (G) §
CD15	Leu M1	Becton-Dickinson	gp105-200 (x-hapten)	G

* According to the 4th International Workshop on leucocyte differentiation antigens (ref. 21); B = B cells, B sub = B cell subset; T = T cells; DRC = dendritic reticulum cells; Macro = macrophages; M = monocytes, G = granulocytes; NK = natural killer cells; act = activated; § to be confirmed by further testing.

Table 1 lists the monoclonal antibodies utilized for the present study, along with their cluster designation (CD), main specificity, and source. Before incubation with saturating concentrations of each antibody, nonadherent cells were preincubated for 30 minutes at 4 °C with occasional gentle shaking in Hanks' balanced saline solution (HBSS) containing 10% rabbit serum (Dakopatts, Glastrup, Denmark) and 0.01% sodium azide to prevent Fc-receptor binding. Indirect and two-colour immunofluorescence tests were performed as described previously [17, 22]. Nonspecific binding of monoclonal antibodies was assessed by labelling cells with purified, fluorescein-treated, or phycoerythrin-treated isotype-matched control mouse immunoglobulins (Coulter).

Viable, antibody-labelled lymphocytes (1×10^4 per sample) were identified according to their forward and right-angle scattering. They were electronically gated and analysed for surface fluorescence on a FACScan flow cytometer (Becton-Dickinson). Antibody staining was considered positive if more than 20% of lymphocytes (remaining monocytes were electronically gated out during analysis) exhibited fluorescence intensity greater than that of 95% of cells stained with negative control antibodies.

Immunohistologic studies and bone marrow biopsy analysis

Immunohistochemical staining was performed on lymph node cryostat sections with the use of avidin-biotin-peroxidase complex (ABC) immunoperoxidase methods or alkaline phosphatase antialkaline phosphatase (APAAP) as previously described [22].

Results of bone marrow histology and immunophenotyping were available in 60 patients. Peripheral blood samples for immunological studies were obtained on the day of bone marrow biopsy or at most one week later. Bone marrow biopsy specimens were processed for histopathological analysis as previously described [23]. All histologic material was independently reviewed by two observers without any information concerning the clinical characteristics of patients and immunophenotypic results. Four different patterns of bone marrow involvement were recognized according to standard criteria [24]: nodular, interstitial, mixed (a combination of nodular and interstitial patterns), and diffuse. For the present analysis the nodular, interstitial, and mixed patterns were considered together and formed the 'nondiffuse' group. Two groups of patients were compared for statistical analysis, those with a nondiffuse and those with a diffuse pattern [25, 26].

Statistical analysis

We analysed the associations of myelomonocytic antigens with the clinical stage (Rai and Binet), the pattern of bone marrow infiltration, and other factors predicting survival in B-CLL, such as age, sex, and lymphocyte counts [27]. The statistical significance of proportions was assessed by the chi-square test [28]. The association between CD13 antigen expression and bone marrow infiltration was estimated by means of the odds ratios (OR) and their 95% confidence intervals (95% CI), with maximum likelihood estimation of the parameter values [29]. In order to control simultaneously for the effect of potential confounding factors, multiple logistic regression equations were fitted. Through analysis of variance [29], the main effects of age (≤ 65 or >65), sex, lymphocyte counts (≤ 40 or $>40 \times 10^9$/L) and of the Rai and Binet systems were separately considered in the model.

Results

Expression of myelomonocytic antigens on B-CLL cells

The expression of B cell and myelomonocytic antigens on leukaemic lymphocytes from our series of B-CLL patients is shown in Figure 1.

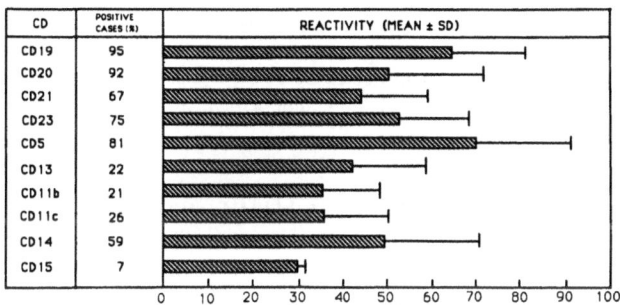

Fig. 1. Expression of B lymphoid and myelomonocytic antigens in B-cell chronic lymphocytic leukaemia. Antigens are defined by their cluster (CD) designation. Histograms show the mean ± SD of the percentage of stained cells in positive samples.

Ninety-seven percent of samples displayed cell surface immunoglobulin with light chain restriction whereas the pan T cell molecule CD5, typically expressed by B-CLL cells, was detected in more than 80% of cases. Pan B antigens (CD19, CD20) were consistently expressed by the vast majority (92–95%) of samples whereas the EBV/C3d receptor CD21 molecule and the B cell activation antigen CD23 were detected in more than 65% and 75% of cases respectively.

The antimonocyte antibody MY4 recognizing an epitope of the CD14 molecule reacted with more than 50% of our B-CLL cases (Fig. 1). A further analysis of CD14 positive cases disclosed a heterogeneous pattern of reactivity of neoplastic lymphocytes with other anti-CD14 monoclonal antibodies such as MO2, CLB-Mon1, UCHM1, M-M42 (data not shown) suggesting an epitopic variability of CD14 expression by B-CLL cells. Expression of CD13 and CD15 antigens was restricted to a smaller subset of patients representing 22% and 7% of our series (Fig. 1). The two antimyelomonocytic cell antibodies, MO1 and LeuM5, recognizing the variant chains of the leucocyte cell adhesion

110

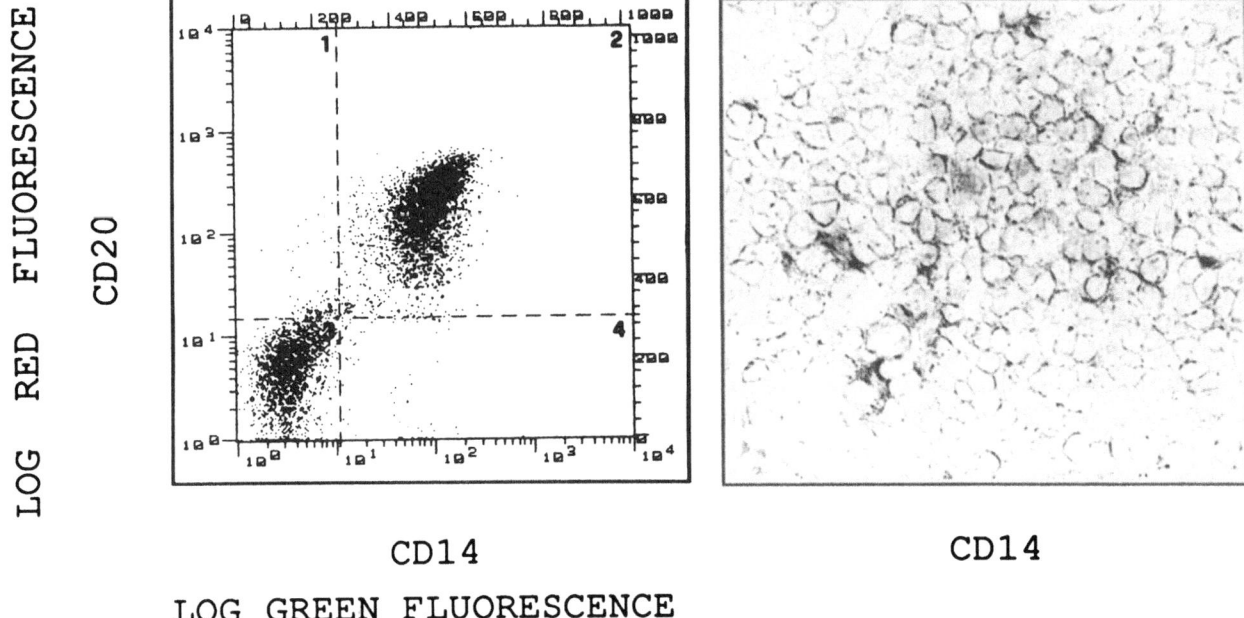

LOG GREEN FLUORESCENCE

Fig. 2. Expression of CD14-MY4 determinants in circulating and lymph nodal B cells from a B-CLL patient. *Left panel:* Two-colour immunofluorescence of peripheral blood lymphocytes showing the simultaneous expression of B lymphoid (CD20-B1) and monocytic (CD14-MY4) antigens by the same leukaemic cells. Region 1 contains cells expressing red fluorescence only; Region 2, cells expressing both red and green fluorescence; Region 4, cells expressing green fluorescence only; Region 3 contains double negative cells. In this case cells in Region 3 have been identified as CD3, CD2-positive T lymphocytes. *Right panel:* immunostaining pattern of a lymph node from the same patient by the anti CD14-MY4 monoclonal antibody (frozen section). Most neoplastic cells show surface and cytoplasmic staining (APAAP × 400).

molecules, Leu-CAMb (CD11b) and Leu-CAMc (CD11c), were reactive with 21 and 26% of our B-CLL samples. Also, as shown in Figure 1, myelomonocytic antigens expressed by cells from only a minor fraction of patients showed a mean reactivity well above the background values. In blood samples from 10 patients the coexpression of CD14 (Fig. 2) and CD13 (data not shown) along with CD20 antigens was demonstrated on more than 50% of leukaemic cells by two-colour immunofluorescence. To assess whether the expression of myelomonocytic antigens was confined to circulating leukaemic cells or involved additional malignant B cells residing in lymphatic tissues, immunohistochemistry studies were performed. Leukaemic B cells expressing CD13 and CD14 antigens were detected in pathologic lymph nodes excised from B-CLL patients during the diagnostic workup. In Figure 2b the immunostaining pattern of the anti-CD14 monoclonal antibody MY4 on frozen sections from a lymph node affected by B-CLL is shown. A definite combined surface and cytoplasmic staining of malignant B cells with the MY4 antibody was evident (Fig. 2).

Correlations with clinicoprognostic factors

The distribution of B-CLL patients according to clinical staging and to the expression of myelomonocytic antigens was then analysed. The presence of CD13 antigen on neoplastic B cells was significantly associated with an advanced clinical stage according to both Rai and Binet systems (Fig. 3). CD13-positive cells

were never detected in patients whose disease was limited to peripheral blood and bone marrow lymphocytosis (Rai 0) as compared to those showing nodal disease and/or organomegaly (Rai I–II and III–IV) (P < 0.01). The differential distribution of CD13-positive cases among early (A) and advanced (B, C) stage patients was maintained when adopting the Binet system (P < 0.05) (Fig. 3). Of the remaining myelomonocytic antigens, only the expression of CD11c and of CD11b showed a significant correlation with the clinical stage (P < 0.01) whereas no statistically relevant dif-

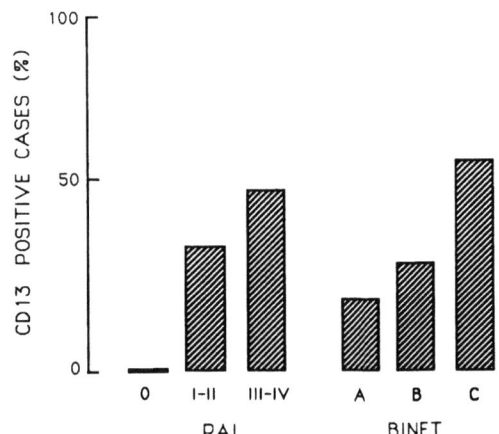

Fig. 3. Distribution of CD13-positive B-CLL cases according to clinical stage (Rai and Binet systems). Differential distribution of CD13-positive cases among early and advanced stages is statistically significant for both staging systems (Rai, P < 0.01; Binet, P < 0.05) (Chi-square test).

ferences in CD14 and CD15 distribution among early and advanced stage patients were observed.

The expression of CD13 was also associated with an older age of patients (>65 years) whilst other known prognostic features of B-CLL, such as sex and lymphocyte counts, had no effect on antigen distribution (data not shown). The correlation between expression of myelomonocytic antigens and the pattern of bone marrow infiltration was then analysed. The distribution of 60 B-CLL patients according to the histologic pattern of bone marrow infiltration and the expression of myelomonocytic antigens is shown in Figure 4. Twenty-nine patients (48.3%) had a nondiffuse involvement (nodular, interstitial, or mixed), and the remaining 31 (51.7%) had a diffuse pattern. The statistical analysis of myelomonocytic antigen distribution among the diffuse and nondiffuse groups revealed a significant association of CD13 (P = 0.0001) and CD11c (P = 0.002) determinants with the histologic pattern of marrow infiltration (Fig. 4).

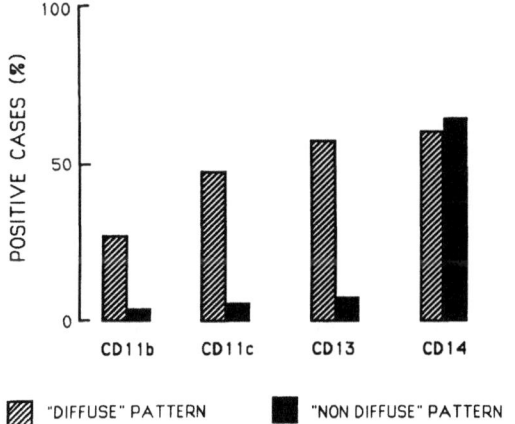

Fig. 4. Distribution of B-CLL patients according to the expression of myelomonocytic antigens and to the histologic pattern of bone marrow infiltration. (CD11b, P = 0.032; CD11c, P = 0.002; CD13, P = 0.0001; CD14, P = 0.61) (Chi-square test).

A weaker but still significant association with the marrow infiltration pattern was demonstrated for CD11b-positive cases (P = 0.032). No relevant differences were found in the distribution of CD14-positive samples (P = 0.61) and CD15-positive samples (P = 0.10) (not shown) among cases with diffuse or nondiffuse bone marrow histology. In agreement with previous reports [24, 25] patients with an advanced clinical stage showed a definite increased prevalence of diffuse patterns (data not shown).

In order to assess the influence of advanced clinical stage on the increased risk of CD13-positive patients to display a diffuse pattern of bone marrow infiltration, a multivariate analysis was performed.

Multiple logistic regression analysis showed that the relative risk of CD13-positive patients presenting a diffuse pattern of bone marrow infiltration was significantly higher (13.7-fold) than that of CD13-negative cases (P = 0.001). In addition, the role of CD13 as a

predictor of the infiltration pattern persisted after correction for the influence of age and stage (Rai, Binet), which themselves confer an increased risk of a diffuse pattern, as shown by univariate analysis in our series and in agreement with previous reports [24, 25]. After such corrections, CD13-positive patients still showed an approximately 10-fold higher risk of a diffuse infiltration pattern than CD13-negative ones (P = 0.001).

Discussion

The availability of monoclonal antibodies to haemopoietic cell surface antigens has greatly enhanced our understanding of phenotypic heterogeneity of haematological malignancies and proven very useful in the clinical evaluation of leukaemia patients [10]. Immunological phenotyping of lymphoid neoplasms has provided new basis for the definition of prognostic subgroups of patients not previously identifiable on conventional cytologic and cytochemical grounds [10]. In this regard the ectopic expression of myelomonocytic antigens (CD13, CD33, and CD11b) in ALL [13] and MM [15, 16] has allowed the identification of a major high-risk group of patients poorly responsive to conventional therapy and with a significantly shorter overall survival. Myelomonocytic antigens that have been so far detected on lymphoid neoplasms are cell surface molecules carrying important functional activities [21]. In this regard CD11b and CD11c molecules, variant chains of the Leu-CAMb and Leu-CAMc complexes, regulate cell adhesion processes and act as soluble factor receptors [30]; CD13 is a cell surface peptidase (aminopeptidase N) able to modify the local concentration of several biologically active peptides [31, 32]; CD33 represents a 67-kd transmembrane glycoprotein showing close structural relationships with the family of neural cell adhesion molecules (N-CAMs) [33]. It is therefore conceivable that the ectopic/inappropriate expression of any one of such molecules by lymphoid leukaemic cells may critically influence their behaviour, resulting in a more aggressive form of disease.

In a previous report we described the expression of CD13, CD14, CD11b, and CD11c antigens on a subset of B-CLL cases [17, 34], and our results were independently confirmed and extended by another group [18]. No conclusions were drawn at that time as to the clinicoprognostic significance of those findings. It was therefore of interest to assess whether, by analogy with ALL and MM, the expression of myelomonocytic antigens might provide an additional tool to dissect B-CLL heterogeneity and identify subsets of patients with different prognoses and clinical courses.

The clinical outcome of B-CLL may in fact show a great variability among different patients and even though the two currently adopted staging systems (Rai and Binet) have been of enormous importance in allocating patients in different prognostic subgroups, they are often unable to predict disease progression. There are in fact patients with advanced-stage disease who have a relatively stable clinical course while others show a rapidly progressive clinical course despite an early-stage disease. More recently the histologic pattern of bone marrow infiltration emerged among other proposed parameters, including age, sex, and lymphocyte counts [24, 27], as one of the most important single prognostic features in B-CLL [24, 25]. Nondiffuse patterns (nodular, interstitial, and mixed) are associated with early stages of the disease, and diffuse patterns with advanced stages (Binet C, Rai III and IV) [24, 26]. In addition, among early-stage patients (0–II or A) the presence of a diffuse pattern of bone marrow infiltration is associated with a poor clinical outcome [25, 35], and a shift from nondiffuse to diffuse pattern has been demonstrated in patients undergoing clinical progression [6, 24].

In the present study we show that the expression of myelomonocytic antigens is a phenomenon occurring with a definite frequency in B-CLL and that the presence of such membrane molecules is significantly associated with clinical stage and the pattern of bone marrow infiltration. About 20–25% of our B-CLL cases expressed one of the myelomonocytic-associated antigens studied (CD13, CD11b, CD11c) whilst less than 10% of samples reacted with anti-CD15 antibodies. Surprisingly the anti-CD14 monoclonal antibody MY4 positively stained cells from almost one half of our cases.

From our data it appears that the cell surface peptidase CD13 (aminopeptidase N) represents a critical molecule among myelomonocytic-associated antigens ectopically expressed by B-CLL cells. It is in fact expressed by a considerable proportion of cases (up to 22%) and almost all cases exhibiting multiple myelomonocytic antigens (two to four myeloid specificities simultaneously expressed on the same B cells) displayed a clear-cut positivity for CD13 (data not shown). In addition, CD13 expression was not confined to previously identified immunological subtypes of B-CLL such as 'bright' SIg or CD5-negative variants, indicating that the detection of selected myeloid-associated molecules could be a further clue to dissect the biological and clinical heterogeneity of B-CLL.

This view is confirmed by the statistically highly significant association of CD13 with the clinical stage and the pattern of bone marrow infiltration. Even though stage and marrow histology in B-CLL are directly related to the increasing tumor load (i.e., a higher leukaemic cell mass corresponds to an advanced clinical stage and a diffuse infiltration pattern), they might also reflect intrinsic biological properties of distinct B-cell subsets sustaining the leukaemic proliferation.

The latter interpretation appears strongly supported by results of our multivariate analysis demonstrating that the increased risk of CD13-positive patients to display a diffuse pattern of marrow infiltration is independent from the clinical stage and from other known unfavourable prognostic features of B-CLL, including

age, sex, and lymphocyte counts. It is therefore tempting to speculate that the ectopic expression of the cell surface peptidase CD13 might confer on the B-CLL lymphocyte additional biological properties resulting in an increased ability to infiltrate and proliferate within bone marrow. For instance, CD13-positive malignant B cells might preferentially activate (or inactivate) by enzymatic cleavage precursor forms of stimulatory (or inhibitory) factors and of other peptides regulating the composition of extracellular matrix within the bone marrow. In that case even a small subpopulation of CD13-positive B-CLL cells could alter the bone marrow microenvironment so as to produce a more advantageous condition for their growth and invasion. Selection of more aggressive clones within the bone marrow would in turn lead, along with an increasing bone marrow failure, to clinical progression. In this regard it was recently reported that bone marrow stromal cells are able to produce several B-cell stimulatory peptides including interleukin-7 [36]. The statistically significant association of CD11b and CD11c determinants with the diffuse pattern of infiltration could also be tentatively explained by the additional interactive properties with marrow stromal components provided by the increased expression of cell adhesion molecules such as Leu-CAMb and Leu-CAMc.

We cannot suggest any hypothesis as to the meaning of CD15 expression in B-CLL owing to the very low number of positive cases, and the functional significance of CD14 determinants on malignant B cells remains an open question. Preliminary data from our group point to the molecular heterogeneity of CD14 expression on B-CLL cells [34]. Antibodies recognizing different epitopes of the molecule react very differently with B-CLL lymphocytes. It could be that epitopes different from those recognized by the MY4 antibody, although expressed to a lesser extent among B-CLL samples, may be found to have some clinicoprognostic importance.

Expression of myelomonocytic-associated antigens might imply a close relationship between B-lymphoid and myelomonocytic lineages of differentiation, as suggested by several authors [12, 15, 17–19]. Alternatively, such expression may reflect an 'activated' state of leukaemic B lymphocytes. In this respect we have demonstrated that in vitro activation/differentiation of B-CLL cells by different stimuli (e.g., phorbol esters, 1,25-dihydroxyvitamin D3, and LPS) may result in the increased expression or de novo induction of several myelomonocytic antigens including CD13, CD14, and CD15 specificities [19]. Similar results have been obtained upon in vitro induction of cells from other B-cell malignancies, including ALL and MM [15], further reinforcing the idea that some myeloid-associated surface molecules may play an important functional role in the activation/differentiation processes of B cells.

The fact that in neoplastic diseases encompassing the whole spectrum of B-cell maturation (ALL, CLL, MM) the presence of myelomonocytic surface antigens is associated with unfavourable clinicopathologic prognostic factors and/or with a poor clinical outcome further points toward a critical role of such molecules in the fine regulation of growth and differentiation of normal and malignant B lymphocytes. In conclusion we propose that the screening of B-CLL samples for myelomonocytic antigen expression provides a clue to dissect the biological and clinical heterogeneity of this lymphoproliferative disorder and to identify subsets of high-risk patients.

Acknowledgements

This work was supported by a grant from the Associazione Italiana per la Ricerca sul Cancro (A.I.R.C.) and by the Associazione 'Lotta contro i Tumori Renzo e Pia Fiorot'. The Authors wish to acknowledge the excellent secretarial assistance of Miss P. Santarossa and Miss E. Montagner.

References

1. Catovsky D. Chronic lymphocytic, prolymphocytic and hairy cell leukaemias. In: Goldman JM and Preisler HD (eds). Haematology I. Leukaemias 1984; 266–98.
2. Freedman AS. Immunobiology of chronic lymphocytic leukemia. Hematology/Oncology Clinics of North America 1990; 4: 405–29.
3. Freedman AS, Boyd AW, Bieber FR et al. Normal cellular counterparts of B cell chronic lymphocytic leukemia. Blood 1987; 70: 418–27.
4. Caligaris-Cappio F, Gobbi M, Bofill M et al. Infrequent normal B lymphocytes express features of B chronic lymphocytic leukemia. J Exp Med 1982; 155: 623–8.
5. Gale RP, Foon KA. Biology of chronic lymphocytic leukaemia. Sem Hematol 1987; 24: 209–14.
6. Rai KR, Montserrat E. Prognostic factors in chronic lymphocytic leukemia. Sem Hematol 1987; 4: 252–5.
7. Hamblin TJ. Chronic lymphocytic leukaemia. Bailliere's Clinical Haematology 1987; 1: 449–91.
8. Rai KR, Sawitsky A, Cronkite EP et al. Clinical staging of chronic lymphocytic leukemia. Blood 1975; 46: 219–34.
9. Binet JL, Catovsky D, Chandra P et al. Chronic lymphocytic leukemia: proposals for a revised prognostic staging system. Br J Haematol 1981; 48: 365–7.
10. Foon KA, Todd RF III. Immunologic classification of leukemia and lymphoma. Blood 1986; 68: 1–31.
11. Maitreyan V, Gale RP. What is hybrid acute leukemia. Leukemia Res 1989; 13: 725–8.
12. Altman AJ. Clinical features and biological implications of acute mixed lineage (Hybrid) leukemias. Am J Pediatr Hematol Oncol 1990; 12: 123–33.
13. Sobol RE, Mick R, Royston I et al. Clinical importance of myeloid antigen expression in adult acute lymphoblastic leukemia. New Engl J Med 1987; 316: 1111–7.
14. Mirro J, Zipft TF, Pui CH et al. Acute mixed lineage leukemia: clinicopathologic correlations and prognostic significance. Blood 1985; 66: 1115–23.
15. Grogan TM, Durie BGM, Spier CM et al. Myelomonocytic antigen positive multiple myeloma. Blood 1989; 73: 763–9.
16. Epstein J, Xiao H, He X-Y. Markers of multiple hematopoietic-cell lineages in multiple myeloma. N Engl J Med 1990; 322: 664–8.
17. Pinto A, Colletta G, Del Vecchio L et al. C-fos expression in human hemopoietic malignancies is restricted to acute leukemias with monocytic phenotype and to subsets of B cell leukemias. Blood 1987; 70: 1450–7.
18. Morabito F, Prasthofer EF, Dunlap NE et al. Expression of myelomonocytic antigens on chronic lymphocytic leukemia B cells correlates with their ability to produce Interleukin 1. Blood 1987; 70: 1750–7.
19. Del Vecchio L, Pinto A, Lo Pardo C et al. Myeloid aspects of B cell differentiation: immunophenotypic analysis of B-leukemic cells exposed in vitro to maturation inducers. In McMichael AJ (ed). 'Leucocyte Typing III'. Oxford University Press 1987; 650.
20. Cheson BD, Bennett JM, Rai KR et al. Guidelines for clinical protocols for chronic lymphocytic leukemia: recommendations of the National Cancer Institute-sponsored working group. Am J Hematol 1988; 29: 152–63.
21. Knapp W (ed.). Leucocyte typing IV. Oxford: Oxford University Press, 1989.
22. Carbone A, Gloghini A, Pinto A et al. Monocytoid B-cell lymphoma with bone marrow and peripheral blood involvement at presentation. Am J Clin Pathol 1989; 92: 228–36.
23. Carbone A, Manconi R, Sulfaro S et al. Practical importance of routine paraffin-embedded bone marrow biopsy in multiple myeloma. Tumori 1987; 73: 315–9.
24. Rozman C, Montserrat E, Rodriguez-Fernandez JM et al. Bone marrow histological pattern. The best single prognostic parameter in chronic lymphocytic leukemia. A multivariate survival analysis of 329 cases. Blood 1984; 64: 642–8.
25. Han T, Barcos M, Emrich L et al. Bone marrow infiltration patterns and their prognostic significance in chronic lymphocytic leukemia: correlations with clinical, immunologic, phenotypic, and cytogenetic data. J Clin Oncol 1984; 2: 562–70.
26. Carbone A, Santoro A, Pilotti S et al. Bone marrow patterns and clinical staging in chronic lymphocytic leukaemia. Lancet 1978; i: 606.
27. Catowsky D, Fooks J, Richards S. Prognostic factors in chronic lymphocytic leukaemia: the importance of age, sex and response to treatment. Br J Haematol 1989; 72: 141–9.
28. Armitage P, Berry G. Statistical methods in medical research. Blackwell Scientific Publications, second edition, London 1987; 125–32.
29. Breslow NE, Day NE. Statistical methods in cancer research IARC Scientific Publication 1980; 32: 192–246.
30. Patarroyo M, Makgoba MW. Leucocyte adhesion to cells in immune and inflammatory responses. Lancet 1989; ii: 1139–41.
31. Look AT, Ashmur RA, Shapiro LH, Peiper SC. Human myeloid plasma membrane glycoprotein CD13 (gp150) is identical to aminopeptidase N. J Clin Invest 1989; 83: 1299–307.
32. Kenny AJ, O'Hare MJ, Gusterson BA. Cell surface peptidase as modulators of growth and differentiation. Lancet 1989; ii: 785–7.
33. Peiper C, Leboeuf RD, Hughes CB et al. Report on the CD33 cluster Workshop: biochemical and genetic characterization of gp67. In: Knapp W (ed.) Leucocyte typing IV. Oxford: Oxford University Press 1989; 814–6.
34. Pinto A, Zagonel V, Carbone A et al. The expression of myelomonocytic antigens on chronic lymphocytic leukaemia B-cells identifies a subset of patients with a 'variant' CLL phenotype and different biological and clinicopathological features. In: Knapp W (ed.) Leucocyte typing IV. Oxford: Oxford University Press 1989; 929–30.
35. Geisler C, Ralfkajer E, Hansen MM et al. The bone marrow histological pattern has independent prognostic value in early stage chronic lymphocytic leukaemia. Br J Haematol 1986; 24: 47–54.
36. Korshkind K. Hemopoietic stem cells and B-lymphocyte differentiation. Immunol Today 1989; 10: 399–401.

Correspondence to:
Antonio Pinto, M.D., Leukemia Unit
Centro di Riferimento Oncologico
Via Pedemontana Occidentale, Aviano
I-33081, Italy

Annals of Oncology, Supplement 2 to Volume 2: 115–122, 1991.
© 1991 *Kluwer Academic Publishers.*

Original article ————————————————————————————

Follicular lymphoma: A model of lymphoid tumor progression in man*

Andrew D. Zelenetz,[1] Michael J. Campbell,[1] David W. Bahler,[1] Shuji Takahashi,[1]
Rachel Oren,[1,5] Laura Esserman,[1,3] Dale T. Umetsu,[2] Larry W. Kwak,[1] David G. Maloney,[1]
Sherri Brown,[1] Thomas T. Chen,[1] Matthew L. Andria,[1] Shoshana Levy,[1] Richard A. Miller[1,4]
& Ronald Levy[1]

[1]*Division of Oncology, Department of Medicine;* [2]*Department of Pediatrics;* [3]*Department of Surgery, Stanford Medical School, Stanford,
CA 94305-5306, USA;* [4]*IDEC Pharmaceuticals Corporation, Mountain View, CA, USA;* [5]*Present address: Department of Biophysics,
Weizmann Institute, Rehovot, Israel*

Summary. Human follicular lymphoma can be viewed as a malignancy in evolution. Since this disease is composed of a clonal population of B lymphocytes all expressing a given immunoglobulin light chain and heavy chain, it seems possible that the initial transforming event, the t(14;18) chromosomal translocation, occurs in a cell already committed to the expression of a particular V_H and V_L gene. A panel of antibodies has been assembled which define a set of idiotypes expressed repeatedly by B-cell lymphomas. Nonetheless, V_H gene usage in follicular lymphoma tumors appears to reflect the normal B-cell repertoire. Growth of follicular lymphoma appears to be partially under normal regulatory control. The expanding malignant B-cell clone grows in follicles with particular apposition to follicular dendritic cells and heavy infiltration with CD4$^+$ T cells. Interaction with T cells can induce the proliferation of follicular lymphoma cells. This tumor eventually evolves into a diffuse large-cell lymphoma which is highly aggressive and lethal. It is now clear that the malignant progression occurs from a single cell within the expanding follicular lymphoma clone. A panel of monoclonal antibodies to cell surface molecules has been generated that inhibit proliferation of diffuse lymphoma cell lines, and some of the target molecules have been partially characterized. Therapeutic application of anti-idiotype monoclonal antibodies has shown a high degree of tumor responsiveness, but ultimately escape of idiotype-negative variant cells occurs. These variants arise as a result of extensive somatic point mutation in the V_H and V_L genes of follicular lymphoma. Active immunization can result in an immune response by patients directed against the idiotype expressed on their own B-cell tumors. It is anticipated that such immune responses will be polyclonal and better able to deal with the problem of tumor heterogeneity.

Key words: anti-idiotype antibodies, immunotherapy, lymphoma, tumor progression, vaccination, variable genes

Development of human follicular lymphoma

Human follicular lymphoma (FL) is a mature B-cell neoplasm characterized by an indolent clinical course with the potential of spontaneous remission [1]. However, with time, this tumor transforms into a more aggressive diffuse lymphoma (DL); the risk for this histologic conversion is approximately 44% at five years [2–3] and 67% at 10 years from initial diagnosis. Our current understanding of the evolution of FL is summarized in Figure 1. A bone marrow origin of this neoplasm is inferred from the finding that 80% of patients with FL have bone marrow involvement at presentation even if the disease is clinically limited to a single lymph node [4]. Normal B cells develop in the bone marrow from stem cells that are committed to lymphoid differentiation. During this process immunoglobulin genes are rearranged such that a J_H segment is joined to a diversity element (D); this is followed by rearrangement of a heavy chain variable gene segment (V_H). Extra nucleotides are often added between the V, D, and J segments during the joining process. When a functional $V_H DJ_H$ rearrangement occurs, the μ protein chain is expressed and light chain gene rearrangement proceeds [5]. FL cells contain an additional DNA rearrangement due to a translocation between chromosomes 14 and 18 which juxtaposes one heavy chain joining segment (J_H) on chromosome 14 to the *bcl*-2

* This work was supported by the National Institutes of Health grants CA-34233 and CA-33399. A. D. Z. is supported by a Clinical Investigator Award, K08 CA01396, from the National Cancer Institute. D. W. B. is supported by a Postdoctoral Fellowship from the American Cancer Society. T. C. is a student in the Medical Scientist Training Program, GM07365. R. L. is an American Cancer Society Clinical Research Professor. Correspondence should be addressed to R. Levy, Stanford Medical School, Department of Medicine/Oncology, Room M211, Stanford, CA 94305-5306. Tel. (415) 725-6453. Fax (415) 725-1420.

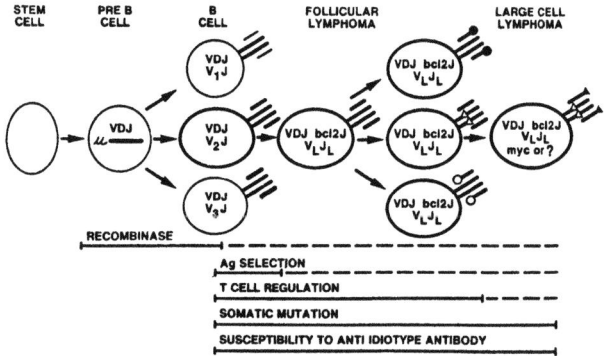

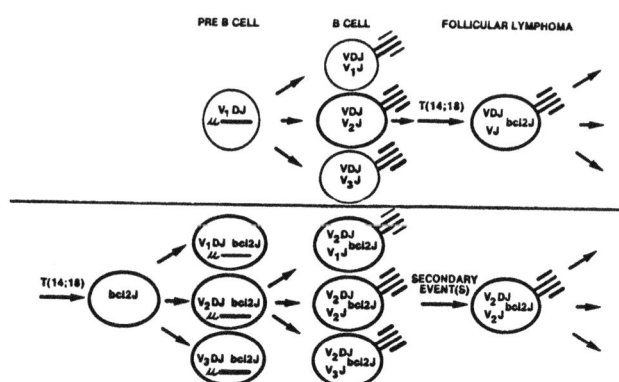

Fig. 1. Evolution of human follicular lymphoma. Though human follicular lymphoma likely arises in the bone marrow [4] the tumor cell is a mature B cell with a concomitant t(14; 18) chromosomal translocation. The role of antigen selection in this disease is unknown (see *Variable gene usage in FL*). The morphology of FL in the lymph node is highly organized and suggests interaction with the host, particularly via the T cells and follicular dendritic cells. In addition, FL can spontaneously regress; thus the host can exert growth modulation via an unknown mechanism(s) (see *Interactions of FL cells with the host*). The development of a transformed large-cell lymphoma is accompanied by aggressive growth reflecting the loss of growth regulation by the host (see *Histologic conversion of FL to tDL*). Since the FL cell is a mature B cell, the surface immunoglobulin molecule is a target for specific immunotherapy (see *Therapy of FL directed against the idiotype*). However, throughout the evolution of FL active somatic mutation remodels the sIg providing a mechanism of escape from anti-idiotype therapy.

Fig. 2. When does the t(14; 18) translocation occur? Two potential models for the timing of t(14; 18) relative to B-cell ontogeny. Upper panel: Late translocation: the t(14; 18) is seen as the final step in the genesis of FL, being both necessary and sufficient to produce the malignant phenotype. In this model both the heavy and light chain genes have been rearranged prior to the development of the tumor. Hence, the basis for conservation of idiotype that is observed throughout the course of this disease [13] is evident. Lower panel: Early translocation: if the t(14; 18) is an error of VDJ joining [51] then it would occur before a functional heavy chain rearrangement has occurred. However, since this pre-B-cell population is proliferating [15] one predicts the existence of an oligoclonal population of pre-B cells, each with the same t(14; 18) and each with a unique VDJ [14]. Furthermore, one would expect multiple light chain rearrangements for each heavy chain rearrangement. Thus, at this stage the tumor would be polyclonal, implying that secondary event(s) are necessary to generate the clinically recognized monoclonal tumor.

proto-oncogene on chromosome 18, t(14; 18) [6–9]. An important issue is the determination of when in relation to normal immunoglobulin gene rearrangements this critical event in the genesis of FL occurs. It has been suggested that the chromosomal translocation occurs in a pre-B cell as a mistake during the normal D-J_H joining process. This is because the J_H-*bcl*-2 joints resemble those formed between V, D, and J segments and contain extra nucleotides [5, 9–10]. However, we have found that mature B-cell lines can also continue to rearrange their immunoglobulin genes and insert extra nucleotides in these new joints [11–12]. This raises the possibility that the t(14; 18) occurs in a B cell which has already made functional heavy and light chain gene rearrangements. Another hallmark of human FL is that all members of the tumor clone express the same immunoglobulin (Ig) genes and proteins; furthermore, this expression is maintained throughout a given patient's remissions, relapses, and tumor progression [13–14]. If the t(14; 18) translocation occurred during D-J_H joining, multiple heavy chain rearrangements should be present in the pre-B cell pool all containing a common t(14; 18) (Fig. 2). Furthermore, with continued replication of the pre-B cells [15] multiple light chain rearrangements would occur for each productive J_H rearrangement; therefore, unless some additional event was required to produce the FL this would lead to tumor cells having multiple different surface Ig (sIg) molecules. Bertoli et al. [14] have reported a patient with FL who had pre-B cells in the bone marrow which contained clones of cells with

different J_H rearrangements. Although there was a *bcl*-2 rearrangement as well, it was not shown to be coincident with any of the J_H bands in the oligoclonal pre-B-cell population. Nonetheless, even in that case a single idiotype was expressed by the tumor cell monitored over a period of 73 months. We suggest the view that the t(14; 18) occurs after selection of both heavy and light chains and thereby represents the critical event in the development of FL. Recently, de Jong et al. [16] analyzed a series of Ig⁻ follicular lymphomas by Southern blot hybridization. In four cases of FL the only heavy chain rearrangement was to the *bcl*-2 locus while all cases had light chain rearrangements. One interpretation of their result is that the functional heavy chain allele rearranged to *bcl*-2 subsequent to the selection of heavy and light chains. This model readily accounts for the constancy of Ig expression in FL.

Variable gene usage in FL

Malignant FL B cells generally express a unique sIg comprising the tumor idiotype. The combinatorial diversity of potential idiotypes is vast [17] though Klpps [18] and Kiyotaki [19] have reported a high incidence of shared idiotypes in patients with chronic lymphocytic leukemia (CLL). To examine the idiotype diversity in FL we analyzed a panel of 199 murine monoclonal antibodies reactive with the idiotype of 67 patients with FL for cross-reactivity [20]. To determine which anti-idiotype monoclonal antibodies were most likely to recognize shared idiotypes (SIDs), the panel of antibodies was first screened for reactivity with a small fraction of normal immunoglobulin [21]. Initially, 20 anti-idiotypic antibodies were selected and found to react with 30 of 110 FL (27%) [20]. These antibodies react with rare cells in normal peripheral blood and in benign follicular hyperplasia tissue. By continued screening this panel has now been expanded to 36 antibodies; individual antibodies reacted with up to 4% of all lymphomas tested. Figure 3 shows the reactivity of this panel of 36 antibodies with 195 cases of FL. This panel of anti-SID antibodies reacts with lymphomas of various subtypes at similar frequency to FL. However, some anti-SID antibodies have a propensity to react with a single histologic subtype, e.g., antibody S011 reacts with 3% of FL and less than 0.5% of nonfollicular lymphoma.

To understand the molecular basis for reactivity with SIDs we have developed a strategy based on the polymerase chain reaction (PCR) which allows us (1) to amplify the immunoglobulin heavy and light chain V region genes expressed by FL cells, (2) to type them as to V region family, and (3) to determine their sequence. Using this approach we have begun to analyze several of the cross-reacting families. Interestingly, there appears to be sharing of V_H family usage between members of cross-reacting groups. Unfortunately, comparison of linear sequences has failed to reveal an obvious basis for cross-reactivity. Three-dimensional analysis using computer modeling, in progress, may shed light on this problem.

The unexpected high frequency of SIDs raised the possibility that there is a bias in variable gene usage in FL as has been described in CLL [22–24]. With the use of the PCR strategy, the V_H gene family was determined for 40 cases of FL. To be certain that the sequences we amplified and sequenced were derived from tumor and not from contaminating normal B cells, the analysis was performed on rescue hybridoma cell lines. In each case the hybridoma is known to be

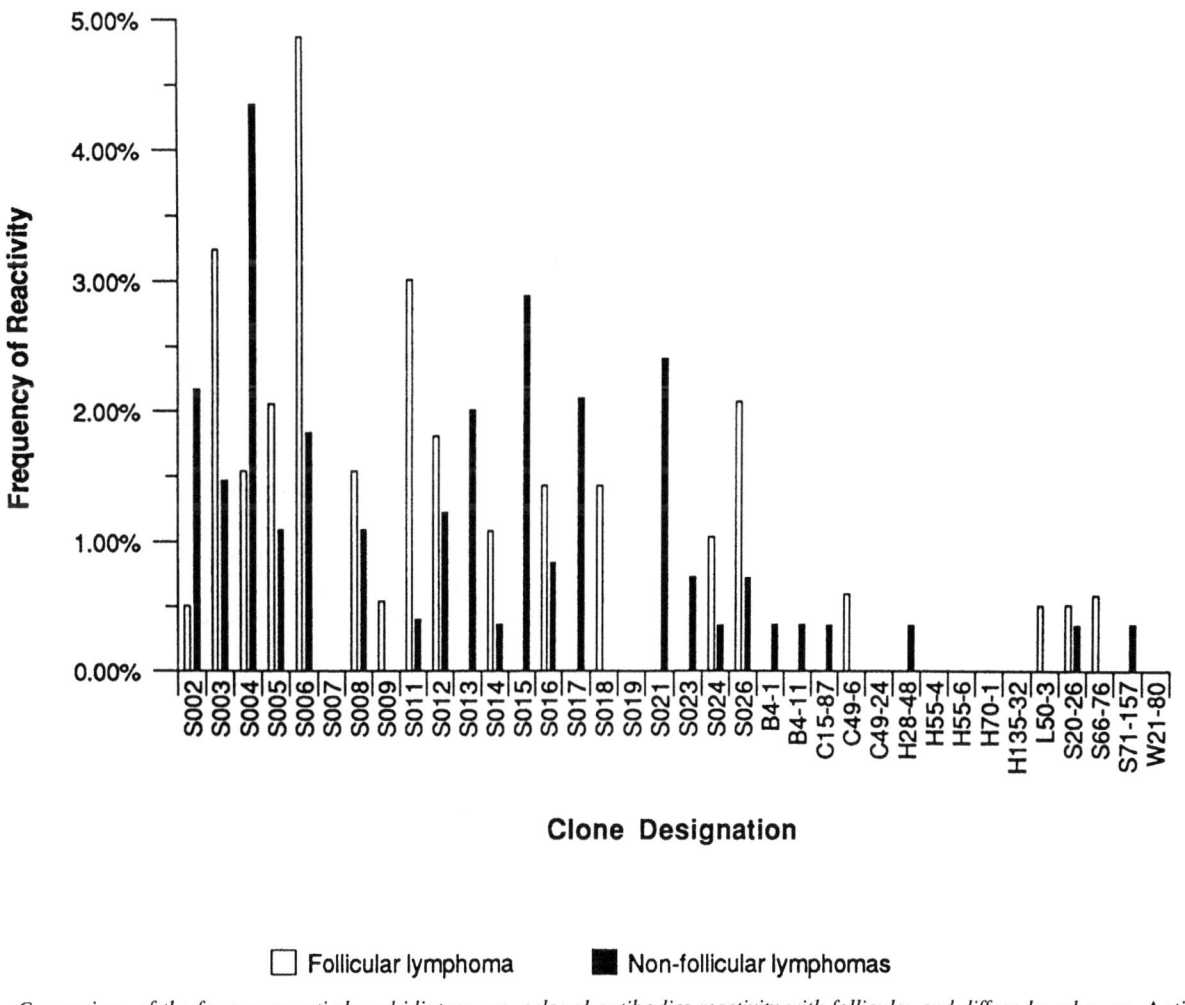

Fig. 3. *Comparison of the frequency anti-shared idiotype monoclonal antibodies reactivity with follicular and diffuse lymphomas.* Anti-idiotype antibodies produced by immunization with tumor idiotype were considered to be directed against shared idiotypes if their binding to tumor idiotype was inhibited by pooled normal human serum [20]. The anti-idiotype selected in this manner were then tested for reactivity to a large panel of human lymphomas of all histologic subtypes [50] by immunohistochemical staining of cryostat sections and/or cell suspensions. Follicular lymphomas included follicular small cleaved cell and follicular mixed large and small cell. The nonfollicular lymphomas included chronic lymphocytic leukemia, small lymphocytic lymphoma, diffuse small cleaved cell, diffuse mixed lymphoma, diffuse large cell lymphoma, and small noncleaved cell lymphoma. Some antibodies which react with shared idiotypes by the assay described failed to react with any of the 400 lymphomas in this panel (e.g., S007, S019).

derived from the tumor because anti-idiotypic monoclonal antibodies made against the idiotype secreted by the rescue fusions bind specifically to the original tumor. Among these 40 cases the heavy chain variable gene family usage appears to be comparable to that of EBV-transformed B cells [25]. Sequence analysis of some of these cases is now being undertaken to determine if there is repeated use of specific variable genes within each family.

Interactions of FL cells with the host

During the clinical evolution of FL, we have observed that tumors can initially progress and then regress spontaneously [1]; this phenomenon remains to be explained. Normal B-cell clones are responsive to antigenic stimulation and are growth modulated, both positively and negatively, by T cells. Within the malignant lymph node, FL cells grow in intimate relationship to follicular dendritic cells and to T cells [26]. The T cells which infiltrate the lymph node are polyclonal and are predominantly CD4$^+$ though a small number of CD8$^+$ T cells are present. In a given patient, the proportion of infiltrating T cells is relatively constant in biopsies from multiple anatomic sites. Furthermore, the number of infiltrating T cells correlated with the

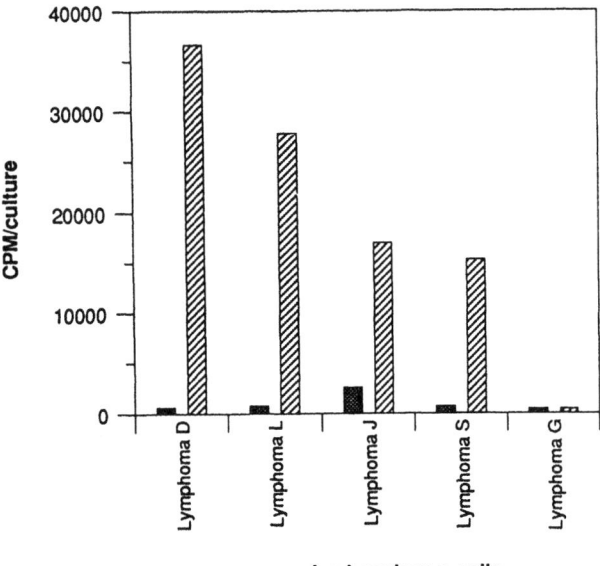

lymphoma alone

lymphoma + H9

Fig. 4. Follicular lymphoma cells are induced to proliferate by coincubation with alloreactive CD4$^+$ T-cell clones. Lymphoma cells were purified from spleens of five patients with follicular lymphoma and were depleted or contaminating T cell by a cocktail of pan-T-cell antibodies and rabbit complement. The alloreactive T-cell clone H9 was irradiated to 1000 cGy to prevent its proliferation in response to the lymphoma cells. Lymphoma cells (10^5) were cultured alone or cocultivated with T cells (5×10^4), labeled with ^{3}[H]thymidine during the last 18 hour of a 72-hour incubation, and proliferation was assessed by incorporation of the radionuclide. (Reproduced from Umetsu et al. [29])

response to therapy with anti-idiotypic antibodies [27–28]. These results suggest that FL cells may be under growth control similar to normal B cells (Fig. 1).

In collaboration with Umetsu [29], we have found that FL cells obtained directly from patient biopsy specimens can be induced to proliferate in vitro by interaction with alloreactive CD4$^+$ human T-cell clones (Fig. 4). This lymphoma growth-stimulating effect was dependent upon contact with the T cells and on their recognition of alloantigens on the tumor. Stimulation could be enhanced by the addition of lymphokines such as interleukin-2 and interleukin-4 to the medium. Karyotypic analysis of the proliferating cells demonstrated that they had the characteristic t(14;18) of the tumor, thus excluding the trivial explanation that proliferation was secondary to contaminating T or normal B cells. In addition, the proliferating cells expressed the immunoglobulin of the input tumor cells. We would like to extend these observations to analyze the role of autologous infiltrating T lymphocytes in the modulation of growth of the FL.

Histologic conversion of FL to tDL

The indolent clinical course of FL is often disrupted by histologic conversion to a diffuse large cell lymphoma [2–3]. The transformed diffuse lymphoma (tDL) has a very poor prognosis and demonstrates aggressive growth in vivo, often involving nonlymphoid sites. The malignant cells in the tDL clone appear to have lost growth modulation by T cells and can be established as cell lines in vitro [30]. Very little is known about the molecular events accounting for tumor progression. To explore the clonal relationship between FL and tDL, we have analyzed 16 paired cases of FL and tDL. In 13 cases anti-idiotypic monoclonal antibodies had been prepared which reacted with a given patient's FL. Anti-idiotype antibodies reacted with both the FL and tDL in 12 of 13 cases (Table 1). In the three cases where anti-idiotype antibodies were unavailable and in the single case of discordant reactivity, clonal evolution was demonstrated by concordant immunoglobulin and *bcl*-2 gene rearrangements. Having established a clonal relationship between FL and tDL, we sequenced repetitive isolates of the heavy and light chain variable genes from two FLs and the paired tDLs. Since light chain rearrangement is the final event in B-cell ontogeny, the finding of the same light chain variable gene used by both members of each pair of tumors demonstrated that they share a common B-cell origin. Furthermore, the sequence of the V_H gene expressed by the tDL demonstrated numerous nonrandom somatic mutations among independent clones implying that they all arose from a common cell. Therefore, progression from FL to tDL likely is the result of a single event.

To identify molecules uniquely expressed in tDL, a panel of monoclonal antibodies was prepared from mice immunized with the tDL of one patient. These

Table 1. Surface immunoglobulin and antiidiotypic mAb reactivity of paired FL and tDL.

Case	Date	Diagnosis[1]	ID[2]	Case	Date	Diagnosis	ID
BH	5/24/84	FML	+	LV	10/15/86	FML	+
	11/4/88	DML	+		10/27/88	F/DLCL	+
BL	1/27/84	FSCL	+	MW	9/19/81	FML	+
	10/6/87	DLCL	+		10/31/83	DML	+
CL	8/23/88	FSCL	+	RF	11/6/86	FML	+
	6/13/89	SNC, nB	+		10/11/88	DL	+
JC	10/6/83	FSCL	+	RS	1/19/88	FSCL	+
	10/9/86	DLCL	+		6/24/88	DLCL	+
BE	9/21/84	FSCL	+	RT	11/15/85	FSCL	+
	6/4/87	FLCL	+		11/22/88	FLC	+
	4/14/88	F/DLCL	+		1/5/90	DLCL	+
EC	3/26/87	FSCL	+	RW	3/27/84	FML	+
	4/6/89	F/DLCL	−		1/8/87	DML	+
	8/23/89	F/DLCL	−		6/21/88	DML	+
SG	11/18/86	FSCL	+				
	4/28/88	DML	+				
	10/7/88	FML	+				

[1] Histologic subtype of non-Hodgkin's lymphoma was made according to the Working Formulation [50]. Abbreviations: DLCL: diffuse large cell lymphoma; DML: diffuse mixed lymphoma; FSCL: follicular small-cleaved cell lymphoma; FML: follicular mixed lymphoma; FLC: follicular large-cell lymphoma (FLCL); SNC, nb: small noncleaved, non-Burkitt's lymphoma.

[2] Reactivity with the tumor specimen was determined by flow cytometry of single cell suspensions of biopsy specimens and/or immunohistochemistry on frozen sections of fresh biopsy material.

antibodies are screened for their ability to distinguish the tDL from the antecedent FL. We isolated one antibody, TRUMP [31], which was found to generally discriminate higher grade and lower grade lymphomas. Molecular analysis of the target of the TRUMP antibody revealed that it reacted with the transferrin receptor. However, the epitope bound by TRUMP was found to be preferentially exposed on the cell surface of higher grade lymphomas.

Cell surface molecules can regulate the growth of lymphoma cells

Compared to FL, diffuse lymphomas have a more aggressive growth pattern. To gain an understanding of this difference, we have developed a methodology to identify cell surface molecules important in growth control. Monoclonal antibodies from mice immunized with human lymphoma cell lines have been screened for their ability to inhibit growth of lymphoma cells in culture [32]. With this strategy, 36 antiproliferative antibodies have been isolated. Thirteen of these antibodies react with molecules previously known to be important in the regulation of growth: transferrin receptor (1 clone); MHC class I (4 clones); MHC class II (4 clones); and Ig (4 clones). The remaining 23 clones react with novel cell surface molecules, 8 of which we have characterized by immunoprecipitation; the remaining 15 react with cell surface molecules that do not readily radiolabel or immunoprecipitate. Table 2 details the characteristics of the 8 antibodies which react with 5 independent cell surface molecules.

Table 2. Characteristics of antiproliferative antibodies to cell surface molecules.

Source of immunizing cells[1]	Histology[2]	Number of isolates	Apparent MW[3] (kd)
B-cell, patient FB	DLCL	1	55
B-cell (OCI-LY8)	DLCL	1	26
B-cell (SU-DHL4)	MF	2	110
T-cell, patient FN	MF	1	28
T-cell, patient JS	CLL	2	110
T-cell (SUP-T13)	ALL	1	110

[1] Hybridomas were produced from mice immunized with the indicated human tumor cells or cell line. They were screened for growth inhibition using the tetrazolium dye MTT as previously described [32]. Hybridomas producing antibodies positive in the initial screen were cloned and then screened on a wider panel of cell lines.

[2] Nomenclature as in footnote 1 of Table 1.

[3] Determined by immunorecipitation of radioiodinated cell surface proteins followed by SDS-PAGE.

We further characterized the 26-kd molecule which we named TAPA-1 (target of an antiproliferative antibody 1). The molecule was found to be expressed on cell lines of hematolymphoid, neuroectodermal, and mesenchymal origin. The antibody induced aggregation of most of these cells though the antiproliferative effect was seen only in a subset of cell lines. TAPA-1 was found to be noncovalently associated with another cell surface molecule, Leu-13. Antibody directed against Leu-13 was also found to cause aggregation of cells and to exert an antiproliferative effect. TAPA-1 cDNA has been cloned by the method of Aruffo and Seed [33–34]. Sequence analysis demonstrated that the protein is highly hydrophobic and contains four putative transmembrane domains and a potential N-terminal myristylation site [35]. The mouse homolog has been cloned and is 92% conserved at the amino acid level. Fifteen of the nineteen residues which differ between the mouse and human TAPA-1 proteins are clustered in one of the putative hydrophilic extracellular domains.

Therapy of FL directed against the idiotype

The sIg molecule of lymphomas can serve as a specific target for therapy [36]. Hopper and Nisonoff [37] found that it was possible to generate antibodies directed to the unique portion of the Ig molecules. We have used this approach to treat human FL [38–40]. To obtain the idiotype immunogen necessary for the generation of murine anti-idiotype antibodies, we produce rescue hybrids between the human tumor cell and a mouse myeloma that has the capacity to secrete high levels of Ig [41–43]. The secreted human Ig is purified and used to immunize mice; immune splenocytes are fused with the mouse myeloma cell line, and hybridomas are selected that secrete antibody that is specifically reactive with the tumor-derived idiotype. These hybridomas, secreting anti-idiotype antibodies, are expanded in bioreactors and pharmacologic quantities (3–10 g) are purified. These antibodies are then infused into patients with FL, generally on an alternating-day regimen, at doses necessary to achieve peak serum concentrations of 100 µg/mL for a period of two weeks. We have completed three trials of murine anti-idiotype monoclonal antibodies in patients with FL (Table 3). The first trial consisted of antibody alone, and dramatic antitumor effects were seen in 8 of 14 patients [39]. Two patients achieved a clinical complete remission. One patient, PK, who had been extensively pretreated with multiple chemotherapeutic regimens, had a durable complete remission that lasted six years. Some patients who had tumor progression following antibody therapy were found to have tumor cell variants which were idiotype negative; these variants have been shown

to arise as a consequence of somatic mutation of their heavy and light chain genes [44]. Based on an animal model [45] and on the independent activity of interferon in patients with B-cell lymphoma [40] we performed a trial of therapy with anti-idiotype antibody in combination with interferon. In this trial, 9 of 11 patients had significant clinical responses, with 2 complete remissions lasting longer than 33 and 36 months. However, idiotype-negative variants again proved to be an obstacle. This was followed by a trial of combined antibody and chlorambucil in an attempt to reduce the problem of tumor escape with idiotype-negative tumor cells. This trial has produced significant clinical responses in 6 of 13 patients, though once again, idiotype-negative variants have limited the utility of the therapy. In an animal model system, we have found potent synergy between anti-idiotype antibody and interleukin-2 [46]. Based on these findings, we are currently conducting a clinical trial of anti-idiotype antibody and interleukin-2.

Idiotype-negative variants have become a drawback to anti-idiotype therapy, since the passively administered antibody is directed to a single epitope. To circumvent this limitation we have investigated the potential of active immunization with purified idiotype to induce a polyclonal response in the tumor-bearing host. A mouse B-cell lymphoma, 38C13, has provided a model system for the study of idiotype vaccination [47]. Studies have revealed that the idiotype protein must be conjugated to a carrier protein such as KLH to induce the production of anti-idiotype antibodies and protect against tumor challenge. Anti-idiotype antibody titers are enhanced 20-fold by the use of an immunoadjuvant; the new adjuvant SAF-1, developed by Syntex, is particularly effective and nontoxic [48]. The immunoprotection experiments were successful even in animals already bearing tumors. It was found that idiotype vaccination after tumor cytoreduction with cyclophosphamide was capable of curing 50% of tumor-bearing animals whereas either therapy alone failed to produce any long-term survival [49]. We have recently extended these findings to idiotype vaccination in man. The tumor idiotype is isolated and purified as described above and conjugated to KLH. Patients have received monthly injections of 500 µg of Id-KLH conjugates in a vehicle emulsion of Pluronic L121 polymer, squalane, and 0.4% Tween-80. Of the 9 patients vaccinated, all have produced either humoral or cellular anti-KLH responses; furthermore, 8 of the 9 patients have generated anti-idiotype antibodies (5 patients) or T cell proliferative responses (5 patients) to the tumor derived idiotype. One patient, ST, developed a relatively high-titer anti idiotype response and also had resolution of a preexisting tumor mass. Though very preliminary, these results are exciting and may herald a new chapter in immunotherapy of lymphoma in man.

Table 3. Development of anti-idiotype antibody clinical trials.

	Anti-idiotype		
	Alone	With α-interferon	With chlorambucil
Number of evaluable patients	14	11	13
Number of responses	10	11	9
Number of CR/PR[1]	2/6	2/7	1/5
Median duration of response	6 mo	7 mo	6 mo
Range	1 mo–6 yr	5 mo–>3 yr	4 mo–32 mo

[1] Includes minor responses (MR, <50% in measurable disease), partial responses (PR, >50% reduction in measurable disease) and complete remissions (CR, complete resolution of detectable disease).

Acknowledgments

The authors would like to thank Deborah Czerwinski, Carol Doss, Sarah Hart, and Vu Nguyen for their expert technical assistance throughout these studies.

References

1. Horning SJ, Rosenberg SA. The natural history of initially untreated low-grade non-Hodgkin's lymphomas. N Engl J Med 1985; 311: 1471–5.
2. Acker B, Hoppe RT, Colby TV et al. Histologic conversion in the non-Hodgkin's lymphomas. J Clin Oncol 1983; 1: 11–6.
3. Ersboll J, Schultz HB, Pedersen-Bjergaard J et al. Follicular low-grade non-Hodgkin's lymphoma: Long-term outcome with and without tumor progression. Eur J Haematol 1989; 42: 155–63.
4. Rosenberg SA. Bone marrow involvement in the non-Hodgkin's lymphomata. Br J Cancer 1975; 31: 261–4.
5. Yancopoulos GD, Alt FW. Regulation of the assembly and expression of variable-region genes. Ann Rev Immunol 1986; 4: 339–368.
6. Yunis JJ, Oken MM, Kaplan ME et al. Distinctive chromosomal abnormalities in histologic subtypes of non-Hodgkin's lymphoma. N Engl J Med 1982; 307: 1231–6.
7. Tsujimoto Y, Finger LR, Ynis J et al. Cloning of the chromosome breakpoint of neoplastic B cells with the t(14;18) chromosome translocation. Science 1984; 226: 1097–9.
8. Bakhshi A, Jensen JP, Goldman P et al. Cloning the chromosomal breakpoint of t(14;18) transcription unit on 18. Cell 1985; 41: 899–906.
9. Cleary ML, Sklar J. Nucleotide sequence of a t(14;18) chromosomal breakpoint in follicular lymphoma and demonstration of a breakpoint cluster region near a transcriptionally active locus on chromosome 18. Proc Natl Acad Sci USA 1985; 82: 7439–43.
10. Lieber MR, Hesse JE, Mizuuchi K et al. Developmental stage specificity of the lymphoid V(D)J recombination activity. Genes Dev 1987; 1: 751–61.
11. Levy S, Campbell MJ, Levy R. Functional immunoglobulin light chain genes are replaced by ongoing rearrangements of germline Vk genes to downstream Jk segments in a murine B cell line. J Exp Med 1989; 170: 1–13.
12. Berinstein N, Levy S, Levy R. Activation of an excluded immunoglobulin allele in a human B lymphoma cell line. Science 1989; 244: 337–9.
13. Kon S, Levy S, Levy R. Retention of an idiotypic determinant in a human B cell lymphoma undergoing immunoglobulin variable-region mutation. Proc Natl Acad Sci USA 1987; 84: 5053–7.
14. Bertoli LF, Kubagawa H, Borzillo GV et al. Bone marrow origin of a B-cell lymphoma. Blood 1988; 72: 94–101.
15. Osmond DG, Park Y-H, Jacobsen K. B cell precursors in bone marrow: in vitro proliferation, localization, stimulation by activated macrophages and implications for oncogenesis. Curr Topics in Micro and Immunol 1988; 141: 2–10.
16. deJong D, Voetdijk BMH, Van Ommen GJB et al. Translocation t(14;18) in B cell lymphomas as a cause for defective immunoglobulin production. J Exp Med 1989; 169: 613–24.
17. Tonegawa S. Somatic generation of antibody diversity. Nature 1983; 302: 575–81.
18. Kipps TJ, Robbins BA, Kuster P et al. Autoantibody-associated cross-reactive idiotypes expressed at high frequency in chronic lymphocytic leukemia relative to B-cell lymphomas of follicular center cell origin. Blood 1988; 72: 422–8.
19. Kiyotaki M, Cooper MD, Bertoli LF et al. Monoclonal anti-Id antibodies react with varying proportions of human B lineage cells. J Immunol 1987; 138: 4150–8.
20. Miller RA, Hart S, Samouszuk M et al. Shared idiotypes expressed by human B cell lymphomas. N Engl J Med 1989; 321: 851–857.
21. Stevenson FK, Wrightam M, Glennie MJ et al. Antibodies to shared idiotypes as agents for analysis and therapy for human B cell tumors. Blood 1986; 68: 430–6.
22. Kipps TJ, Fong S, Romhave E et al. High frequency expression of a conserved K light chain variable region gene in chronic lymphocytic leukemia. Proc Natl Acad Sci USA 1987; 84: 2916–20.
23. Logtenberg T, Schutte MEM, Inghirami G et al. Immunoglobulin VH gene expression in human B cell lines and tumors: Biased VH gene expression in chronic lymphocytic leukemia. Int Immunol 1989; 1: 362–6.
24. Kipps TJ, Tomhave E, Pratt LF et al. Developmentally restricted immunoglobulin heavy chain variable region gene expressed at high frequency in chronic lymphocytic leukemia. Proc Natl Acad Sci USA 1989; 86: 5913–7.
25. Mayer R, Togtenberg T, Strauchen J et al. CD5 and immunoglobulin V gene expression in B-cell lymphomas and chronic lymphocytic leukemia. Blood 1990; 75: 1518–24.
26. Dvoretsky P, Wood GS, Levy R et al. T lymphocyte subsets in follicular lymphomas compared to those in non-neoplastic lymph nodes and tonsils. Human Pathol 1982; 13: 618–25.
27. Garcia CF, Lowder J, Meeker TC et al. Differences in host infiltrates among lymphoma patients treated with anti-idiotype antibodies: Correlation with treatment response. J Immunol 1985; 135: 4252–60.
28. Lowder J, Meeker T, Campbell M et al. Studies on B lymphoid tumors treated with monoclonal anti-idiotype antibodies: Correlation with clinical responses. Blood 1987; 69: 199–210.
29. Umetsu DT, Esserman L, Donlon TA et al. Induction of proliferation of human follicular (B-type) lymphoma cells by cognate interaction with a CD4$^+$ T cell clones. J Immunol 1990; 144: 2550–7.
30. Tweeddale ME, Lim B, Jamal N et al. The presence of clonogenic cells in high-grade malignant lymphoma: a prognostic factor. Blood 1987; 69: 1307–14.
31. Esserman L, Takahashi S, Rojas V et al. An epitope of the transferrin receptor is exposed on the cell surface of highgrade but not lowgrade human lymphomas. Blood 1989; 74: 2718–29.
32. Vaickus L, Levy R. Antiproliferative monoclonal antibodies: Detection and initial characterization. J Immunol 1985; 135: 1987–97.
33. Aruffo A, Seed B. Molecular cloning of a CD28 cDNA by a high-efficiency COS cell expression system. Proc Natl Acad Sci USA 1987; 84: 8573–7.
34. Seed B, Aruffo A. Molecular cloning of the CD2 antigen, the T-cell erythrocyte receptor, by a rapid immunoselection procedure. Proc Natl Acad Sci USA 1987; 84: 3365–9.
35. Oren R, Takahashi S, Doss C et al. TAPA-1, the target of an antiproliferative antibody, defines a new family of transmembrane proteins. Molec Cell Biol 1990; in press.
36. Stevenson GT, Stevenson FK. Antibody to a molecularly-defined antigen confined to a tumour cell surface. Nature 1975; 254: 714–6.
37. Hopper JE, Nissonoff A. Individual antigenic specificity of immunoglobulins. Adv Immunol 1971; 13: 57–99.
38. Miller RA, Maloney DG, Warnke R et al. Treatment of B cell lymphoma with monoclonal anti-idiotype antibody. N Engl J Med 1982; 306: 517–22.
39. Meeker TC, Lowder J, Maloney DG et al. A clinical trial of anti-idiotype therapy for B cell malignancy. Blood 1985; 65: 1349–63.
40. Brown SL, Miller RA, Horning SJ et al. Treatment of B cell lymphoma with anti-idiotype antibodies alone and in combination with alpha interferon. Blood 1989; 3: 651–61.
41. Levy R, Dilley J. Rescue of immunoglobulin secretion from human neoplastic lymphoid cells by somatic cell hybridization. Proc Natl Acad Sci USA 1978; 75: 2411–5.

42. Brown SL, Dilley J, Levy R. Immunoglobulin secretion by mouse × human hybridomas: an approach for the production of anti-idiotype reagents useful in monitoring patients with B cell lymphoma. J Immunol 1980; 125: 1037–43.

43. Carroll WL, Thielemans K, Dilley J et al. Mouse × human heterohybridomas as fusion partners with human B cell tumors. J Immunol Methods 1986; 89: 61–72.

44. Levy R, Levy S, Cleary ML et al. Somatic mutation in human B cell tumors. Immunol Rev 1987; 96: 43–58.

45. Basham TY, Kaminski M, Kitamura K et al. Synergistic antitumor effect of interferon and anti-idiotype monoclonal antibody in murine lymphoma. J Immunol 1986; 137: 3019–24.

46. Berinstein N, Starnes CO, Levy R. Specific enhancement of the therapeutic effect of anti-idiotype antibodies on a murine B cell lymphoma by IL-2. J Immunol 1988; 140: 2839–45.

47. Kaminski MS, Kitamura K, Maloney DG et al. Idiotype vaccination against murine B cell lymphoma. Inhibition of tumor immunity by free idiotype protein. J Immunol 1987; 138: 1289.

48. Allison AC, Byars NE. An adjuvant formulation that selectively elicits the formation of antibodies of protective isotypes and of cell-mediated immunity. J Immunol Methods 1986; 95: 157–

49. Campbell MJ, Esserman L, Levy R. Immunotherapy of established murine B cell lymphoma. Combination of idiotype immunization and cyclophosphamide. J Immunol 1988; 141: 3227–33.

50. The Non-Hodgkin's Lymphoma Pathologic Classification Project. National Cancer Institute Sponsored Study of Classifications of Non-Hodgkin's Lymphomas. Cancer 1982; 49: 2111–35.

51. Tsujimoto Y, Gorham J, Cossman J, Jaffe E, Croce CM. The t(14;18) chromosome translocations involved in B cell neoplasms result from mistakes in VDJ joining. Science 1985; 229: 1390–3.

Annals of Oncology, Supplement 2 to Volume 2: 123–129, 1991.
© 1991 *Kluwer Academic Publishers*.

Orginal article

Follicular lymphomas: Assessment of prognostic factors in 127 patients followed for 10 years

Yves Bastion,[1] Françoise Berger,[2] Paul-André Bryon,[3] Pascale Felman,[4] Martine Ffrench[5] & Bertrand Coiffier[1]

[1]*Service d'Hématologie, Centre Hospitalier Lyon-Sud, Pierre-Bénite;* [2]*Service d'Anatomie Pathologique, Hôpital Edouard-Herriot, Lyon;* [3]*Laboratoire de Cytologie Analytique, Université Claude-Bernard, Lyon;* [4]*Laboratoire d'Hématologie, Centre Hospitalier Lyon-Sud, Pierre-Bénite;* [5]*Service d'Hématologie, Hôpital Edouard-Herriot, Lyon, France*

Summary. Response to treatment, histologic progression, and survival of 127 patients with follicular lymphoma were analyzed according to histologic, clinical, and biological parameters. Histologic parameters were percentage of large cells (<10%, 41 patients; 10–25%, 38 patients; 25–50%, 11 patients; ≥50%, 30 patients), percentage of diffuse areas, presence of intrafollicular proliferation or fibrosis, and mitotic scale. Eighty percent of the patients achieved complete remission (CR) with radiotherapy for localized stages and various chemotherapy regimens for disseminted stages. Three patients did not respond to treatment, and 23 were in partial remission (PR) at the end of treatment. Median survival time was 9.25 years. A constant death rate of 8% per year was observed without plateau. Histologic progression was observed in 32 patients; it occurred at a constant rate during the first six years and plateaued thereafter. Factors associated with low response rate were stage IV, B symptoms, high tumor mass, and two or more extranodal sites. Factors associated with histologic progression were bone marrow involvement and two or more extranodal sites. Factors associated with poor survival were advanced stage, two or more extranodal sites, bone marrow involvement, high lactate dehydrogenase level, and absence of interfollicular fibrosis. The percentages of large cells and diffuse areas had no influence on prognosis, nor had the type of treatment. Median survival has not been reached for CR patients and was four years for PR patients (P < 0.0001). The LNH-84 prognostic index for aggressive lymphomas, based on tumor mass, number of extranodal sites, stage, and LDH level, is a clear-cut indicator of prognosis in follicular lymphomas too. This study shows that the prognosis of follicular lymphoma patients is related to clinical and biological parameters of a high tumor mass and to response to treatment, but not to classical histologic parameters.

Key words: follicular lymphomas, histology, histologic progression, prognostic factors

Follicular lymphomas are defined by the presence of a nodular pattern of proliferation and are derived from normal follicular center cells [1]. According to the Working Formulation [2], three subtypes of follicular lymphomas exist with increasing percentages of large cells: group B, predominantly small cleaved cells; group C, mixed, small and large cleaved cells; and group D, predominantly large cells. Groups B and C are considered low-grade malignant lymphomas, but group D belongs to the intermediate grade and is considered more aggressive. Most patients are asymptomatic at presentation [3], and evolution is characterized by a relatively indolent course; but histologic progression to a more aggressive lymphoma often occurs and bears a poor prognosis [4, 5, 6].

Localized follicular lymphomas can be cured by radiation therapy [7]. However, disseminated disease represents more than 80% of the cases and is rarely curable [3, 8]. No therapeutic approach appears better than others in terms of survival. Follicular mixed lymphomas have been treated with some success with Adriamycin-containing regimens [9, 10, 11], but these results have been debated [12]. Follicular large-cell lymphomas are less frequent but are considered more curable by intensive therapy [13, 14, 15]. The diagnosis of subtype in follicular lymphomas raises problems [16, 17], and it is difficult to decide on a treatment solely on the basis of the histologic subtype. Some patients have been treated with high-dose therapy and bone marrow transplantation [18, 19], but indications for this treatment remain unclear. This emphasizes the importance of prognostic factors in follicular lymphomas in defining prognostic subgroups and their appropriate treatment. Classical prognostic factors are age, tumor mass, B symptoms, and lactate dehydrogenase (LDH) level [7, 15, 20]. Two histologic factors have been described as important for survival: number of large cells [13, 17, 21] and the degree of follicularity [22, 23, 24], but their significance has not been confirmed in all studies [13, 20].

This retrospective study was undertaken to define the prognostic significance of clinical, biological, and histological parameters in 127 patients with follicular lymphoma followed in our department for a median of 10 years.

Material and methods

Patients

From January 1975 to June 1985, 164 patients with a diagnosis of follicular lymphoma have been treated in our department. Thirty-seven patients were not included in this analysis for the following reasons: histologic documentation not available (8 patients); inadequate histologic material (3 patients); lymphoma not follicular after review (26 patients: 4 MALT lymphoma, 22 diffuse pattern). Biopsy sites were a lymph node in 120 patients, a salivary gland in 3, and thyroid, soft tissue, amygdala, and gut in 1 patient each.

All patients had clinical evaluation and chest x-rays. Bone marrow aspiration was performed in 123 patients (97%) and bone marrow biopsy in 120 (94%). All but 4 patients had investigations for periaortic disease: 65% bipedal lymphography, 50% echotomography or CT scan, and 19% laparotomy. Patients were staged according to the Ann Arbor system. The diameter of the largest tumoral mass was divided into 3 categories: <5 cm, 5–10 cm, and >10 cm. Biologic examinations were complete blood count, protein and serum albumin levels, erythrocyte sedimentation rate (ESR), and hepatic enzyme levels in all the patients; serum LDH level was determined in 65% and β2-microglobulin level in 31%.

Histologic parameters

All slides were reviewed for confirmation of diagnosis of follicular lymphoma and complementary analyses (FB, PAB). Percentages of large cleaved and non-cleaved cells were divided subjectively into four classes: <10%, 10 to 25%, 25 to 50%, and >50%. When the cellular composition was heterogeneous from one neoplastic follicle to another, areas with the greatest number of large cells were considered, as proposed by Nathwani [17]. Degree of follicularity was evaluated by the extent of diffuse areas (<10%, 10 to 25%, 25 to 50%, >50%). The presence or absence of intrafollicular pattern of proliferation [1, 24], as well as fibrosis was evaluated. Mitotic activity was subjectively evaluated in 10 high-power fields and was graded from 1 to 3.

Treatment and assessment of response

Patients with stage I or II and a tumor ⩽10 cm were treated with radiotherapy alone (23 cases) or with radiotherapy plus chemotherapy (15 cases). Patients with advanced stage were treated with various chemotherapy regimens (Table 1). From 1981 to 1984, patients received procarbazine, cyclophosphamide, vincristine, and prednisone (PCOP) or procarbazine, Adriamycin, cyclophosphamide, vincristine, and prednisone (PACOP) as part of a prospective randomized trial [25]. Response to treatment was assessed at the end of therapy. Complete response (CR) was defined as the disappearance of all clinical evidence of disease and the normalization of bone marrow. Partial response (PR) was defined as a greater than 50% reduction of the largest dimension of each site of measurable disease or as persistence of bone marrow involvement without other evidence of disease. Failure comprised progressive disease and death during induction therapy.

Table 1. Influence of treatment in the 127 follicular lymphoma patients on response to treatment and survival.

	Number of patients (%)	Percentage of			Expected 10 year survival
		CR	Relapse	Transformation	
All patients	127 (100)	80	47	26	0.49
Radiotherapy	23 (18)	100	52	17	0.62
Chemotherapy					
Clorambucil	7 (6)	100	43	14	0.00
CVP	14 (11)	86	58	21	0.48
PCOP	16 (13)	75	42	19	0.71
CHOP	43 (34)	67	41	35	0.49
PACOP	20 (16)	80	44	25	0.48
Others	4 (3)	50	50	25	–

Statistical methods

Duration of remission was calculated for CR patients from the onset of treatment to the first evidence of relapse or the date when the patient was last known to be free of disease. Survival duration was calculated from the date of the diagnostic biopsy to death or last date known alive. Survival curves were estimated by the method of Kaplan and Meier [26]. Univariate analyses were performed using the χ^2 test and log-rank tests [27]. Statistically significant factors were included in a proportional hazards model regression analysis of survival [28].

Results

Clinical features at presentation

Seventy patients were male and 57 female with a median age of 50.5 years (range 26 to 85). Initial parameters are shown in Table 2. Eighty-nine patients (70%) had stage III or IV disease. Among the 57 patients (45%) with bone marrow involvement, 20 had a bone marrow aspiration considered normal. Fifteen patients had evidence of peripheral blood involvement.

Liver was considered involved in 15 cases: positive biopsy in 7 cases, conjunction of clinical, biological and echotomographic evidence in 8 cases. Splenomegaly or histologic evidence of splenic localization was found in 34 cases (27%).

Histologic parameters

Forty-one patients had less than 10% of large cells, 38 patients 10–25% of large cells, 11 patients had 25–50%, and 30 patients had more than 50% of large cells. Six patients had a mantle-zone lymphoma [29]. Large cleaved cells were predominent in 7 patients and present in 5 others. Fifty-seven patients (48%) had a pure follicular pattern of proliferation, and 20 patients had more than 50% of diffuse areas. A diffuse pattern was more common with increasing percentage of large cells but the association was not statistically significant. An intrafollicular pattern of proliferation was seen in 35 patients (28%) without any correlation with the percentage of large cells. Mitotic rate was determined in 115 patients. A highly significant correlation was found between a high mitotic activity and the percentage of large cells ($\chi^2 = 38.6$, $P < 0.0001$) or the percentage of diffuse areas ($\chi^2 = 14.41$, $P < 0.05$). Interfollicular fibrosis was present in 65 cases and was not correlated with percentage of large cells, diffuse areas, or mitotic rate. Mitotic rate was the only morphologic parameter correlated with clinical or biological parameters: a high mitotic rate was associated with high LDH level ($\chi^2 = 6.1$, $P < 0.05$) and large tumor mass ($\chi^2 = 11.8$, $P < 0.05$).

Response to treatment

One hundred one patients (80%) achieved CR; 23 patients (18%) were in PR; and 3 patients failed to respond to treatment. No real difference was seen in response rate according to type of treatment (Table 1). Table 2 shows the response rate according to some initial clinical parameters. Factors statistically associated with a low response rate were stage IV, presence of B symptoms (particularly weight loss), large tumor mass, or more than one extranodal site (particularly bone marrow involvement with a high percentage of lymphoma cells). None of the morphological parameters studied was associated with a lower response rate (Table 3).

Survival

The median survival time was 9.25 years. Figure 1 shows that no plateau was obtained, with a constant death rate of 8% each year. Four patients were lost to follow-up before five years. Five patients died in CR (3 from myelodysplastic syndrome or secondary acute leukemia, 2 from solid tumor). Clinical and biological parameters staistically associated with poorer survival were B symptoms, advanced stage, two or more extra-

Table 2. Influence of initial clinical and biological parameters in the 127 follicular lymphoma patients on response to treatment and survival.

	Number of patients (%)	Percentage of			Expected 10 year survival
		CR	Relapse	Transformation	
Age					
<50 y	62 (49)	79	43	50	0.58
50–65 y	36 (28)	81	55	34	0.46
≥65 y	29 (23)	79	43	16	0.33
Stage					
I	18 (14)	100	50	6	0.55
II	20 (16)	100	40	16	0.63
III	26 (20)	92	42	9	0.76
IV	63 (50)	62[c]	51	35	0.32[c]
B symptoms	15 (12)	47[c]	29	40	0.27[a]
Weight loss					
≥10%	14 (11)	43[c]	17	43	0.34
Tumor mass					
<5 cm	67 (54)	90	48	22	0.53
5–10 cm	39 (32)	72	43	33	0.54
≥10 cm	17 (14)	53[b]	44	18	0.22
Number of extranodal sites					
0–1	103 (81)	87	48	21	0.57
≥2	24 (19)	46[c]	36	42[a]	0.18[c]
Bone marrow localization					
Yes	57 (48)	60[c]	47	35[a]	0.33[c]
Percentage of lymphoma cells in bone marrow					
<5	96 (76)	86	47	24	0.55
5–20	20 (16)	75	40	25	0.45
≥20	11 (9)	27[c]	67	36	0.15
LDH level					
Normal	65 (79)	83	37	25	0.59
>normal	17 (21)	59	50	29	0.00[c]
Serum albumin level					
<35 g/L	15 (14)	47	71	40	0.12
≥35 g/L	89 (86)	84[b]	33	22	0.55[c]
β2-microglobulin level					
<3 mg/L	28 (76)	89	40	32	0.69
≥3 mg/L	9 (24)	56	60	33	0.22[b]

[a] $P < 0.05$, [b] $P < 0.01$, [c] $P < 0.001$.

nodal sites, bone marrow involvement, high LDH level, and low serum albumin level (Table 2). Neither the percentage of large cells and of diffuse areas nor the type of treatment influenced overall survival (Tables 1 and 3, Fig. 2). This was not explained by a difference in therapy for patients with a greater percentage of large cells. Interfollicular fibrosis was associated with a longer survival (log-rank test $\chi^2 = 7.48$, $P = 0.006$). Median survival has not been reached for patients in CR after treatment and was four years for patients in PR (Fig. 3). This advantage for CR patients persisted after stratification for other significant prognostic factors (stage, B

Table 3. Influence of morphologic parameters in the 127 follicular lymphoma patients on response to treatment and survival.

	Number of patients (%)	Percentage of			Expected 10 year survival
		CR	Relapse	Transformation	
Percentage of large cells					
<10	41 (34)	73	50	24	0.47
10–25	38 (32)	87	48	26	0.49
25–50	11 (9)	82	56	36	0.53
≥50	30 (25)	77	43	23	0.49
Percentage of diffuse areas					
<10	58 (48)	78	47	22	0.53
10–25	20 (17)	90	50	30	0.43
25–50	23 (19)	78	44	26	0.53
≥50	20 (17)	75	60	35	0.27
Intrafollicular proliferation					
Yes	35 (28)	86	23	14	0.63
No	92 (72)	77	56[b]	29	0.43
Mitotic scale					
1	48 (42)	77	43	15	0.47
2	54 (47)	81	61	41	0.44
3	13 (11)	77	40	23	0.50
Fibrosis					
No	62 (49)	77	60	32	0.38
Yes	65 (51)	82	34[a]	18	0.58[b]

[a] $P < 0.05$, [b] $P < 0.01$, [c] $P < 0.001$.

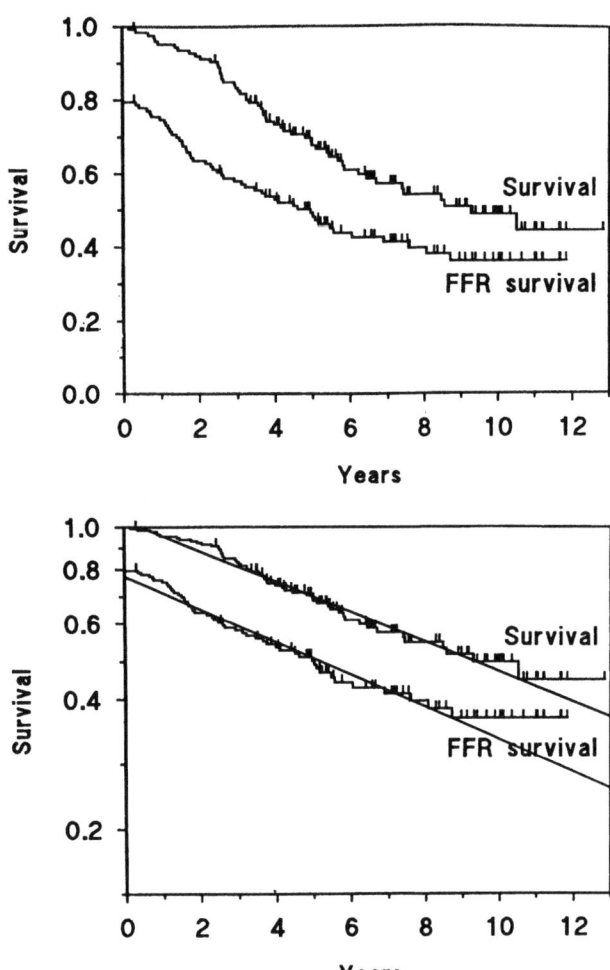

Fig. 1. (A) Survival and freedom-from-relapse (FFR) of the 127 patients with follicular lymphoma. (B) The same data expressed in semilogarithmic scale showing the constant death and relapse rates.

symptoms, tumor mass, number of extranodal sites, LDH level, and fibrosis).

Relapse and histologic progression
Forty-seven patients relapsed (47%) with a median freedom from relapse (FFR) survival of 7.5 years (Fig. 1). None of the clinical or biological parameters was associated with a higher relapse rate (Table 2). An intrafollicular pattern of proliferation was associated with a lower relapse rate (Table 3) and a longer FFR survival (log-rank test $\chi^2 = 9.92$, $P = 0.0016$). A higher relapse rate was associated with a high mitotic scale or absence of interfollicular fibrosis (Table 3).

Progression to a more aggressive lymphoma was diagnosed in 24 patients, 19 on histologic and 5 on cytologic grounds. Such a progression was thought likely to be present in 8 other patients because of a rapidly growing tumor with high LDH level and impaired performance status or extranodal location, but it was not documented. These 32 patients represent 26% of all the patients and 46% of the patients who progressed. Transformation occurred in 52% of the PR patients and in 20% of the CR patients ($\chi^2 = 11.45$, $P = 0.003$). The probability of transformation was constant during the first six years of follow-up then decreased rapidly (Fig. 4). Seventy-five percent of these transformations occurred before four years, and none was observed after nine years (30 patients at risk). Factors affecting

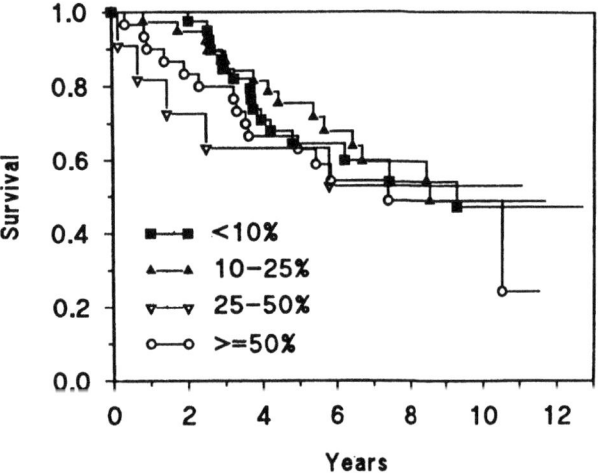

Fig. 2. Survival of the patients with follicular lymphoma according to the percentage of large cells. The 6 patients with mantle-zone lymphoma are not included. No statistical difference exists between the four groups of patients (log-rank test $\chi^2 = 0.9$).

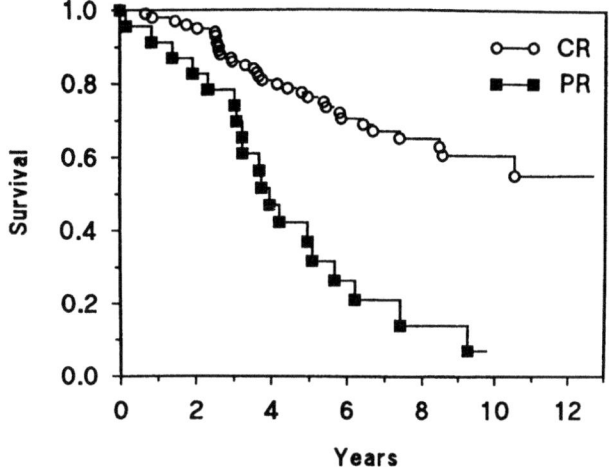

Fig. 3. Survival of the 124 patients with follicular lymphoma according to response to treatment (log-rank test χ^2 = 25.20, P < 0.0001). Response was determined at the end of treatment whatever its duration. The 3 patients who did not respond are not included.

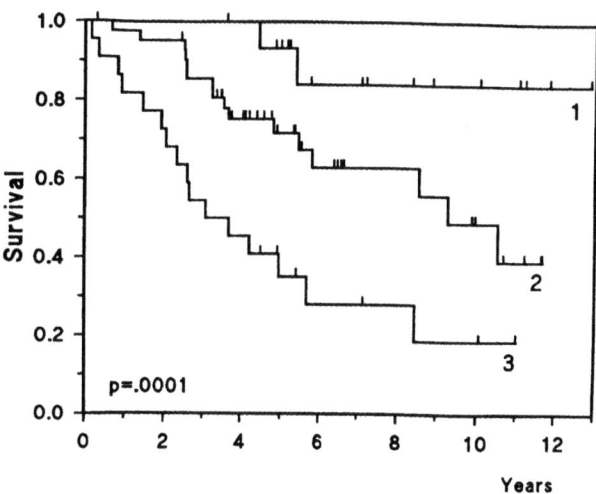

Fig. 5. Survival of the 127 patients with follicular lymphoma according to the prognostic index described for aggressive lymphomas based on stage, tumor mass, number of extranodal sites and LDH level (30) (log-rank test χ^2 = 18.19, P = 0.0001).

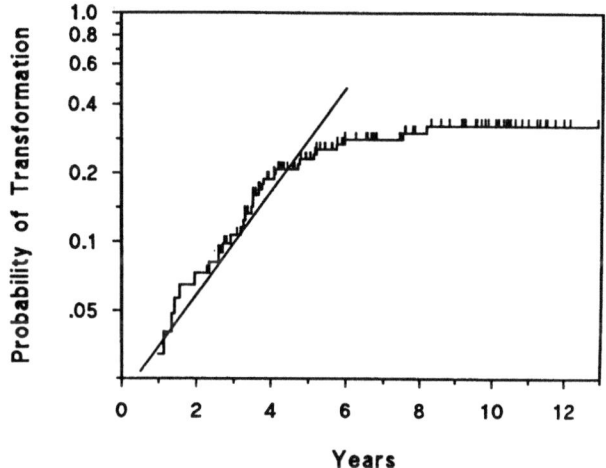

Fig. 4. Probability of histologic progression in the 127 patients with follicular lymphomas. The semilogarithmic scale shows the constant probability during the first years of follow-up.

the occurrence of histologic progression were bone marrow involvement and two or more extranodal sites (Table 2). Initial treatment did not influence the rate of transformation.

After transformation, the median survival was 5.5 months. Two patients are still alive in subsequent CR with a follow-up of 11 and 35 months after transformation (1 received massive chemotherapy and autologous bone marrow transplantation).

Multiparametric studies

Parameters statistically associated with poor survival in multiparametric regression analyses were high LDH level (P = 0.0002), absence of fibrosis (P =0.0004), two or more extranodal sites (P = 0.0239), and stage IV (P = 0.0743). A high risk of histologic progression was

associated with absence of fibrosis (P = 0.0003) and two or more extranodal sites (P = 0.0006). The index described for aggressive lymphoma patients [30] based on LDH level, stage, tumor mass and number of extranodal sites was very useful in discriminating high-risk patients (Fig. 5).

Discussion

Clinical characteristics and evolution of our patients are consistent with other series of follicular lymphomas. Median survival is not radically different from the six- to eight-year range generally observed [2, 7, 9, 11, 15]. The absence of a difference between therapeutic approaches was largely confirmed in advanced follicular small cleaved cells by randomized studies [8, 31]. These results are more controversial in follicular mixed lymphomas where prolonged remissions have been reported [10,11] but not confirmed in randomized studies [12]. This study confirms that patients who reached a CR have a longer survival [11, 20, 25] and have a lower risk of histologic progression. Although it was not confirmed by randomized studies, this point favors the intensification of treatment in subgroup(s) of patients.

Histologic subclassification of follicular lymphomas is often subjective. There is no agreement among pathologists, and in the Working Formulation, this subclassification is based on estimates of the percentage of large cells [2]. Actual counts of large cells have been proposed [17, 32] but their reproducibility is uncertain. In our study, subclassification was based on subjective assessment of the percentage of large cells within follicles with thresholds at 10%, 25%, and 50%. The absence of statistical correlation between the percentage of large cells and the outcome is one of the most striking results, but has already been described by others [17]. We found more patients with large cell lymphoma than other series [2, 7, 19] probably because we analyzed the percentage of large cells in follicles with the higher proportion of large cells, as proposed by Nathwani [17]. Ezdinli [22] found that the presence of diffuse areas implied a poor prognosis specimens, but we and others [12, 33] did not verify these results. Moreover, when two or more biopsies were obtained in the same patient, the percentage of diffuse areas varied from one location to another [23]. An intrafollicular pattern of proliferation probably reflects a new lesion and is correlated with a longer FFR survival. A computer-based analytic and morphometric study of lymphoma cells is currently in progress to see if any histologic prognostic parameters can be found.

The reported frequency of histologic progression ranges from 10% to 60% depending on the duration of follow-up, frequency of rebiopsies, and inclusion of autopsy data. Some results are reported for patients who had a new biopsy and others for patients with progressive disease, making comparisons difficult. None of the previous studies found a constant rate for transformation or a decrease in frequency after six years of follow-up. A higher rate of histologic progression in PR patients has been reported [11]. Although we did not observe any plateau for overall survival, the decrease of transformation rate after six years and the small plateau observed for FFR survival after nine years are tiny promisis for cure in a subgroup of patients. A longer follow-up would confirm this point.

Our study identified a subgroup of patients with a shorter survival and a higher risk of histologic progression. These patients are characterized by two or more extranodal sites (particularly bone marrow), stage IV with B symptoms, high LDH level, absence of fibrosis, and partial response to treatment. The prognostic index described for aggressive lymphomas [30] can identify these patients with poorer outcome. New strategies, particularly intensive chemotherapy with autologous bone marrow rescue [18, 19], must be tested for patients with these characteristics.

Acknowledgements

Supported by grants from the Comité Départemental du Rhône de la Ligue Nationale contre le Cancer.

References

1. Lukes RJ, Collins RD. Immunologic characterization of human malignant lymphomas. Cancer 1974; 34: 1488–1503.
2. The non-Hodgkin's lymphoma pathologic classification project. National Cancer Institute sponsored study of classifications of non-Hodgkin's lymphomas. Summary and description of a Working Formulation for clinical usage. Cancer 1982; 49: 2112–2135.
3. Jones SE. Follicular lymphoma. Do no harm. Cancer Treat Rep 1986; 70: 1055–1058.
4. Acker B, Hoppe RT, Colby TV et al. Histologic conversion in the non-Hodgkin's lymphomas. J Clin Oncol 1983; 1: 11–16.
5. Garvin AJ, Simon RM, Osborne CK et al. An autopsy study of histologic progression in non-Hodgkin's lymphomas. 192 cases from the National Cancer Institute. Cancer 1983; 52: 393–398.
6. Coiffier B, Sebban C, Berger F et al. Transformation histologique des syndromes lymphoprolifératifs de faible malignité. Etude clinique et évolutive de 32 cas. Presse Med 1985; 14: 1229–1236.
7. Gospodarowicz MK, Bush Rs, Brown TC et al. Prognostic factors in nodular lymphomas: a multivariate analysis based on the Pricess Margaret Hospital experience. Int J Radiat Oncol Biol Phys 1984; 10: 489–497.
8. Hoppe RT, Kushlan P, Kaplan HS et al. The treatment of advanced stage favorable histology non-Hodgkin's lymphoma: A preliminary report of a randomized trial comparing single agent chemotherapy, combination chemotherapy and whole body irradiation. Blood 1981; 58: 592–598.
9. Anderson T, Bender RA, Fisher RI et al. Combination chemotherapy in non-Hodgkin's lymphoma: results of long-term follow-up. Cancer Treat Rep 1977; 61: 1057–1066.
10. Ezdinli EZ, Costello WFG, Icli F et al. Nodular mixed lymphocytic histiocytic lymphoma. Response and survival. Cancer 1980; 45: 261–267.
11. Longo DL, Young RC, Hubbard SM et al. Prolonged initial remission in patients with nodular mixed lymphoma. Ann Intern Med 1984; 100: 651–656.
12. Glick JH, Barnes JM, Ezdinli EZ et al. Nodular mixed lymphoma: results of a randomized trial failing to confirm prolonged disease-free survival with COPP chemotherapy. Blood 1981; 58: 920–925.
13. Osborne CK, Norton L, Young RC et al. Nodular histiocytic lymphoma: An aggressive nodular lymphoma with potential for prolonged disease-free survival. Blood 1980; 56: 98–103.
14. Horning SJ, Weiss LM, Nevitt JB et al. Clinical and pathologic features of follicular large cell (nodular histiocytic) lymphoma. Cancer 1987; 59: 1470–1474.
15. Kantarjian HM, McLaughlin P, Fuller LM et al. Follicular large cell lymphoma: analysis and prognostic factors in 62 patients. J Clin Oncol 1984; 2: 811–819.
16. Metter GE, Nathwani BN, Burke JS et al. Morphological subclassification of follicular lymphoma: variability of diagnoses among hematopathologists. A collaborative study between the Repository Center and Pathology Panel for Lymphoma Clinical Studies. J Clin Oncol 1985; 1: 25–38.
17. Nathwani BN, Metter GE, Miller TP et al. What should be the morphologic criteria for the subdivision of follicular lymphomas? Blood 1986; 68: 837–845.
18. Takvorian T, Canellos GP, Ritz J et al. Prolonged disease-free survival after autologous bone marrow transplantation in patients with non-Hodgkin's lymphoma with a poor prognosis. N Engl J Med 1987; 316: 1499–1505.
19. Schouten HC, Bierman PJ, Vaughan WP et al. Autologous bone marrow transplantation in follicular non-Hodgkin's lymphoma before and after histologic transformation. Blood 1989; 74: 2579–2584.
20. Glick JH, McFadden E, Costello W et al. Nodular histiocytic lymphoma: factors influencing prognosis and implications for aggressive chemotherapy. Cancer 1982; 49: 840–845.
21. Anderson T, DeVita VT, Simon RM et al. Malignant lymphoma. II. Prognostic factors and response to treatment of 473 patients at the National Cancer Institute. Cancer 1982; 50: 2708–2721.
22. Ezdinli EZ, Costello WG, Kucuk O et al. Effect of the degree of nodularity on the survival of patients with nodular lymphomas. J Clin Oncol 1987; 5: 413–418.
23. Warnke RA, Kim H, Fuks Z et al. The coexistence of nodular and diffuse patterns in nodular non-Hodgkin's lymphomas. Significance and clinicopathologic correlation. Cancer 1977; 40: 1229–1233.

24. Schultz HB, Ersboll J, Hougaard P. Prognostic significance of architectural patters in non-Hodgkin's lymphomas. Scand J Haematol 1985; 35: 270–283.

25. Lepage E, Sebban C, Gisselbrecht C et al. Treatment of low-grade non-Hodgkin's lymphomas: assessment of doxorubicin in a controlled trial. Hematol Oncol 1990; 8: 31–39.

26. Kaplan EL, Meier P. Nonparametric estimation for incomplete observations. J Amer Stat Assoc 1958; 53: 157–181.

27. Cox DR. The analysis of binary data. New York, Chapman and Hall, 1970.

28. Cox DR. Regression models and life tables. J Roy Stat Soc [B] 1972; 34: 187–202.

29. Weisenburger DD, Kim H, Rappaport H. Mantle-zone lymphoma: A follicular variant of intermediate lymphocytic lymphoma. Cancer 1982; 49: 1429–1438.

30. Coiffier B, Gisselbrecht C, Vose JM et al. Prognostic factors in aggressive malignant lymphomas: description and validation of a prognostic index that could identify patients requiring a more intensive therapy. J Clin Oncol 1990: to be published.

31. Jacobs P, King HS. A randomized prospective comparison of chemotherapy to total body irradiation as initial treatment for the indolent lymphoproliferative diseases. Blood 1987; 69: 1642–1646.

32. Mann RB, Berard CW. Criteria for the cytologic subclassification of follicular lymphomas: a proposed alternative method. Hematol Oncol 1983; 1: 187–192.

33. Hu E, Weiss LM, Hoppe RT et al. Follicular and diffuse mixed small-cleaved and large-cell lymphoma. A clinicopathologic study. J Clin Oncol 1985; 3: 1183–1187.

Correspondence to:
Professeur B. Coiffier
Hematology Service
Centre Hospitalier Lyon-Sud
69310 Pierre-Bénite, France

Annals of Oncology, Supplement 2 to Volume 2: 131–135, 1991.
© 1991 *Kluwer Academic Publishers.*

Original article ⎯⎯⎯⎯⎯⎯⎯⎯⎯⎯⎯⎯⎯⎯⎯⎯⎯⎯

The management of follicular lymphoma

T. A. Lister

Department of Medical Oncology, St. Bartholomew's Hospital, London, United Kingdom

Introduction

Fifty years ago, when irradiation was the only treatment available, Symmers recorded that giant follicular lymphadenopathy (Brill-Symmers Disease) could be manifest in four ways [1]. It could follow a relatively benign remitting-recurring course, without change in histology; a leukaemic picture could develop; or evolution into a sarcomatous form, or even Hodgkin's disease, could occur. Shortly thereafter, Gall and Mallory showed the median survival to be five years [2]. It is clear today, that despite the introduction of an array of cytotoxic chemicals into the therapeutic armamentarium, the two main patterns of persistent follicular lymphoma and blastic transformation still dominate the clinical course of the disease.

Few patients have been cured, even though the median survival has been extended to nine years [3] with the approaches adopted during the last two decades. The experience at a single centre over this period is presented below, to provide the background against which to evaluate the most recent trials and reflect upon their chances of success.

Patterns of survival at St. Bartholomew's Hospital

All patients

One hundred forty-seven previously untreated adults, presenting to St. Bartholomew's Hospital between 1972 and 1983, with follicular lymphoma diagnosed by Dr. A. G. Stansfeld, form the basis of the most recent analysis. Clinical stage was determined by conventional methods, and treatment recommended according to the protocols of the day, as previously described. Fifty-three patients are still alive, with 94 having died, only 18 of causes unrelated to lymphoma. The overall survival cure is shown in Figure 1, with a minimum follow-up of seven years. Survival according to initial stage is shown in Figure 2, deaths due to other causes (n = 18) having been excluded. A significant difference in survival pattern between 'early' and 'late' stage is demonstrated. This difference is not apparent, or significant, if all causes of death are included.

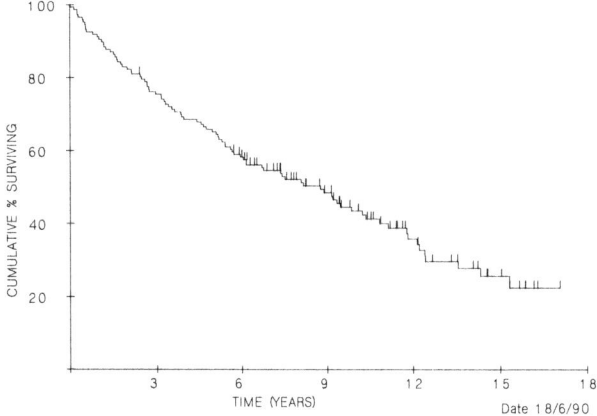

Fig. 1. Survival of 147 previously untreated adults with follicular lymphoma.

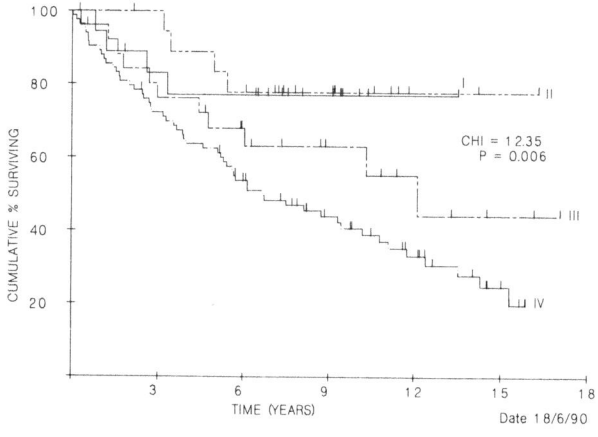

Fig. 2. Correlation between survival and stage (censored for 18 'other' causes of death).

Stage III + IV only

(i) Patients and therapy. One hundred ten patients (75%) had stage III or IV disease, for which chemotherapy was the treatment of choice; the remainder of the analysis including the figures, refers only to them. There were three 'eras' of therapy. During the first, chlorambucil was compred with cyclical combination chemotherapy using cyclophosphamide, vincristine,

and prednisone (CVP); during the second, chlorambucil was allocated according to risk factors determined previously, and during the third chlorambucil was the treatment for all but a few patients who received experimental treatment before chlorambucil. All treatment was short term and the survival for the patients treated during these eras was the same. They have accordingly been presented as a single group. A management policy of short-term therapy followed by observation with rebiopsy and restaging at relapse to determine further therapy was pursued throughout. Response to therapy was defined as previously described [3].

(ii) Response to therapy and duration of response. It was possible to induce repeated remission with a high frequency [3]. The duration of first and subsequent remission is shown in Figure 3. This confirms the remitting and recurring patterns of the disease, provided that the histology is unchanged, with the results only deteriorating significantly after three remissions. It is important to note, however, that a small proportion remain in continuous remission, even with the relatively modest treatment prescribed.

(iii) Survival according to response to first and second therapy. Survival correlated closely with response to both first (Figure 4) and second therapy (not shown):

on neither occasion was there any difference between survival of patients for whom complete remission (CR) or good partial remission (GPR) was achieved.

(iv) Survival from first and subsequent relapse, provided that the histological pattern remained follicular, is shown in Figure 5. This pattern of survival may be contrasted with that following transformation at any time (Figure 6); survival from remission (after initial therapy or subsequent therapy at relapse) is shown in Figure 7.

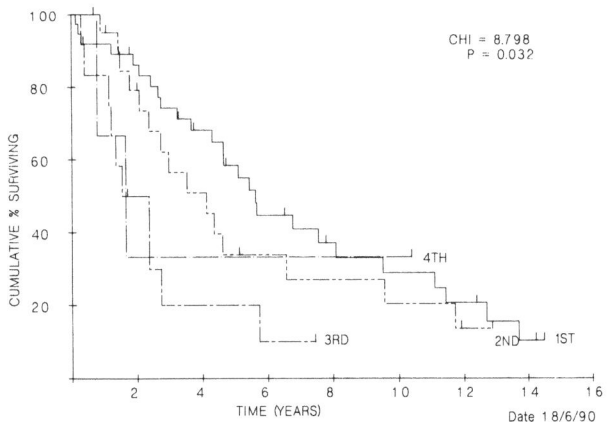

Fig. 5. Survival from first and subsequent relapse (follicular lymphoma only).

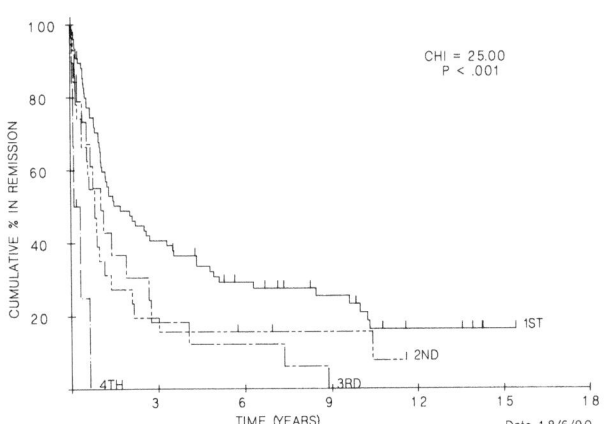

Fig. 3. Duration of first and subsequent remissions (CR and GPR).

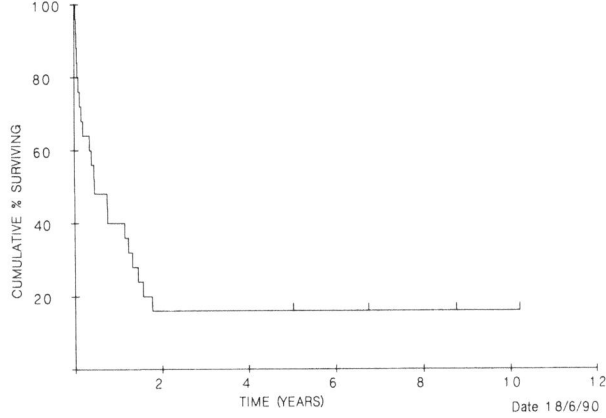

Fig. 6. Survival from transformation at any time.

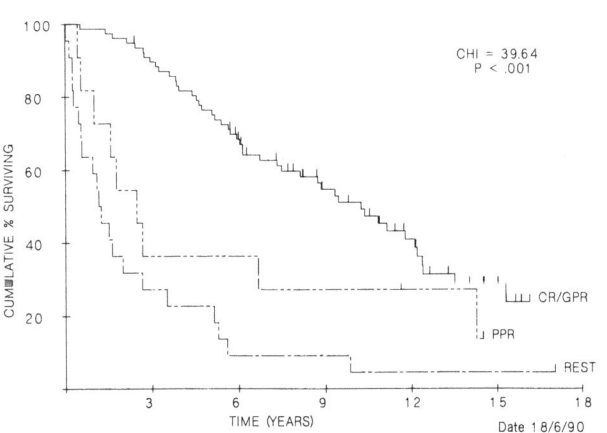

Fig. 4. Correlation between survival and response to initial therapy.

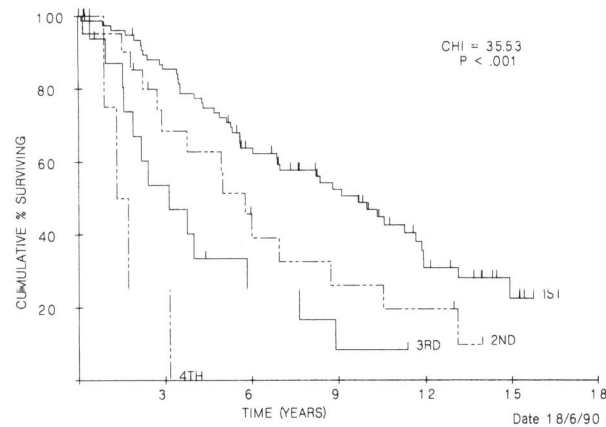

Fig. 7. Survival from first and subsequent remission (CR and GPR).

These results suggest strongly that the effect of the treatments was relatively modest and that for most patients the natural history of the disease was changed only marginally. This does not of course mean that the treatment was not to the benefit of the patients, but indicates that better could be done. Studies conducted elsewhere tend to confirm this interpretation. A randomized trial conducted at Stanford [4] yielded higher remission rates with longer administration of single-agent chemotherapy (cyclophosphamide) or CVP, but no statistical difference between the two treatments. The survival curves were identical to those shown above, and similar results have been achieved by others [5]. Prolonged administration of chlorambucil as 'maintenance' of remission achieved with CVP increased remission duration, but had no influence on survival in a trial conducted at the Christie Hospital, Manchester [6]. The introduction of anthracycline antibiotics into combination chemotherapy did not yield significantly higher CR rates (77%) [7] than reported for others treated with CVP. More important, the survival patterns, overall, are no better following cyclophosphamide, Adriamycin, vincristine, and prednisone (CHOP) as initial therapy than for any less intensive treatment except possibly for the small group of patients whose lymphomas contain a relatively high proportion of blast cells [8, 9, 10].

All these results argue strongly in favour of the 'watch and wait' policy emanating from Stanford, whereby treatment is only instituted if there is a strong clinical indication [11]. Since cure is the primary objective and since obvious regressions are achieved relatively easily for the majority of patients, it is tempting to ask whether the patients predicted to do best (who are not treated de horo) might be the group to treat most intensively. The trial testing this hypothesis is in progress at the National Cancer Institute, Bethesda and compares a watch-and-wait policy with intensive chemotherapy using prednisone, methotrexate, Adriamycin, cyclophosphamide, and etoposide (VP-16) plus nitrogen mustard, vincristine, procarbazine, and prednisone (ProMACE-MOPP) at initial presentation [12]. The preliminary analysis revealed an advantage in terms of freedom from recurrence for those treated intensively at presentation. There was no overall survival advantage, but accrual to the study and follow-up continue. The result will obviously be of great importance.

Alternatives

(i) Interferon, interferon and chlorambucil. Alpha-Interferon (IFNα) has been shown to cause regression of lymphadenopathy with minimal toxicity in patients with follicular lymphoma when given over a prolonged period in low doses. The response rate (CR plus PR) is approximately 40%, being highest for previously untreated patients [13–16].

Based on data suggestive of synergy between interferon and cytotoxic chemotherapy for treatment of murine leukaemia and lymphoma, as well as human cancer in nude mice [17–21], and given the possibility of extrapolation to lymphoma in humans, a phase II trial was conducted at St. Bartholowmew's Hospital to test the feasibility of administering the combination of IFNα and chlorambucil [22]. The result was considered promising enought to warrant the initiation of a randomized trial in which chlorambucil is compared with chlorambucil and IFNα as initial therapy for stage III and IV follicular lymphoma, with a further randomisation to IFNα or no further therapy for those patients for whom remission is achieved. Interim results from this collaborative trial between St. Bartholomew's Hospital, the Christie Hospital and the Queen Elizabeth Hospital, Birmingham, into which 120 patients have been entered, indicate that the response rates are the same but that there is a significant advantage in terms of remission duration for patients receiving maintenance IFNα. No survival advantage has yet emerged [23].

(ii) Bone marrow ablative therapy. It may be postulated that the administration of very high doses of treatment known to cause regression of lymphoma, and theoretically highly active against resting cells, might be the best way to consolidate remission and possibly cure patients whose remission and subsequent survival would otherwise be brief. Since cyclophosphamide and total body irradiation are a well-tried combination, and autologous bone marrow transplantation has been shown to be able to rescue patients from such therapy, it was selected as the treatment of choice. Since in vitro treatment of bone marrow with antibody and complement directed against potential residual lymphomatous infiltration had been shown to be safe [24] and since it confers an obvious potential advantage, it was incorporated into the treatment programme, regardless of the fact that its efficacy would be hard to prove. It was elected to test the treatment, not in first remission (at which point the median survival was 12 years) but at second, or subsequent remission. Thirty-eight patients have been treated to date, in complete remission or in a maximum response, minimal disease state. Recurrence has occurred in 8 so far, with a median follow-up of two years, and a treatment-related mortality of 5–10% [25].

Much longer follow-up is required to determine whether either of these approaches will result in a change in the overall survival pattern of patients with follicular lymphoma, by their incorporation into its management either early or late in the course of the disease.

Other treatments are being tested in patients with refractory disease to determine whether they have enough 'activity' to warrant further study. Perhaps the most promising new chemotherapy agent is fludarabine, known to cause complete remission of chronic lymphatic leukaemia. Several studies [26–28] have shown remissions to be induced in approximately 40%

of patients with follicular lymphoma, the treatment being well tolerated. Antibody therapy alone or conjugated to radioisotope or immunotoxins is being evaluated in phase I and II trials, and benefit has been reported for selected patients [29–32]. α-Calcidol has been shown to induce remissions and is being tested as maintenance therapy [33].

It may not be possible to demonstrate a potential major role for such new treatments without their being tested at specific points in the course of the disease, prior to the developments of resistance to conventional therapy.

New studies

The major trials recently conceived to test new ways of influencing the survival pattern of patients with follicular lymphoma by modifying the nature of their initial treatment are shown in Tables 1, 2, and 3. They reveal a polarisation of interest from very intensive therapy on the one extreme to a biological approach on the other. Studies addressing the management of initial (refractory) or later (recurrent) disease are not easy to identify.

Table 1. More is better (and needs to be).

1. CVP	→ CY/TBI + ABMT	STANFORD
2. CHOP	→ CY/TBI + ABMT	DFCI (Nadler)
3. ProMACE-MOPP	↗ CY/TBI + ABMT ↘ RT	MSKI

Table 2. Biology is beautiful.

1. CYCLO ± IFNα		CALGB
2. COPA		ECOG
	→ IFNα vs 0	
3. CVP		EORTC
4. PDM		LOW GRADE GERMAN GROUP

Table 3. The Texas solution (SWOG).

ProMACE-MOPP → CR	↗ IFNα ↘ 0

The rationale and the justification for these trials may be debated. They must be seen as applying to selected patients by virtue of their toxicities and within the context of other studies in progress and their differing relevance to those at the extremes of the age range of the population at risk. They will be judged on their design and perceived chances of providing an unequivocal answer, and finally whether or not they result in a change in the clinical course of the disease described by Symmers [1].

All treatment, however, is not administered with curative intent. The palliative role of all therapeutic options at the different points of the natural history of the disease and the potential benefits must also be evaluated fully to enable the physician to select the best therapy for any given patient.

Acknowledgements

I am grateful to Jackie Lim for providing the data and Sian Evans for typing the manuscript.

References

1. Symmers D. Giant follicular lymphadenopathy with or without splenomegaly. Arch Path 1938; 26: 603.
2. Gall EA, Mallory TB. Malignant lymphoma: A clinicopathological survey of 618 cases. Am J Path 1942; 18: 381.
3. Gallagher CJ, Gregory WM, Jones AE et al. Follicular lymphoma: Prognostic factors for response and survival. J Clin Oncol 1986; 4: 1470–1480.
4. Portlock CS, Rosenberg SA, Glatstein E, Kaplan HS. Treatment of advanced non-Hodgkin's lymphoma with favorable histologies: Preliminary results of a prospective trial. Blood 1976; 47, 5: 747.
5. Kaufman JH, Ezdinli E, Aungst CW, Stutzman L. Lymphosarcoma: A comparison of extended to conservative therapy. Cancer 1976; 37: 1283.
6. Steward WP, Crowther D, McWilliam LJ et al. Maintenance Chlorambucil after CVP in the management of advanced stage, low grade histologic type non-Hodgkin's lymphoma. Cancer 1988; 61, 3: 441–447.
7. McKelvey EM, Gottlieb JA, Wilson HE et al. Hydroxydaunomycin (Adriamycin) combination chemotherapy in malignant lymphoma. Cancer 36; 2: 428.
8. Dana B, Dahlberge S, Miller T et al. Long-term follow-up of patients with low grade lymphoma treated with CHOP (Cyclophosphamide, Doxorubicin, Vincristine, Prednisolone)-based chemotherapy or chemoimmunotherapy on southwest oncology group studies. Proc ASCO (1989), abstract 1001.
9. Fisher RI, Dahlberg S, Miller TP et al. Long term survival of patients with nodular histiocytic diffuse poorly differentiated lymphocytic diffuse mised and diffuse unditferentiated lymphoma treated with CHOP chemotherapy. ASO Proceedings (1989), abstract 1002.
10. Peterson BA, Anderson JR, Frizzera G et al. Combination chemotherapy prolongs survival in follicular mixed lymphoma (FML). ASCO Proceedings (1990), abstract 1004.
11. Portlock CS, Rosenberg SA. Chemotherapy of the non-Hodgkin's lymphomas: The Stanford Experience. Cancer Treatment Report 1977; 61, 6: 1049.
12. Young RC, Longo DL, Glatstein E et al. The treatment of indolent lymphomas: Watchful waiting vs aggressive combined modality treatment. Sem Hem 1988; 255 2 Suppl. 2, 11.
13. Gutterman JU, Blumenschien GR, Alexanina R et al. Leucocyte interferon-induced tumor regression in human metastatic breast cancer, multiple myeloma and malignant lymphoma. Ann Intern Med 1980; 93: 388.
14. Louie AC, Gallagher JG, Sikora K et al. Follow-up observations of the effect of human leucocyte interferon in non-Hodgkin's lymphoma. Blood 1981; 58: 712.
15. Ozer H, Leavitt R, Ratanatharathern V et al. Experience in the use of DNA alpha interferon in the treatment of malignant lymphomas. Blood 1983; 62, 1: 2149.
16. Wagstaff J, Lynds P, Crowther D. A phase II study of human recombinant DA α2 interferon in patients with low-grade non-Hodgkin's lymphoma. Cancer Chemoth and Pharmacol 1986; 18: 54.

17. Chirigos MA, Pearson JW. Cure of murien leukaemia with drug and interferon treatment JNCI 1973; 51: 1367.
18. Gresser I, Muary C, Tovery M. Efficacy of combined interferon cyclophosphamide therapy after diagnosis of lymphoma in AKR mice. Eur J Cancer 1978; 14: 97.
19. Slater WM, Wetzel MW, Cesario T. Combined interferon-antimetabolite therapy of murine L1210 leukaemia. Cancer 1981; 48: 5.
20. Mowshowitz SL, Chin-Bow ST, Smith GD. Interferon and Cis-DPP: Combination chemotherapy for P388 leukaemia in CDFI mice. J Inf Res 182; 2: 587.
21. Balkwill FR, Moodie EM. Positive interactions between human interferon and cyclophosphamide or adriamycin in a human tumor model system. Cancer Res 1984; 44: 904.
22. Rohatiner AZS, Richards MA, Barnett MJ et al. Chlorambucil and Interferon for low-grade non-Hodgkin's lymphoma. Brit J Canc 1987; 55: 437.
23. Price CGE, Rohatiner AZS, Steward W et al. Interferon-α_{2b} as initial therapy in combination with Chlorambucil and as maintenance therapy in follicular lymphoma. Annals of Oncology, 1990; (in press).
24. Nadler LM et al. Anti-B1 monoclonal antibody and complement treated autologous bone marrow transplantation for relapsed B cell non-Hodgkin's lymphoma. Lancet 1984; ii: 427.
25. Rohatiner AZS, Price CGA, Arnott S et al. Myeloablative therapy with autologous bone marrow transplantation as consolidation of remission in patients with follicular lymphoma. Annals of Oncology 1990; (in press).
26. Leiby JM, Snier KM, Fraut EH et al. Phase II Trial of 9-B-D Arabinofuranosyl-2-fluoroadenine 5'Monophosphate in non-Hodgkin's lymphoma: prospective comparison of response with deoxyxytidine kinase activity. Cancer Res 1987; 47, 10: 2719–2722.
27. Reman J, Cabanillas F, McLaughlin P. Fludarabine Phosphate: A new agent with major activity in low grade lymphoma. Proc AACR 1988; 29: 211.
28. Hochest H, Kim K, Green M et al. Fludarabine is highly active in refractory low grade lymphoma. Results of ECOG 4484 – A randomized Phase II study. Proc ASCO 1989.
29. Levy R, Miller RA. Therapy of lymphoma directed at idiotypes. Journal of the National Cancer Institute Monographs 1990; 10: 61–68.
30. Press OW, Appelbaum F, Ledbetter JA et al. Monoclonal antibody 1F5 (anti-CD20) serotherapy of human B cell lymphomas. Blood 1987; 69: 584–591.
31. Press OW, Eary JF, Badjer CC et al. Treatment of refractory non-Hodgkin's lymphoma with radiolabeled MB-1 (Anti-CD37) antibody). J Clin Oncol 1989; 7, 8: 1027–1039.
32. Hale G, Dyer MJS, Hayhoe FGJ et al. Effects of ACAMPATH-1 antibodies in vivo in patients with lymphoid malignancies: Influence of antibody isotype. Lancet 1988; 2: 1394–1399.
33. Cunningham D, Gilchrist NL, Cowan GJ et al. Alfacalcidol as a modulator of growth of low grade non-Hodgkin's lymphomas. BMJ 1985; 295: 1153–1155.

Correspondence to:
T. A. Lister
Dept. of Medical Oncology
St. Bartholomew's Hospital
London, United Kingdom

Annals of Oncology, Supplement 2 to Volume 2: 137–140, 1991.
© 1991 *Kluwer Academic Publishers*.

Original article

Stage I–II low-grade lymphomas: A prospective trial of combination chemotherapy and radiotherapy

P. McLaughlin, L. Fuller,[1] J. Redman,[2] F. Hagemeister,[1] E. Durr,[2] P. Allen,[2] L. Holmes,[2]
W. Velasquez,[2] F. Swan[2] & F. Cabanillas[2]
From the Departments of [1]*Radiotherapy and* [2]*Hematology, The University of Texas MD Anderson Cancer Center, Houston, Texas 77030, USA*

Summary. Between 1984–1989, 44 patients with stage I–II low grade lymphoma were treated prospectively with sequential chemotherapy and involved-field radiotherapy. The chemotherapy was cyclophosphamide, vincristine, prednisone, and bleomycin (COP-Bleo); doxorubicin was included (CHOP-Bleo) for patients with adverse prognostic features (high LDH; extranodal sites; bulky nodes). Of the 44 patients, 37 had measurable disease and all have responded. With a median follow-up of 32 months, the 5-year survival and failure-free survival were 89% and 74%, respectively. Compared to past experience with involved-field radiotherapy alone, the failure-free survival is significantly better with COP-Bleo plus radiotherapy. The potentially cured fraction has risen from 40% to 74%.

Key words: stage I–II low grade lymphoma; chemotherapy-radiotherapy

Approximately half of all patients with stage I–II low-grade lymphoma (LGL) appear to be curable with current therapies [1–6]. Numerous trials have reported this potential for cure, many employing involved-field radiotherapy (IF XRT) only. Virtually all of the larger reported series were retrospective, employed nonuniform staging, and included patients with a variety of management approaches, including IF XRT, extended-field XRT, total lymphoid irradiation (TLI), and combined chemotherapy-radiotherapy.

Unresolved issues in the management of stage I–II LGL include the role of surgical staging and the optimum therapy for patients who are not laparotomy candidates. For patients with clinical stage (CS) I–II with upper torso presentations, occult abdominal disease is present in 40–60% [7, 8]. But for many patients, treatment planning is and will continue to be based on clinical staging alone, since intercurrent illness and age in this population make many patients unsuitable candidates for laparotomy.

In theory, comprehensive therapy for clinically staged patients should include more than IF XRT, to account for the possibility of occult disease. Both TLI and the inclusion of chemotherapy have been reported, with some encouraging results [2, 3, 6]. However, each is associated with more morbidity than IF XRT. TLI has been noted by some to be associated with fairly severe gastrointestinal and marrow toxicity, including myelodysplasia [4]. Chemotherapy complications vary with different regimens. In the current prospective trial, we report preliminary results with a relatively mild chemotherapy regimen (cyclophosphamide, vincristine,

prednisone, and bleomycin) in conjunction with IF XRT for patients with stage I–II LGL.

Material and methods

Between February 1984 and August 1989, patients with previously untreated stage I–II LGL (follicular small cleaved cell, follicular mixed, or diffuse small lymphocytic) were entered on a protocol of chemotherapy with cyclophosphamide, vincristine, prednisone, and bleomycin (COP-Bleo) and IF XRT. Fifty-two patients were registered, of whom 44 were evaluable and are included in this report. Exclusions included 2 with incorrect histology, 2 with incorrect stage, and 4 patients who were inevaluable because of refusal of chemotherapy and follow-up after zero to three cycles of therapy.

Staging was assigned according to the Ann Arbor system. Staging evaluation included either computed tomography of the abdomen and pelvis or a lymphangiogram, or both, for all patients, and bone marrow biopsies for all. Staging laparotomy was performed in only 1 patient.

Clinical features of the 44 patients are listed in Table 1. The median age was 57 years (range 28–77). Also listed are the clinical features of 42 patients with stage I–II follicular low-grade lymphoma treated with IF XRT alone between 1974–1981, who served as historical controls.

Table 1. Patient characteristics.

Feature	By cell type				Histor-ical controls (N=42)
	DSL (N=4)	FSC (N=26)	FM (N=14)	Total (N=44)	
Gender					
Male	4	10	10	24	19
Female	0	16	4	20	23
Stage I	2	9	3	14	15
II contiguous	1	3	3	7	9
II discontig-uous	1	14	8	23	18
'B' symptoms	0	3	1	4	4
'E' sites	4	6	3	13	7
Upper torso	2	9	3	14	14
Lower torso	2	17	11	30	28
Bulky abdominal disease	1	6	2	9	9
Periph. LN's >5 cm	0	2	0	2	4
Elevated LDH	0	3	2	5	3

Table 2. Radiation fields and chemotherapy.

Chemo-therapy	Radiation field					No XRT
	Upper torso	Upper 2/3 abd.	Pelvis	Hemi-pelvis	Upper 2/3 + pelvis	
COP	4	–	1	–	–	–
COP-Bleo	5	–	3	2	7	–
CHOP	2	2	–	–	2	1
CHOP-Bleo	3	5	–	–	5	2

Therapy

The therapy sequence started with three cycles of COP-Bleo, followed by IF XRT, then resumption of COP-Bleo for seven more cycles (total 10), as shown in Figure 1. If a second XRT field was needed, this occurred after the sixth cycle of COP-Bleo. COP-Bleo consisted of cyclophosphamide 1000 mg/m² IV, vincristine 2 mg IV, prednisone 100 mg by mouth daily for five days, and bleomycin 15 units IV, with repeat cycles every three weeks. For patients with high-risk clinical features (high LDH, extranodal involvement, or bulky adenopathy) and for all patients with small lymphocytic lymphoma, doxorubicin 50 mg/m² IV was included (i.e., CHOP-Bleo) and cyclophosphamide was decreased to 750 mg/m². Doxorubicin was deleted after a total dose of 450 mg/m², or if any cardiac symp-

toms occurred. Bleomycin was not given to patients over age 60 and was deleted if any pulmonary symptoms occurred. The combinations of XRT fields and chemotherapy are shown in Table 2.

Radiation was administered to involved fields. Upper torso fields were limited to affected lymph node-bearing regions. The mantle was not used unless the mediastinum was involved. In general, the peripheral areas and the midplane of the upper mediastinum were treated to a tumor dose of 40 Gy in 20 fractions over four weeks, through parallel opposed anterior and posterior fields.

Treatment to the abdomen was delivered through anterior and posterior fields, which extended from the dome of the diaphragm to the iliac crests. In treating the pelvis, the inguinal and femoral nodes were included. The overall dose to the upper abdomen and to the pelvis was limited to 30 Gy in 20 fractions over four weeks. The right lobe of the liver was shielded anteriorly and posteriorly with one half-value layer (HVL) of lead. The kidneys were shielded posteriorly with two HVL of lead to reduce their dose to approximately 18 Gy. Residual disease in the para-aortic and pelvic regions received additional boost treatment of up to 10 Gy through reduced anterior and posterior parallel opposed fields.

The choice of radiotherapy equipment was based on the average maximum AP/PA diameter of the region to be treated. Involved sites with average diameters of 22 cm or greater were treated with a 6-meV linear accelerator. All others were treated with cobalt 60.

Data analysis

Survival curves were calculated according to the method of Kaplan and Meier [9]. Comparisons of outcomes were made using Gehan's modification of the generalized Wilcoxon test for survival [10].

Complete remission was defined as the disappearance of all signs and symptoms of disease both clinically and radiographically. Partial remission was defined as a >50% reduction in the sum of the products of the two greatest perpendicular diameters of all measurable lesions. The category 'probable complete remission' (PCR) was used for responding patients with stable

TREATMENT SCHEMA

COP - Bleo x 3

↓

XRT (Involved Field)

↓

COP - Bleo x 7

- CHOP-Bleo was used for high risk patients ("E" sites; high LDH; bulky abdominal disease)

- XRT: involved field 4500 cGy for upper torso sites, 3000 cGy for lower torso; for whole abdomen, XRT delivered in 2 sessions (upper 2/3; pelvis) in sandwich fashion, after the 3rd and 6th chemotherapy cycles

Fig. 1. Treatment schema.

minimal residual radiographic abnormalities who were otherwise free of disease [11].

Survival and failure-free survival (FFS) were measured from the date of initial therapy to the time of death or treatment failure, respectively. Two patients in complete remission who died of other causes were carried as alive and free of disease at the time of death in the corrected survival analysis.

Results

Response

Seven patients with stage I disease had no measurable disease following their diagnostic biopsies; the other 37 all responded, with 34 CR (92%), and 3 PCR (8%).

Survival

At the time of this analysis, the median follow-up for the group of 44 patients was 32 months. The overall survival was 89% at five years (Fig. 2). Of the three deaths, two were unrelated to disease or therapy (automobile accident at 11 months; myocardial infarction at 10 months; both occurred when the patients were off therapy and free of disease). One death, at 38 months, was due to myelodysplasia attributed to the COP-Bleo and radiotherapy and occurred in a patient without evidence of active lymphoma. Counting this one death as treatment related, the corrected survival was 95% at five years. At the time of this analysis, freedom from tumor mortality was 100%.

When the overall survival figure was compared to the survival results for 42 historical control patients treated with XRT only between 1974–1981, there was a trend for superior survival with the current combined modality program (89% vs. 76% at five years, P = 0.16).

Failure-free survival

The failure-free survival was 74% at five years (Fig. 2). Of the seven relapses, five were transdiaphragmatic, one was in lymph nodes on both sides of the diaphragm, and one was at a site of previous disease (bowel) that was not irradiated. Of the seven relapses, three occurred in patients who had received doxorubicin (two because of extranodal involvement, and one because of bulky abdominal disease at presentation), and two others occurred in patients who had bulky peripheral nodes (>5 cm) at presentation; only two relapsed patients, a man with stage I-A follicular mixed cell lymphoma and a woman with stage II-A follicular small cleaved cell lymphoma, had no apparent adverse pretreatment clinical features.

When FFS was compared to the FFS results for 42 historical control patients treated with XRT only, there was a significantly better FFS for the combined-modality program (74% vs. 40% at five years, P < 0.01; Fig. 3).

Complications

The regimen was generally well tolerated. Neutropenia was the most common toxicity, and it was modest. Of over 300 evaluable chemotherapy cycles, the WBC nadir was <2000/mm^3 in 28%, and the absolute granulocyte count was <1000/mm^3 in 30%, while the platelets were <100 000/mm^3 in only 2%. There were 3 infectious episodes, only 1 in the setting of neutropenia, and all were managed with oral antibiotics. The most common nonhematologic toxicity was nausea and vomiting, which occurred in 11 patients, but this was severe for only 3. Parasthesias occurred in 10 patients, stomatitis in 5, diarrhea in 3, and hematuria, hypothyroidism, and catheter thrombosis in 1 each. Localized herpes zoster occurred in 2. Mild dyspnea occurred in 2 and prompted the early discontinuation of bleomycin. One patient developed myelodysplasia 21 months after completion of COP-Bleo plus XRT of the

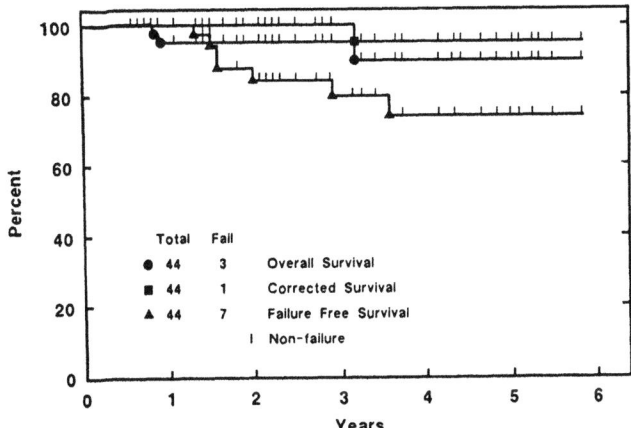

Fig. 2. Overall survival, corrected survival, and failure-free survival.

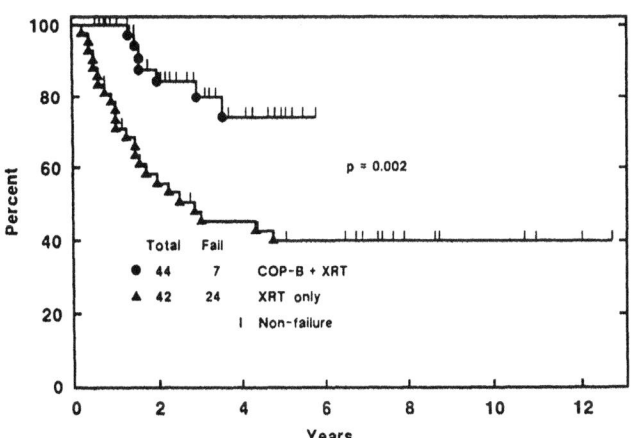

Fig. 3. Failure-free survival of 44 study patients, compared with 42 historical control patients treated with IF XRT only.

abdomen and pelvis, and subsequently died at 38 months.

Six patients did not complete all therapy as planned. Three patients with primary small bowel presentations did not receive any XRT, because of concern about postoperative adhesions and bowel tolerance of radiation therapy. One patient with known atherosclerotic heart disease and a history of coronary artery bypass graft surgery had CHOP-Bleo changed to COP-Bleo after one cycle because of an episode of angina and concern about incipient congestive heart failure. Two patients had early discontinuation of chemotherapy because of poor tolerance, after a total of three and six cycles, respectively. One of these patients had excessive nausea and vomiting and weight loss, and the other had prolonged pancytopenia following pelvic XRT.

Discussion

This preliminary report demonstrates that the inclusion of chemotherapy along with IF XRT can result in a high failure-free survival rate for patients with stage I–II LGL. Longer follow-up will be needed to know if this strategy ultimately results in more cures. We are hopeful of this, since 43% of patients in the current trial have already been followed longer than 36 months, by which time 92% of relapses had already occurred in the control group (Fig. 3). Several previous reports have indicated a decreasing risk of failure beyond five years, so the five-year failure-free survival percentage should approximate the cure rate.

Intensive therapy, or any initial therapy at all, is a matter of controversy for patients with advanced-stage LGL, largely because of valid questions about their potential curability [12, 13]. The same basis for controversy should not exist for patients with stage I–II disease, since investigators at many centers agree that a large fraction are curable. Implicit in this observation of potential curability is a mandate to act; watchful waiting is not appropriate for these patients. In fact, efforts at early diagnosis should be emphasized, in the hope of treating more patients at a time when they have stage I–II disease, since patients who progress to stage III–IV are generally considered incurable with current therapies.

Besides the addition of chemotherapy, as in the current report, another way to attempt to improve on results with IF XRT is to employ more extensive XRT. Paryani and coworkers reported superior freedom from relapse for patients who received TLI compared to those who received IF or extended-field XRT. The patterns of failure revealed notably fewer marginal relapses with TLI than with IF or extended-field XRT. In our early experience with combined-modality therapy, the pattern of failure appears to be mainly out of field and in patients with bulky or extranodal disease at presentation. Three of the seven relapses in the current report occurred in patients who had received doxorubi-

cin because of adverse pretreatment features, but the total number of failures to date is too small to reveal any statistically significant differences among patient subsets. As methods for stratifying prognostic groups become more refined [14], the strategy of tailoring therapy to pretreatment clinical features will likely permit more intensive therapy to be reserved for those at highest risk. The current report suggests that a relatively modest intensification of therapy, the inclusion of COP/CHOP-Bleo, can significantly improve the failure-free survival results attained with IF XRT alone for patients with stage I–II LGL.

References

1. Gospodarowicz MK, Bush RS, Brown TC, Chua T. Prognostic factors in nodular lymphomas: A multivariate analysis based on the Princess Margaret Hospital experience. Int J Radiat Oncol Biol Phys 1984; 10: 489–97.
2. Paryani SB, Hoppe RT, Cox RS, Colby TV, Rosenberg SA, Kaplan HS. Analysis of non-Hodgkin's lymphomas with nodular and favorable histologies, stage I and II. Cancer 1983; 52: 2300–7.
3. McLaughlin P, Fuller LM, Velasquez WS, Sullivan-Halley JA, Butler JJ, Cabanillas F. Stage I–II follicular lymphoma. Treatment results for 76 patients. Cancer 1986; 58: 1596–602.
4. Gomez GA, Barcos M, Krishnamsetty RM, Panahon AM, Han T, Henderson ES. Treatment of early stages I and II nodular, poorly differentiated lymphocytic lymphoma. Am J Clin Oncol 1986; 9: 40–4.
5. Lawrence TS, Urba WJ, Steinberg SM et al. Retrospective analysis of stage I and II indolent lymphomas at the National Cancer Institute. Int J Radiation Oncology Biol Phys 1988; 14: 417–24.
6. Richards MA, Gregory WM, Hall PA et al. Management of localized non-Hodgkin's lymphoma: the experience at St. Bartholomew's hospital 1972–1985. Hemal Oncol 1989; 7: 1–18.
7. Heifetz LJ, Fuller LM, Rodgers RW et al. Laparotomy findings in lymphangiogram-staged I and II non-Hodgkin's lymphomas. Cancer 1980; 45: 2778–86.
8. Goffinet DR, Warnke R, Dunnick NR et al. Clinical and Surgical (Laparotomy) Evaluation of Patient with Non-Hodgkin's Lymphomas. Cancer Treat Rep 1977; 61: 981–92.
9. Kaplan EL, Meier P. Non-Parametric estimation from incomplete observations. J Am Stat Assoc 1958; 53: 457–81.
10. Gehan EA. A generalized Wilcoxan test for comparing arbitrarily singly-censored samples. Biometrika 1965; 52: 203–23.
11. Zuckerman KS, LoBuglio AF, Reeves JA. Chemotherapy of intermediate and high grade non-Hodgkin's lymphomas with a high-dose doxorubicin-containing regimen. J Clin Oncol 1990; 8: 248–56.
12. Cabanillas F, Freireich EJ. Intensive treatment of nodular non-Hodgkin's lymphoma. In: Wiernik PH (ed.). Controversies in Oncology. John Wiley & Sons, New York, 1982; pp 31–43.
13. Rosenberg SA. Is intensive treatment of favorable non-Hodgkin's lymphoma necessary? In: Wiernik PH (ed.). Controversies in Oncology. John Wiley & Sons, New York, 1982; pp 45–60.
14. Romaguera JE, McLaughlin P, North L et al. Multivariate analysis of prognostic factors in stage IV follicular low grade lymphoma: A risk model. J Clin Oncol (in press).

Reprint requests to:
Peter McLaughlin, M.D.
Department of Hematology
UT M.D. Anderson Cancer Center
1515 Holcombe, Houston, Texas 77030, USA

Annals of Oncology, Supplement 2 to Volume 2: 141–145, 1991.
© 1991 Kluwer Academic Publishers.

Original article

Interferon-α_{2b} in the treatment of follicular lymphoma: Preliminary results of a trial in progress

C. G. A. Price, A. Z. S. Rohatiner, W. Steward,[1] D. Deakin,[2] N. Bailey,[3] A. Norton,[4] G. Blackledge,[3] D. Crowther[1] & T. A. Lister

ICRF Dept of Medical Oncology, & Dept of Histopathology,[4] St. Bartholomew's Hospital, London EC1; CRC Dept of Medical Oncology,[1] & Dept of Radiotherapy,[2] Christie Hospital & Holt Radium Institute, Manchester; CRC West Midlands Clinical Trials Unit,[3] Queen Elizabeth Hospital, Birmingham, United Kingdom

Summary. Since 1985 the combination of chlorambucil (10 mg daily, initially for six weeks, then alternating fortnights for 12 weeks) and interferon-α_{2b} (Schering-Plough; 2×10^6 U/m^2 three times weekly by subcutaneous injection for 18 weeks) has been compared in a randomised trial with chlorambucil alone in previously untreated patients with stage III or IV follicular lymphoma. Responding patients have subsequently been randomised to receive maintenance interferon-α_{2b} or no further treatment. Of the 124 treated patients, 108 are evaluable for response with a median follow-up of 30 months. The major toxicity was myelosuppression which was more frequent with chlorambucil and IFNα_{2b} in combination than with chlorambucil alone (P < 0.01). There was no treatment-related mortality. Actuarial survival at three years is 75% for all patients, regardless of therapy. There was no significant difference in response rate according to initial therapy. For the 60 patients achieving a good response to initial therapy who have entered the second part of the trial, there has been a significant prolongation of remission duration in favour of maintenance IFN-α_{2b} (median not yet reached versus two years for the 'no treatment' arm, P < 0.015). Fewest relapses have been seen in patients who received IFN-α_{2b} throughout. Accrual to this trial continues; this preliminary analysis indicates that maintenance IFN-α_{2b} may extend remission duration in follicular lymphoma.

Introduction

Follicular lymphoma is highly responsive to chemotherapy, remission being achieved in the majority of patients with standard therapy, although few patients are cured [1]. Several studies have shown that combination chemotherapy is not superior to single-agent therapy in the durability of remissions induced, or in consequent survival [2, 3, 4], although a recent report suggests that the nodular-mixed subgroup may differ in this respect [5]. Chlorambucil (CB) is a commonly used single agent, being well tolerated and conveniently administered on an outpatient basis. Response rates of 70% (complete response [CR] 30%) are typical with a median duration of remission of two years [6]. Nevertheless, the majority of patients eventually die of lymphoma and new approaches to treatment are required.

The activity of alpha-interferon in low-grade non-Hodgkin's lymphoma (NHL), and follicular lymphoma in particular, has been demonstrated in several clinical trials [7, 8, 9]. An overall response rate of at least 30% in previously treated patients, and 50% in untreated patients [10], can be inferred from the published data. Studies in murine models [11, 12] and human tumour xenografts [13] have shown synergism between alpha-interferon and a variety of cytotoxic agents. Against

this background a study was undertaken at St. Bartholomew's Hospital to evaluate the combination of CB and interferon-α_{2b} (IFN-α_{2b}) in patients with relapsed low-grade NHL. It was concluded that the treatment was feasible in terms of toxicity and at least as effective as CB alone [14]. These results encouraged the instigation of a randomised trial comparing CB alone with CB and IFN-α_{2b} (Schering-Plough) as primary therapy for patients with follicular lymphoma stages III and IV. Experience with alpha-interferon in other haematological malignancies such as hairy cell leukaemia [15] and chronic myeloid leukaemia [16] suggests that prolonged administration of this agent may confer an advantage. Accordingly the trial included a second randomisation after completion of the first phase, patients either receiving no further therapy or maintenance IFN-α_{2b}. A preliminary analysis of the results of this trial which commenced in 1985, and to which patients are still being accrued, forms the basis of this report.

Materials and methods

Patient population

Previously untreated patients referred to one of the

Table 1. Patient characteristics.

Patients entered (M : F):	124 (68 : 56)
No. evaluable for response:[1]	108
Median age in years (range):	52 (26–81)
Stage:	
III	32
IV (BM + ve : BM − ve)	92 (71 : 21)

[1] 16 patients remain on treatment.

three participating centres were eligible for the study conditional upon their informed consent and (1) local histological review confirming the diagnosis of follicular lymphoma; (2) stage III or IV disease after full staging investigations (including physical examination, chest x-ray, CT scans of abdomen and chest (if chest x-ray was normal), biochemical assessment of liver function and bone marrow biopsy); and (3) a clinical indication for treatment. Entry to the study was deferred in asymptomatic patients with stable disease, who were mangaged expectantly until there was evidence of disease progression. Characteristics of patients entered into the study are shown in Table 1.

Treatment

The treatment regimen is shown in Figure 1. Entry to the second (maintenance) part of the study was dependent on a response being achieved with CB or CB + IFN-α_{2b}, and randomisation was stratified according to the quality of this response. IFN-α_{2b} was administered by subcutaneous injection by the patient, a relative or a district nurse. Maintenance IFN-α_{2b} was continued for seven months in patients treated in two of the three

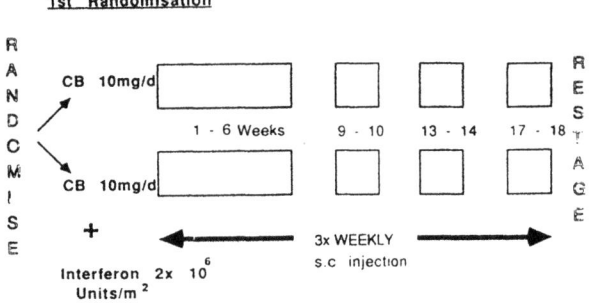

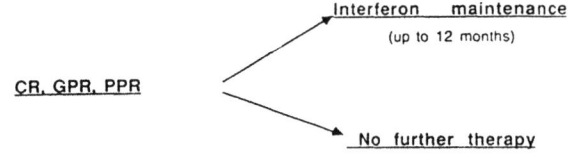

Fig. 1. Treatment.

centres (Manchester and Birmingham) and for one year in the third (St. Bartholomew's Hospital).

Treatment modifications

Treatment was discontinued for two weeks in patients with treatment-related cytopenia (neutrophil count $<1 \times 10^9/L$; platelet count $<100 \times 10^9/L$) and was restarted in full dosage after recovery of the count. Persistent or recurrent cytopenia provoked a 50% reduction in CB dose or discontinuation of therapy. Persistent intolerable subjective side effects of interferon were managed by 50% dose reduction or cessation of that agent alone.

During the trial period the policy was changed for patients in whom only a poor partial response (PPR; reduction $>50\%$ in any measurable lesion associated with improvement in nonmeasurable involvement) was achieved, such that some of the latter were not entered into the second part of this trial but went on to receive more intensive chemotherapy in an attempt to achieve CR. Patients in whom the response is classified as PPR are therefore considered separately.

Assessment of response

Response to therapy was first assessed at one month after completion of CB or CB + IFN-α_{2b} and again after the maintenance period, whether or not IFN-α_{2b} was received.

Definitions

Response was defined as either complete remission (CR; no evidence of residual disease), good partial remission (GPR; clinical complete response with minimal residual abnormality on radiographic or bone marrow examination), poor partial remission (PPR; reduction $>50\%$ in any measurable lesion associated with improvement in nonmeasurable involvement, i.e., less than GPR) or failure to respond (Fail). Duration of remission was recorded from the time of reassessment at five months; relapse was defined as recurrent or progressive disease and was confirmed histologically.

Statistical Methods

Survival and remission duration curves were plotted according to the method of Kaplan and Meier [17], and the log rank method was used to test for significance of differences in distributions.

Results

Response to initial treatment

Table 2 shows response according to initial treatment (CB or CB + IFN-α_{2b}). Major responses (CR + GPR)

Table 2. Response according to initial treatment.

	CB	CB + IFN
CR	15	8
GPR	27	19
PPR	9	11
FAIL	8	11
total	59	49
CR + GPR	71%	55% (N.S.)

were seen in 71% of those who received CB alone and 55% of those receiving the combination.

Randomisation and response to maintenance interferon

Eighty-one patients were eligible for entry into the second part of the trial. Ten patients were withdrawn either because (1) the response to initial therapy was PPR (see above) (2) patients' wishes, or (3) protocol violation. Five of 27 patients with initially incomplete responses (GPR + PPR) who then received IFN-α_{2b} maintenance demonstrated an improvement in response.

Survival

Survival is shown in Figure 2. Twenty-eight patients have died and 96 remain alive with a median follow-up

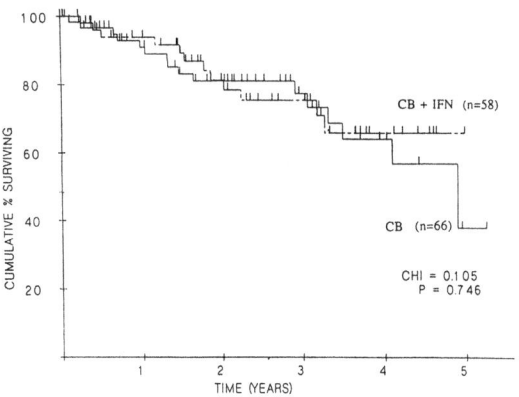

Fig. 2. Survival according to initial therapy.

of 32 months. Actuarial survival at three years is 75% with no difference between the two initial therapy arms.

Duration of remission

Duration of remission according to initial treatment, maintenance therapy, and overall treatment are shown in Figures 3a, b, and c, respectively, for patients achieving a major response (CR + GPR) to initial therapy. The median remission duration for this group has not yet been reached, whereas that for patients receiving no maintenance is two years (P < 0.013). Among patients

randomised to IFN-α_{2b} maintenance, 7 of 35 (20%) relapsed while receiving the drug, while 10 of 25 (40%) of those receiving no therapy relapsed during the maintenance period. The length of remission is currently the same for the patients in the maintenance IFN-α_{2b} arm regardless of whether it was continued for seven months or one year. Response duration for patients in whom a PPR was achieved and who were randomised in the second part of the study is shown in Figure 4.

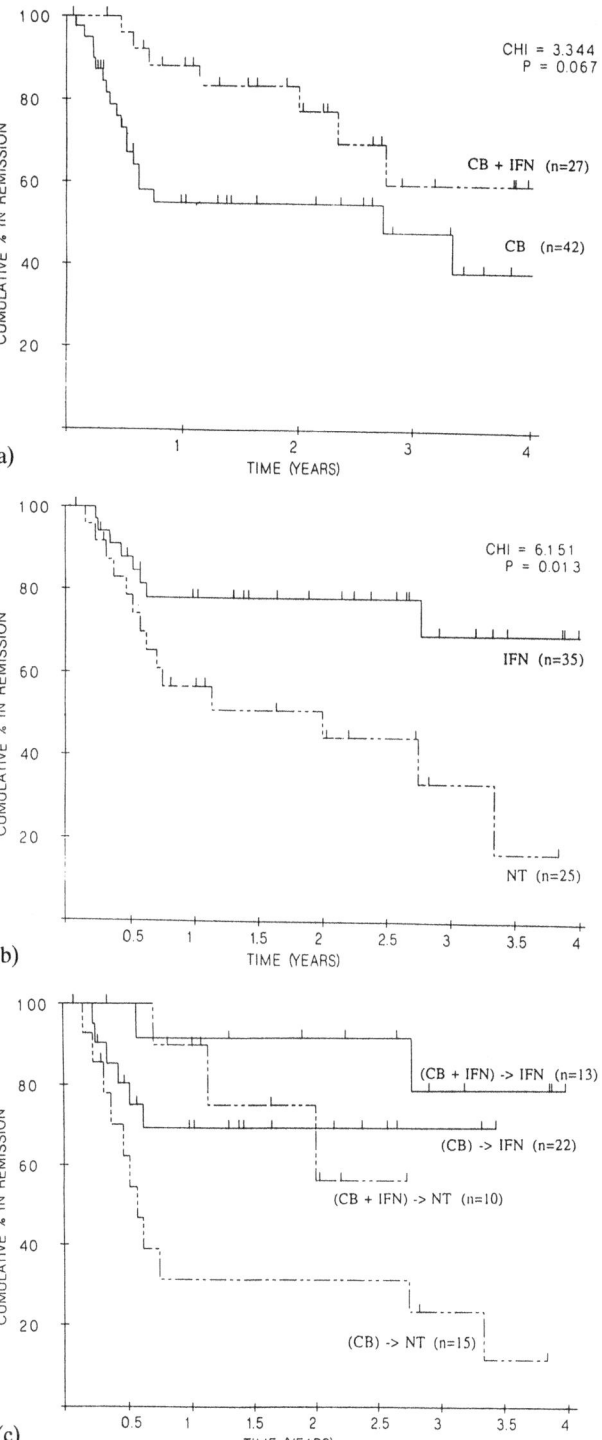

Fig. 3. Duration of remission (CR + GPR only). (a) Initial therapy: CB vs CB + IFN; (b) Second randomisation: 'Maintenance IFN' versus 'No Rx'; (c) Treatment overall (4 treatment arms).

144

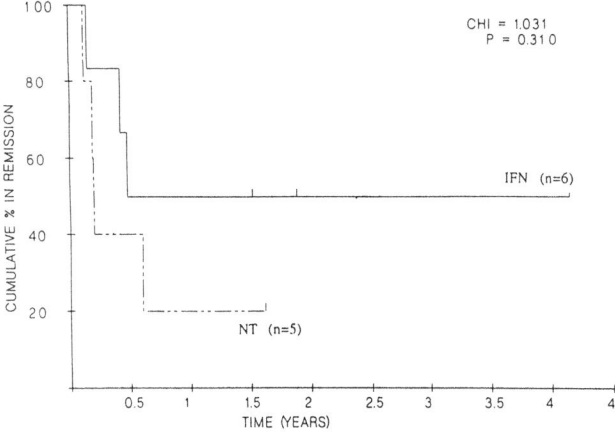

Fig. 4. Second randomisation: PPR to initial therapy.

Toxicity

Most patients initially experienced subjective systemic symptoms from IFN-α_{2b} as previously described [18]; these were insufficient to interfere with daily activities in the majority, but led to discontinuance of the drug in 6 patients (8%). One patient developed haemolytic anaemia within two weeks of starting IFN-α_{2b} (as maintenance). IFN-α_{2b} was also possibly associated with the exacerbation of angina in one patient, and an epileptiform seizure in another. Three patients suffered skin rashes attributable to CB. Among patients receiving CB + IFN-α_{2b}, 31 of 49 (62%) had periods of cytopenia sufficient for their treatment to be delayed compared to 9 of 59 (16%) who received CB alone ($P < 0.01$).

Discussion

This preliminary report is based on analysis of outcome for the first 120 patients entered into the study over a period of 56 months. These data confirm that low-dose, thrice-weekly subcutaneous IFN-α_{2b} can be administered on an outpatient basis and is well tolerated by the majority of patients, though with the expected early subjective symptoms. Haemolysis, which occurred in 1 patient soon after starting IFN-α_{2b}, is an unusual consequence of treatment with the alpha-interferons, but has been reported previously [19, 20]. The most important side effect encountered was myelotoxicity, which was seen significantly more often with the combination of CB and IFN-α_{2b} than with CB alone, and led to delays in treatment for the majority of patients receiving the combination. Speculatively, these delays may have abrogated any potential enhancement of the efficacy of remission induction associated with the addition of IFN-α_{2b} and might explain the lower response rate for the combination.

A significant prolongation of remission duration was seen with maintenance IFN-α_{2b}, but follow-up is not sufficient as yet to know whether survival is being influenced. This will clearly be of importance when the benefits of treatment are being weighed against the inconvenience of thrice-weekly injections of IFN-α_{2b}. Moreover, assessment of the effect of IFN-α_{2b} maintenance is currently based on a small number of patients and these observations should be regarded with caution.

As previously discussed, the benefit of IFN-α_{2b} in other haematological malignancies has been most apparent in the context of prolonged therapy and low-volume disease. If the present findings are confirmed after further patient accrual and longer follow-up, these observations will have been extended to follicular lymphoma. Further questions regarding the optimal dose and duration of maintenance IFN-α_{2b} in this disease will then need to be addressed.

Acknowledgements

Interferon-α_{2b} was kindly supplied by Schering-Plough. Data was collected and analysed by J. Wright, J. Matthews & M. Carter (SBH), V. Sykes (Birmingham) and D. Brown (Manchester). We thank all the physicians who have referred patients for inclusion in this study.

References

1. Anderson T, DeVita VT, Simon SM et al. Malignant lymphoma II. Prognostic factors and response to treatment of 473 patients at the National Cancer Institute. Cancer 1982; 50: 2708.
2. Lister TA, Cullen MH, Beard MEJ et al. Comparison of combined and single agent chemotherapy in non-Hodgkin's lymphoma of favourable histological type. Br Med J 1978; i: 533.
3. Portlock CS, Rosenberg SA, Glatstein E, Kaplan HS. Treatment of advanced non-Hodgkin's lymphomas with favourable histologies: Preliminary results of prospective trial. Blood 1976; 47 5: 747.
4. Glick JH, Barnes JM, Ezdinli EZ et al. Nodular mixed lymphoma: Results of a randomized trial failing to confirm prolonged disease-free survival with COPP chemotherapy. Blood 1981; 58: 920.
5. Peterson BA, Anderson JR, Frizzera G et al. Combination chemotherapy prolongs survival in follicular mixed lymphoma. Proc ASCO 1990; 9: 259.
6. Gallagher CJ, Gregory WM, Jones AE, Stansfeld AG, Richards MA, Dhaliwal HS, Malpas JS, Lister TA. Follicular lymphoma: Prognostic factors for response and survival. J Clin Oncol 1986; 4: 1470.
7. Foon KA, Sherwin SA, Abrams PG et al. Treatment of advanced non-Hodgkin's lymphoma with recombinant leukocyte A interferon. N Engl J Med 1984; 311: 1148.
8. Roth MS, Foon KA. Alpha interferon in the treatment of hematologic malignancies. Am J Med 1986; 81: 871.
9. O'Connell MJ, Colgan JP, Oken MM et al. Clinical trial of recombinant leucocyte A interferon as initial therapy for favourable histology non-Hodgkin's lymphoma and chronic lymphocytic leukaemia: An ECOG pilot study. J Clin Oncol 1986; 4: 128–36.
10. Wagstaff J, Loynds P, Crowther D. A phase II study of human rDNA alpha-II interferon in patients with low grade non-Hodgkin's lymphoma. Cancer Chemother Pharmacol 1986; 18: 54.

11. Chirigos MA, Pearson JW. Cure of murine leukaemia with drugs and interferon treatment. JNCI 1973; 14: 97.
12. Gresser I, Maury C, Tovey M. Efficacy of combined interferon cyclophosphamide therapy after diagnosis of lymphoma in AKR mice. Eur J Cancer 1978; 14: 97.
13. Balkwill FR, Moodie EM. Positive interactions between human interferon and cyclophosphamide or adriamycin in a human tumor model system. Cancer Res 1984; 44: 904.
14. Rohatiner AZS, Richards MA, Barnett MJ et al. Chlorambucil and interferon for low-grade non-Hodgkin's lymphoma. Brit J Can 1987; 55: 437.
15. Quesada JR, Reuben JR, Manning JT et al. Alpha interferon for induction of remission in hairy cell leukemia. N Engl J Med 1984; 310: 15.
16. Talpaz M, Kantarjian HM, McCredie K. Hematologic remission and cytogenetic improvement induced by recombinant human interferon alpha A in chronic myelogenous leukemia. N Engl J Med 1986; 314: 1065.
17. Kaplan EL, Meier P. Nonparametric estimation from incomplete observations. J Am Stat Assoc 1958; 53: 457–481.
18. Spiegel RJ. The alpha interferons: Clinical overview. Seminars in Oncology 1987; 14: (2) suppl. 2 1–12.
19. Akard LP, Hoffman R, Elias L, Saiers J. Alpha-interferon and Immune Haemolytic Anaemia. Ann Int Med 1986; 105: 306.
20. Braathen LR, Stavem P. Autoimmune haemolytic anaemia associated with interferon alfa-2a in a patient: with mycosis fungoides. Brit Med J 1989; 298: 1713.

Correspondence to:
Professor T. A. Lister, MD, FRCP
ICRF Department of Medical Oncology
St Bartholomew's Hospital
London EC1A 7BE
England

Annals of Oncology, Supplement 2 to Volume 2: 147–150, 1991.
© 1991 Kluwer Academic Publishers.

Original article

Myeloablative therapy with autologous bone marrow transplantation as consolidation of remission in patients with follicular lymphoma

A. Z. S. Rohatiner, C. G. A. Price, S. Arnott, A. Norton, M. L. Evans, F. Cotter, E. Dorey, C. L. Davis, P. Clark, J. Sterlini, J. Lim, M. Horton & T. A. Lister
ICRF Dept of Medical Oncology and Depts of Radiology, Haematology & Histopathology, St. Bartholomew's Hospital, London, EC1A 7BE, UK

Summary. A study has been in progress since June 1985 to evaluate the use of myeloablative therapy (cyclophosphamide [60 mg/kg × 2] and total body irradiation [200 cGy × 6]) followed by reinfusion of autologous bone marrow in patients in second or subsequent remission of B-cell non-Hodgkin's lymphoma. The marrow mononuclear cell fraction is being treated in vitro with three cycles of the monoclonal antibody anti-CD20 (anti-B1, Coulter Immunology) and baby rabbit complement (Pel-Freez).

Thirty-eight patients with follicular lymphoma (age range 29–61 years, median 43) have been treated to date. At the time of treatment, 28 patients were in second remission, 7 were in third, and 3 were in more than third remission. Twenty-three patients were in complete remission, 15 had residual disease (7 had lymph nodes <2 cm diameter, 4 had <10% bone marrow infiltration, 1 had involvement of lymph nodes and bone marrow, and 3 had involvement at other sites). Of the 38 study patients, 32 are alive; 6 have died, 4 in remission. Two of the deaths were treatment related: 1 resulted from cerebral haemorrhage at 29 days; 1 resulted from systemic fungal infection at three months). One patient died from secondary acute myelogenous leukaemia at four years, and another from an unrelated cause. Two patients died following relapse. The median time to engraftment was 28 days (range 15–45 days) for neutrophils >0.5×10^9/L and 28 days (range 15–46 days) for platelets >20×10^9/L.

Twenty-six patients continue in remission between one month and five years (median follow-up 22 months); 8 have relapsed, 2 with transformation to high-grade histology. In the context of the natural history of follicular lymphoma these results are preliminary but encouraging. It remains to be established whether such intensive therapy is curative.

Key words: ablative therapy, ABMT, follicular lymphoma

Introduction

The majority of patients with follicular lymphoma die as a consequence of the disease despite responsiveness to both chemotherapy and irradiation. Repeated remissions can usually be achieved but are hardly ever more than temporary, the continuous relapse pattern making death from lymphoma virtually inevitable [1–4].

Recently, attention has focused on the use of very intensive therapy supported by autologous bone marrow transplant (ABMT) in patients with high-grade histology in whom conventional therapy has failed. The results in a heterogeneous group suggest that this approach results in long-term survival for approximately one third of patients with otherwise incurable disease [5–11], provided that they are selected on the basis of responsiveness to conventional treatment [6, 8–11]. In view of the incurability of follicular lymphoma and data suggesting that intensive therapy prolongs duration of remission [12–14], these principles were applied to younger patients. The rationale for the choice of

cyclophosphamide (CY) and total body irradiation (TBI) is based on their known efficacy at inducing remission in follicular lymphoma, together with the hope that using both treatment modalities at maximum dose, as consolidation, might prolong remission duration and hence survival.

In view of the frequency of bone marrow involvement in follicular lymphoma, it was decided to treat the marrow in vitro with a monoclonal antibody directed against the CD20 (B1) antigen and rabbit complement as previously described [15].

Patients and methods

1. Patients

Thirty-eight patients have been treated to date. Their clinical characteristics at diagnosis and at the time of receiving CY + TBI are shown in Table 1; 23 patients were in complete remission, and 15 had 'minimal'

148

Table 1. Clinical characteristics of the patients at diagnosis and at the time of receiving CY + TBI + ABMT.

Stage	No. of pts
I	2
II	5
III	9
IV	22
BM + ve	20
BM − ve	18 (7)[a]

[a] BM + ve at some point in disease.

Age and remission status at time of CY + TBI + ABMT

Median age:	43 (Range 28–61 yr)	
Remission:	2nd:	28
	3rd	7
	>3rd:	3
K.P. Status	90%–100%	

residual disease, which was defined as <10% infiltration of the intratrabecular space on a trephine biopsy (5 patients), lymph nodes <2 cm in diameter (7 patients), or involvement of other sites (3 patients). All had a Karnofsky performance status of 90–100%.

All patients had received multiple previous treatments (median 3, range 2–7) since the time of diagnosis. In 13 of 38 patients, more than one treatment was required to achieve remission prior to administering CY + TBI + ABMT; 15 of 38 patients needed an Adriamycin-containing regimen. Reactivity with anti-CD20 was demonstrated by indirect immunofluorescence and flow cytometric analysis of bone marrow, or by immunoperoxidase staining of lymph node or other tissue, in all but two cases where fresh biopsy material was not available.

2. Collection, in vitro treatment, and reinfusion of bone marrow

At least 1 L of bone marrow was harvested under general anaesthetic, the cells were washed three times on an IBM 2991 red cell washer, and the mononuclear cell (MNC) fraction from the first 50 ml isolated over Ficoll-Hypaque. The MNCs were treated in vitro with three cycles of anti-CD20 (Coulter Clone anti-B1, Coulter Immunology, Hialeah, Fla) and baby rabbit complement (Pel Freez, Wisconsin) as described by Nadler et al. [15] prior to cryopreservation. The cells were phenotyped as described previously [16] before and after the in vitro treatment and were analysed using a Coulter EPICS C flow cytometer. Within 24 hours of the last dose of TBI, the bone marrow was thawed and reinfused.

3. Treatment

Cyclophosphamide, 60 mg/kg (with MESNA), was

administered as a one-hour intravenous infusion on two consecutive days. TBI was given as six fractions of 200 cGy each, over three days. Three patients who had clinical evidence of residual lymph node enlargement and one with residual skin involvement received additional radiotherapy concurrent with the TBI.

4. Supportive care

Patients were looked after in single rooms until the absolute neutrophil count exceeded 0.5×10^9/L. Oral nonabsorbable antibiotics (Framycetin, Nystatin, and Colistin) [17] were prescribed although not always consistently taken, and prophylactic Acyclovir was continued for one year. Intravenous Gentamycin and Ceftazidime were commenced empirically in patients who became pyrexial (38 °C); the combination was altered on the basis of bacteriological isolates when appropriate. Single-donor platelets were administered when the platelet count fell below 20×10^9/L or when clinically indicated. HLA-matched donors were used if alloimmunisation was suspected or demonstrated. Cytomegalovirus (CMV)-negative blood products were used in patients who were demonstrated to be CMV-negative. All blood products were irradiated with 2000 cGy.

Results

1. In vitro treatment of bone marrow

The number of MNCs reinfused and the effect of the in vitro treatment on CD20 expression are shown in Table 2.

Table 2. Number of MNC reinfused and the effect of the in vitro treatment on the % of CD20 + ve cells.

No. of MNC reinfused:	
Mean:	2.6×10^7/kg
Range:	$1.1 - 6.9 \times 10^7$/kg

% of CD 20 + ve cells before and after in vitro treatment
CR

	Pre	Post
Median:	5	1
Range:	1–2	0–5
Minimal residual disease (BM)		
Median:	7	1
Range:	3–20	1–6

2. Clinical toxicity

The early toxicity and late complications are shown in Table 3.

Table 3. Toxicity.

Mortality		Early toxicity		Late complications	
Cer. haem	1	Fever	All	Cataracts	2
Sys. fung.		Septicaemia	22	H. zoster	1
Infection	1	Pneumonia	2	2° AML	1
		Mucositis	7	Raeb	1

3. Haematological recovery

The majority of patients left the hospital after 4 weeks (range 3–8.5 weeks). The median number of red cells and platelet transfusions required was 8 units and 7 units respectively (range 2–48 and 2–54). Five patients required HLA-identical platelets.

4. Immunological recovery

Reduced levels of immunoglobulin were observed for up to 18 months.

T cell recovery: A relative excess of circulating T8+ (T suppressor cells) was observed for approximately one year.

5. Duration of remission

Twenty-six patients continue in remission between two months and five years with a median follow-up of 22 months. Eight have relapsed, 6 with follicular lymphoma and 2 with transformation to high-grade histology. None of the 5 patients who were treated with minimal residual disease in the bone marrow have relapsed (maximum follow-up two years). Details of time and site of relapse and subsequent survival are shown in Table 4.

Table 4. Outcome after recurrence.

Follicular lymphoma
Cyclophosphamide + TBI + ABMT

Outcome after recurrence

Years from diagnosis	Rem	Dur of rem	Site of rel	Survival since rel	Current situation
1	2nd	3 m	LN	8 m	PD, died
2	2nd	7 m	LN	4 m	Well
2.5	2nd	18 m	LN	11 m	PD + Rx
2	2nd	20 m	LN+BM	39 m	Well + Rx
2	2nd	27 m	BM	21 m	Well
13	5th	28 m	LN	17 m	Well
10	4th	10 m	Liver & Bone	1 m	PD, died
8	2nd	22 m	S/Cut	26 m	Well + Rx

6. Survival

Thirty-two patients are alive, 6 have died, and 4 are in remission. Two deaths were a consequence of the transplant procedure (1 cerebral haemorrhage at 29 days, 1 systemic fungal infection at three months); 1 patient died from secondary acute myelogenous leukaemia at four years, having presented eight years prior to receiving CY + TBI + ABMT, and another died from an unrelated cause. Two patients died of progressive lymphoma following relapse despite further treatment.

Discussion

The median survival for patients with follicular lymphoma at St. Bartholomew's Hospital is nine years, with a conservative approach comprising observation, short courses of chlorambucil given to achieve clinical remission, and repeat biopsy on relapse to determine subsequent management [4]. In patients presenting with stage III and stage IV disease, the median survival from second remission is six years but decreases with each subsequent remission thereafter. Thus in the younger patient with follicular lymphoma an experimental approach is justified.

Several studies have investigated the use of intensive therapy in follicular lymphoma: the first in newly diagnosed patients compares an expectant policy of observation until such time as symptoms supervene with an intensive drug regimen (ProMACE-MOPP) followed by total nodal irradiation. A preliminary analysis shows no difference in overall survival between the two groups of patients; however, disease-free survival at four years is significantly different in favour of the patients receiving intensive initial therapy [12]. The results of another study, in patients with stage III disease who received intensive chemotherapy and radiotherapy sequentially, show a difference in survival in comparison with a historical control group [13]. A Cancer and Leukemia Group B trial in patients with nodular mixed lymphoma shows longer survival for patients receiving an intensive multidrug regimen as compared to cyclophosphamide alone [14].

Myeloablative therapy with ABMT has only recently been considered in the management of patients with follicular lymphoma following the demonstration of its apparent value in patients with sensitive relapse [6] of high-grade lymphoma. The frequent occurrence and persistence of bone marrow infiltration in follicular lymphoma have in general precluded the use of such marrow to support very intensive therapy. In vitro treatment of the marrow might circumvent the problem to some extent. The morbidity and potential mortality of the treatment has also contributed to a reluctance to use it in patients who might otherwise remain well for a meaningful period of time, together with a degree of complacency about the indolent nature of a disease, the mortality of which is without question.

The treatment-related mortality in the study to date (2 of 38 patients) is lower than that reported in most series [5, 6, 8–10] and probably reflects the degree of selection of the patients in terms of remission status and therefore by definition very good performance status. Haematological recovery was not appreciably different from that reported for patients in whom the marrow was not treated in vitro [5–10]. The delayed recovery of immunoglobulins consequent upon B-cell depletion of the marrow and the preponderance of T8+ cells for a prolonged period of time confirms the experience of Anderson et al. [18].

The question of whether reinfusion of morphologically undetectable (or detectable) lymphoma contributes to relapse remains to be resolved. Only a randomised comparison would definitively answer the question of efficacy of the in vitro treatment. However, a quantitative adaptation of the polymerase chain reaction to detect the presence of bone marrow cells containing the t(14;18) translocation, before and after the in vitro treatment, has shown a 5- to 50-fold reduction in all 10 patients in this study investigated to date [19]. Although reduced in number, cells containing the t(14;18) translocation were still detectable, but their significance is at present uncertain.

The results presented above are preliminary and raise a number of questions: Is the combination of cyclophosphamide and TBI the best ablative regimen? What, if any, is the role of the in vitro treatment? Should such therapy be used in first remission? Will such intensive therapy be curative in follicular lymphoma? Longer follow-up is obviously required, but the results to date are encouraging and warrant further evaluation.

Acknowledgements

We are indebted to the nursing staff of Annie Zunz and Dalziel Wards at St. Bartholomew's Hospital and Gordon Hamilton Fairley Ward at Homerton Hospital and the staff of the Radiotherapy Department at St. Bartholomew's Hospital. Anti-CD20, complement and the EPICS C Flow Cytometer were generously provided by Coulter Immunology, Hialeah Florida. We thank Claire Parfitt for preparing the manuscript.

References

1. Kennedy T et al. Combination vs successive single agent chemotherapy in lymphocytic lymphoma. Cancer 1978; 41: 23.
2. Lister TA et al. Comparison of combined and single agent chemotherapy in non-Hodgkin's lymphoma of favourable histological type. Br Med J 1978; 1: 533.
3. Hoppe RT, Kushalan P, Kaplan HS et al. The treatment of advanced stage favourable histology non-Hodgkin's lymphoma: A preliminary report of a randomised trial comparing single agent chemotherapy, combination chemotherapy and whole body irradiation. Blood 1981; 58: 592.
4. Gallagher CJ et al. Follicular Lymphoma: Prognostic factors for response and survival. J Clin Oncol 1986; 4: 1470.
5. Armitage JO, Gingrich RD, Klassen LW et al. Trial of high dose Cytarabine, Cyclophosphamide, total body irradiation and autologous bone marrow transplantation for refractory lymphoma. Cancer Treat Rep 1986; 70: 871.
6. Philip T, Armitage JO, Spitzer G et al. High dose therapy and autologous bone marrow transplantation after failure of conventional chemotherapy in adults with intermediate grade or high grade non-Hodgkin's lymphoma. N Engl J Med 1987; 316: 1493.
7. Gulati SC, Shank B, Black P et al. Autologous bone marrow transplantation for patients with poor prognosis lymphoma. J Clin Oncol 1988; 1303.
8. Goldstone AH, Linch DC, Gribben JG et al. Experience of autologous bone marrow transplantation in the first 100 lymphomas. Bone Marrow Transplant 1988; 3: 65.
9. Colombat P, Gorin NC, Lemonnier MP et al. The role of autologous bone marrow transplantation in 46 adult patients with non-Hodgkin's lymphoma. J Clin Oncol 1990; 8 (4): 630.
10. Petersen FB, Appelbaum FR, Hill R et al. Autologous transplantation for malignant lymphoma. A report of 101 cases from Seattle. J Clin Oncol 1990; 8 (4): 638.
11. Freedman AS, Takvorian T, Anderson KC et al. Autologous bone marrow transplantation in B cell non-Hodgkin's lymphoma: very low treatment mortality in 100 patients in sensitive relapse. J Clin Oncol 1990; (in press).
12. Young RC, Longo DL, Glatstein E et al. The treatment of indolent lymphomas; watchful waiting vs aggressive combined modality treatment. Sem Hem 1988; 25 (2): 11.
13. McLaughlin P, Fuller L, Velasquez W et al. Stage III Follicular Lymphoma: durable remissions with combined chemotherapy and radiotherapy regime. J Clin Oncol 1987; 5: 867.
14. Peterson BA, Anderson JR, Frizzera CD et al. Combination chemotherapy prolongs survival in follicular mixed lymphoma (FML). Proc ASCO 1990; 9: 259.
15. Nadler LM, Takvorian T, Botnick L et al. Anti-B1 monoclonal antibody and complement treatment in autologous bone marrow transplantation for relapsed B cell non-Hodgkin's lymphoma. Lancet 1984; 2: 427.
16. Dorey EL, Outram SV, Holder A et al. Assessment of bone marrow infiltration in B cell non-Hodgkin's lymphoma. Br J Cancer 1989; 59: 772.
17. Storring RA, McElwain TJ, Jameson B et al. Oral non-absorbed antibiotics prevent infection in acute non-lymphoblastic leukaemia. Lancet 1977; ii: 837.
18. Anderson KC, Ritz J et al. Haematologic engraftment and immune reconstitution post-transplantation with anti-B1 purged autologous bone marrow. Blood 1987; 69: 597.
19. Price CGA, Rohatiner AZS, Cotter FE et al. Minimal residual disease and the efficacy of in vitro bone marrow (BM) purging in follicular lymphoma measured by an adapted polymerase chain reaction technique. Proc ASCO 1990; 9: 258.

Correspondence to:
Dr. A. Z. S. Rohatiner
Dept of Medical Oncology
St. Bartholomew's Hospital
London, EC1A 7BE, UK

Annals of Oncology, Supplement 2 to Volume 2: 151–155, 1991.
© 1991 *Kluwer Academic Publishers*.

Original article

Expression of growth-related genes and drug-resistance genes in HTLV-I-positive and HTLV-I-negative post-thymic T-cell malignancies*

Ih-Jen Su, Inn-Chuun Chang & Ann-Lii Cheng
Department of Pathology and Hematology/Oncology, National Taiwan University Hospital and College of Medicine, Taipei, Taiwan, R.O.C.

Summary. This study was designed to investigate the biologic and molecular basis of the aggressive behavior of high-grade post-thymic T-cell malignancies. Freshly frozen tumor tissues from (1) human T-cell leukemia/lymphoma virus type I (HTLV-I)-positive adult T-cell lymphoma (ATL) (7 cases), (2) HTLV-I-negative aggressive T-cell lymphoma (12 cases), and (3) HTLV-I-negative nonaggressive T-cell lymphoma (11 cases) were studied for the expression of several growth-related genes or proliferation antigens including interleukin-2 receptor (IL-2R), Ki-67, transforming growth factor-β (TGF-β), topoisomerase, and the multidrug resistance (MDR) gene by immunohistochemistry and Northern blot hybridization. Our results showed that tumor cells associated with HTLV-I and anaplastic morphology had an enhanced expression of Ki-67, TGF-β, and topoisomerase, as compared to nonaggressive T-cell lymphoma. The expression of IL-2R was limited to ATL and one Ki-1 lymphoma. The MDR gene was frequently expressed in ATL, but only infrequently in other, HTLV-I-negative, malignancies. Clinical progression or relapse was associated with the expression of MDR, in addition to an increased expression of Ki-67. We therefore conclude that the aggressive clinical behavior of high-grade T-cell lymphoma may result mainly from the high proliferative activity of tumor cells, but the association with HTLV-I and clinical relapse is further complicated by the development of drug resistance.

Key words: growth factor, drug resistance, T cell lymphoma

Post-thymic T-cell malignancies encompass an increasingly wide spectrum of neoplasms with diverse clinicopathologic features [1, 2]. Although the prognosis of these T-cell malignancies still remains controversial, several factors have been implicated as indicative of a poor prognosis, including infection with human T-cell leukemia/lymphoma virus type I (HTLV-I), blastic transformation, and anaplastic morphology [2, 3]. The common features of these aggressive T-cell lymphomas are the failure to achieve remission or the short remission duration and rapid development of resistance to conventional chemotherapy after clinical relapse [4].

One of the several factors that may be responsible for the failure of lymphoma therapy is a high proliferative activity of the tumor cells probably associated with the activation of growth factors and oncogenes such as interleukin-2 receptor (IL-2R) and transforming growth factor type β (TGF-β) [5]. The expression of Ki-67 antigen in the nuclei has been noted to correlate well with the growth fraction of the tumor cells and has been applied to predict the tumor prognosis [6]. Recently, a DNA topoisomerase which modulates the topological state of DNA has been shown to be essential for the replication of cellular as well as viral DNA,

and the activity of topoisomerase may be regarded as a marker of cellular proliferation [7].

A second factor that may contribute to the failure of lymphoma therapy is the development of multidrug resistance (MDR) particularly after chemotherapy [8]. The expression of the MDR gene has been shown to play an important role in predicting the failure of cancer chemotherapy in some human cancers.

In this study, we investigated the expression of several growth-related genes or proliferation-associated antigens and MDR genes in a spectrum of T-cell lymphomas to explore the possible biological and molecular basis of the rapid clinical course and poor prognosis of these aggressive T-cell lymphomas.

Materials and methods

Specimens

Freshly frozen lymphoma tissues are selected for this study. The specimens included the following three groups of post-thymic T-cell malignancies (Table 1): Group A, 7 cases of HTLV-I-positive ATL, including 2 medium-cell type, 2 large-cell, and 3 pleomorphic type;

* Supported by a research grant from the National Science Council, Taiwan, R.O.C. (NSC 78-0412-B002-162).

Table 1. A summary of the expression of growth-related genes and drug resistance genes in HTLV-1-positive and HLTV-1 negative post-thymic T cell malignances.

| | No. of cases studied | No. of cases positive | | | | | | |
| | | Immunohistochemistry | | | Transcripts | | | |
		IL-2R	Ki-67[b]	MDR	IL-2R	TGF	Top	MDR-1
(A) HTLV-1 (+) ATL	7	6	5	4	4	7	6	3
(B) HTLV-1 (−) aggressive PTL	12	1	5	2[a]	1	8	8	2
(C) HTLV-1 (−) nonaggressive PTL	11	0	0	1	0	3	4	0

[a] Both cases had a low proportion of Ki-67-positive cells.
[b] The number representing cases in which Ki-67-positive cells account for more than 30% of the total neoplastic cells.

Abbreviations: IL-2R, interleukin-2 receptor; MDR, multidrug resistance, P-glycoprotein; TGF, transforming growth factor-beta; Top, topoisomerase; ATL, adult T cell lymphoma; PTL, peripheral T cell lymphoma.

Group B, 12 cases of HTLV-I-negative aggressive or high-grade peripheral T-cell lymphoma (PTL). All cases had large-cell or immunoblastic morphology; Group C, 11 cases of HTLV-I-negative nonaggressive T-cell lymphoma, including 3 mixed cell type, 2 angioimmunoblastic lymphadenopathy (AILD)-like lymphoma, 3 small/medium type lymphoma, and 3 mycosis fungoides. Five paired specimens from 5 patients were separately included to compare the expression of Ki-67 and the MDR gene before and after chemotherapy.

Immunophenotypic studies

For immunophenotypic study, thin 6-μm sections of lymphoma tissues were cut, briefly fixed in cold acetone for five minutes, and immunostained by the avidin-biotin-complex (ABC) method. Monoclonal antibodies Ki-67 (Dako) defining proliferative activity, IL-2 receptor (IL-2R, CD25) (Dako) defining the T-cell growth factor receptor, and P-glycoprotein (P-glycoCHEK C219, Centocor) defining the product of the MDR gene were applied.

RNA isolation and northern blot hybridization analysis

Total cellular RNA from tumor was isolated by a modified rapid method [5]. Briefly, the tumor tissues were lysed in a solution containing 0.05 M sodium acetate (pH 5.2) and 1.0% sodium dodecyl sulfate, and extracted with phenol saturated with 0.05 M sodium acetate at 65 °C for 15 min, followed by an ice bath for another 15 min. The solution was centrifuged in Eppendorf tubes for five min. The upper aqueous layer was harvested, and the RNA was dissolved in DEPC (diethyl-pyrocarbonate)-treated water containing RNAsin (RNAse inhibitor; 1 U/μg, Promega, Madison, Wis.) and kept at −70 °C. For Northern blot hybridization,

40 μg of the extracted RNA were size-fractionated by electrophoresis on a 1.4% agarose gel containing formaldehyde, transferred to a nylon membrane, and then baked, prehybridized, and hybridized with the appropriate probes, as the manufacturer suggested.

cDNA probes

To study the expression of growth-related genes and the MDR gene in post-thymic T-cell malignancies, DNA fragments specific for the following genes were used: IL-2R (320 bp, 4th exon, Oncor, Gaithersburg, Md.), TGF-β (320 bp, kindly provided by Dr. R. Derynck, Genentech, South San Francisco, Cal.), topoisomerase I and II (kindly provided by Dr. Huang in Academia Sinica, R.O.C.) and MDR-1 (kindly provided by Dr. Gottesman, National Institutes of Health, Bethesda, Md., USA). The DNA probes were synthesized with P[32]-dCTP by the random oligonucleotide primer method, and highly radioactive probes were used for the hybridization. An actin probe (Oncor) was used for the quantitative control of loaded cellular RNAs.

Results

Immunohistochemical Studies

The results of immunohistochemistry studies are shown in Table 1 and Figure 1.

Ki-67
Ki-67 immunoreactivity was found in the nuclei of a variable proportion of cells in all cases of ATL and high-grade T-cell lymphoma in group B ranging from 5% to more than 50%. In nonaggressive T-cell lymphoma or mycosis fungoides, the Ki-67 staining was

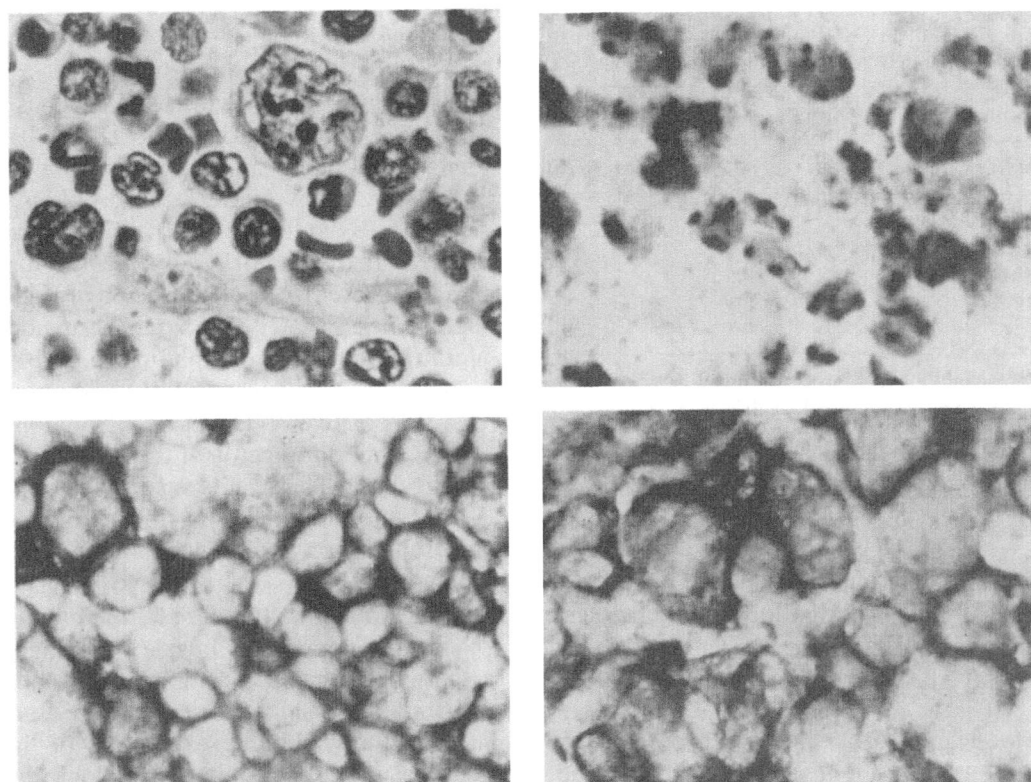

Fig. 1. (top left) The histology of a pleomorphic type HTLV-1-positive adult T cell lymphoma (H-E, × 400). (top right) The immunostaining of Ki-67 in the same ATL case. Most cells are positive for Ki-67 in the nuclei (ABC immunoperoxidase, × 400). (bottom left) The expression of IL-2 receptor (Tac). (bottom right) The expression of P-glycoprotein in the cell membrane.

only sporadic, usually less than 5%. The percentage of Ki-67-positive cells was more than 30% in 5 of 7 ATL (Fig. 1b), in 5 of 12 group B cases, and in none of 11 low-grade T-cell lymphomas in group C.

IL-2R
The expression of IL-2R was limited to 6 of 7 ATL (Fig. 1c) and 1 Ki-1 lymphoma in group B. The majority of HTLV-T-negative T-cell lymphoma cases were negative for IL-2R.

P-glycoprotein (MDR)
The expression of P-glycoprotein (MDR) was unusually high in ATL (4 of 7) (Fig. 1d). The staining is on the cell membrane. However, a faint cytoplasmic expression cannot be neglected. In HTLV-T-negative high-grade T-cell lymphoma, the expression of P-glycoprotein was present in only 2 of 12 cases; both cases showed a low percentage (<10%) of Ki-67-positive cells. Therefore, there is a discordant expression of Ki-67 and MDR.

Studies on paired biopsy specimens obtained before and after chemotherapy

Morphologic and immunohistochemical studies were performed on 5 HTLV-I-negative paired lymphoma specimens removed from 5 patients before and after chemotherapy. The results are shown in Table 2. A significant morphologic progression from mixed-cell morphology to large-cell/immunoblastic lymphoma was demonstrated in 3 patients. There is also a significant increase of the proportion of Ki-67-positive cells in the relapse specimens. The most remarkable finding was the acquired expression of P-glycoprotein in 2 relapse specimens.

Northern blot hybridization

The results of Northern blot studies are shown in Table 1 and Figure 2.

IL-2R
Two transcripts were noted at approximately 3.5 kb and 1.5 kb in 4 of 7 ATL and in one Ki-1 lymphoma in group B. The remaining cases showed no detectable transcripts.

TGF-β
The transcripts of TGF-β were detected at 2.5 kb in all 7 cases of ATL, in 8 of 12 high-grade PTL in group B, and in 3 of 11 low-grade T-cell lymphomas in group C.

Topoisomerase
The transcripts of topoisomerases I and II were detected at around 6 and 7 kb, respectively; 6 of 7 ATL, 8 of

Table 2. A comparison of the morphologic change and expression of Ki-67 and P-glycoprotein (MDR) in 5 paired specimens from 5 patients biopsied separately before and after chemotherapy.

	Morphology		Ki-67[a]		P-glycoprotein	
	Before	After	Before	After	Before	After
Case 1	mixed cell	large	–	+++	–	–
Case 2	mixed cell	large	+	+	–	+
Case 3	AILD-like	IBL	–	++	–	–
Case 4	large	large	++	+++	–	–
Case 5	large	large	++	++	–	+

[a] The immunoreactivity of Ki-67 was expressed as '–', 0–10%; '+' 10–20%; '++', 20–50%; '+++', more than 50%.

Abbreviations: AILD, angioimmunoblastic lymphadenopathy; immunoblastic lymphoma; MDR, multidrug resistance, P-glycoprotein.

12 high-grade PTL in group B, and 4 of 11 low grade T cell lymphomas in group C had detectable transcripts of topoisomerase I or II.

MDR-1

Detectable levels of MDR-1 transcript were noted in 3 of 7 ATL, in 2 of 12 high-grade PTL, and in none of the 11 low-grade T-cell lymphomas.

Discussion

Our study demonstrates high-level expression of a combination of growth-related genes in HTLV-I-positive T-cell lymphoma and HTLV-1-negative high-grade T-cell malignancies, but only low-level or absent expression in low-grade T-cell lymphoma. The expression of Ki-67 antigen, TGF-β, and topoisomerase is increased in the majority of cases of high-grade lymphoma. Therefore, the expression of Ki-67, TGF-β and topoisomerase can be regarded as an index of high proliferative activity of lymphoma [5, 9, 10]. The expression of IL-2R, however, is more type-specific, limited to HTLV-I-positive ATL and Ki-1 lymphoma [5] and may not be a good indicator of the proliferative activity for practical use. The results suggest that different types of T-cell lymphoma may use different growth factors for the proliferation and growth of neoplastic cells.

The high expression of the MDR gene in ATL may help to explain the frequent failure of lymphoma therapy in these patients, besides the high proliferative activity of these neoplasms. All but one of the specimens of ATL in this series were sampled before chemotherapy, and the expression of the MDR gene therefore may be an inherent biological feature of the neoplastic cells. Since the samples we used in this study

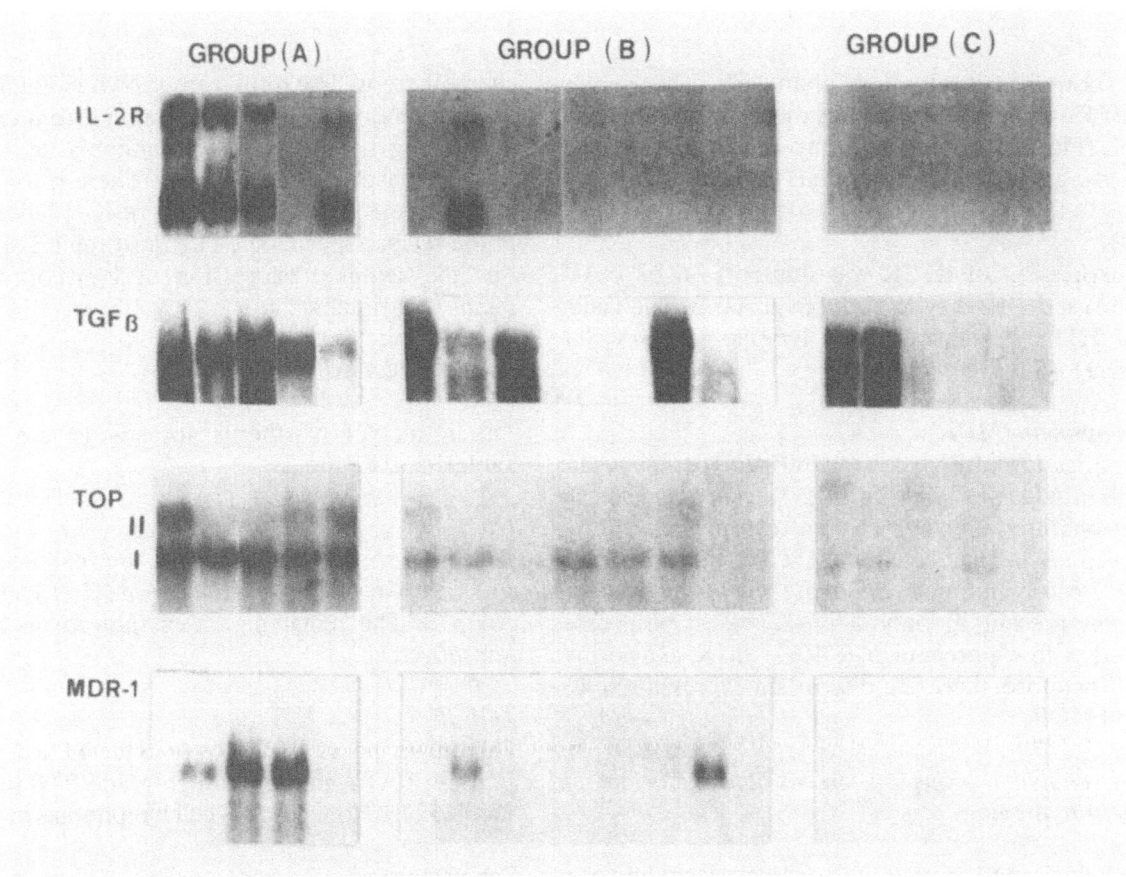

Fig. 2. Northern analysis of several growth-related genes and multidrug resistance gene (MDR-1) in some representative cases of HTLV-1-positive (Group A), HTLV-1-negative aggressive (Group B), and HTLV-1-negative nonaggressive (Group C) T cell lymphoma.

were limited, this observation should be further clarified. The expression of MDR in other groups of T-cell lymphomas is only sporadic. In the two cases of high-grade PTL in group B which showed expression in MDR-1, the staining of Ki-67 was, however, only of low percentage (<10%), suggesting that complex factors may co-operate to determine the prognosis of these aggressive T cell lymphomas.

Clinical relapse is an important feature of T-cell lymphoma and usually indicates a poor prognosis [4, 11]. The observations we made from the five paired biopsy specimens examined separately before and after chemotherapy from five patients revealed significant morphologic progression from a mixed cell type to a more homogeneous large-cell/immunoblastic lymphoma in three cases. There is also a remarkable increase of the proportion of Ki-67-positive cells. The acquisition of MDR gene expression in 2 of them may explain the frequent resistance to chemotherapy in relapsing T-cell lymphoma. The same observations have been noted in acute leukemia and myeloma [12, 13]. Therefore, clinical relapse of T-cell lymphoma carries the risk of blastic transformation, an increase in proliferative activity, and the possible development of drug resistance.

The operative mechanisms contributing to the failure of lymphoma therapy are complex. Besides the proliferative activity of tumor cells and the expression of the MDR gene mentioned in this study, other factors such as immune escape and the released lymphokines may also play important roles contributing to the biologic behavior and clinical course of T-cell lymphoma and finally resulting in the failure of lymphoma therapy.

References

1. Jaffe ES. Pathologic and clinical spectrum of post-thymic T-cell malignancies. Cancer Invest 1984; 2: 413–26.
2. Suchi T, Lennert K, Tu LY, Kikuchi M, Sato E, Stansfeld AG, Feller EC. Histopatholoty and immunohistochemistry of peripheral T-cell lymphomas: A proposal for their classification. J Clin Pathol 1987; 40: 995–1015.
3. Su IJ, Wang CW, Cheng AL et al. Characterization of the spectrum of postthymic T-cell malignancies in Taiwan – A clinicopathologic study of HTLV-1-positive and HTLV-1-negative cases. Cancer 1988; 61: 2060–70.
4. Cheng AL, Chen YC, Wang CH et al. Direct comparisons of peripheral T cell lymphoma with diffuse B cell lymphoma of comparabel histologic grades. Is PTCL a unique entity of lymphoma which warrants separate considerations. J Clin Oncol 1989; 7: 715–23.
5. Su IJ, Kadin M. Expression of growth factor/receptor genes in postthymic T cell malignancies. Am J Pathol 1989; 135: 439–45.
6. Hall PA, Crocker J, Watts A, Stansfeld AG. A comparison of nucleolar organizer region staining and Ki-67 immunostaining in non-Hodgkin's lymphoma. Histopathology 1988; 12: 373–81.
7. Uemura T, Yanagida M. Isolation of type I and II DNA topoisomerase mutants from fission yeast: single and double mutants show different phenotypes in cell growth and chromatin organization. EMBO J. 1984; 3: 1737–44.
8. Weinstein RS, Kuszak JR, Kluskens LF, Coon JS. P-glycoproteins in pathology. The multidrug resistance gene family in humans. Human Pathol 1990; 21: 34–49.
9. Gerdes J, Dallenbach F, Lennert K, Stein H. Growth fractions in malignant non-Hodgkin's lymphomas as determined in situ with the monoclonal antibody Ki67. Haematol. Oncol. 1984b; 2: 365–71.
10. Tandau G, Mirambeau G, Lavenot C, der Garabedian A, Vermeersch J, and Duguet M. DNA topoisomerase activities in concanavalin A-stimulated lymphocytes. FEBS Lett. 1984; 176: 431–5.
11. Armitage JO, Greer JP, Levine AM et al. Peripheral T cell lymphoma. Cancer 1989; 63: 158–63.
12. Fojo AT, Ueda K, Slaman DJ et al. Expression of a multidrugresistance gene in human tumors and tissues. Proc Natl Acad Sci USA 1987; 84: 3004–8.
13. Cairo MS, Siegel S, Anas N et al. Clinical trial of continuous infusion verapamil, bolus vinblastine, and continuous infusion VP-16 in drug-resistant pediatric tumors. Cancer Res 1989; 49: 1063–6.

Correspondence to:
Dr. Ih-Jen Su
Department of Pathology
National Taiwan University Hospital
1, Chang-Teh Street, Taipei, Taiwan, R.O.C.

Annals of Oncology, Supplement 2 to Volume 2: 157–162, 1991.
© 1991 *Kluwer Academic Publishers*.

Original article

Peripheral T-cell lymphoma in Japan: Recent progress*

Masanori Shimoyama

Hematology-Oncology and Medical Oncology Division, National Cancer Center Hospital, Tokyo, Japan

Summary. T-lymphoma, including adult T-cell leukemia-lymphoma (ATL) accounted for 75% of non-Hodgkin's lymphoma in the Kyushu district of Japan and for 43% in the nation as a whole. Human T-cell leukemia/lymphoma virus type I (HTLV-I) is closely associated with ATL; however, 11 (7.5%) of 147 patients with ATL were HTLV-I negative. The cumulative percentage incidence of anti-HTLV-I seropositive ATL patients can be simply described by a Weibull model of the typical tear-off type, suggesting that ATL leukemogenesis may be the result of accumulation of approximately five critical events, most likely somatic mutations within HTLV-I-infected T-cells. ATL is still a difficult disease to treat successfully, while peripheral non-ATL T-lymphoma responded to standard chemotherapy in the same way as B-lymphoma. The disease entity of immunoblastic lymphadenopathy (IBL)-like T-lymphoma was also described. Morphological recognition of focal or sheetlike proliferation of atypical neoplastic pale cells and immunoblasts of T-cell nature were important findings for the diagnosis. Major prognostic factors differed greatly among ATL, peripheral non-ATL T-lymphoma and B-lymphoma. Pathology was not associated with treatment outcome and survival in T-cell diseases. These results indicate that the terms ATL, peripheral non-ATL T-lymphoma, and B-lymphoma should be used instead of the all-inclusive term non-Hodgkin's lymphoma, because of differences in cellular origin, clinical features, treatment outcome, prognosis, prognostic factors, chromosomal aberrations, and etiology.

Key words: AILD, ATL, EBV, HTLV-I, IBL-like T-lymphoma, prognostic factor

Introduction

Recent lymphoma research has revealed that non-Hodgkin's lymphoma consists of T-lymphoma and B-lymphoma. T- and B-lymphomas are different in cellular origin, clinical features, treatment response, prognosis, prognostic factors, chromosomal aberrations, and etiology. Also, there are many differences in the characteristics of adult non-Hodgkin's lymphomas between the East and the West. The prognosis of patients with non-Hodgkin's lymphoma in Japan is generally poorer than that in Western countries. Unfavorable peripheral T-cell lymphomas such as adult T-cell leukemia-lymphoma (ATL) are more frequently observed in Japan than in the West, while incidence of favorable B-cell lymphomas is much less in Japan than in Western countries [1, 2]. Our previous study revealed that one of the most important prognostic factors of adult patients with advanced non-Hodgkin's lymphomas was surface marker [3], and that prognostic factors were greatly different between T- and B-lymphomas, indicating that T- and B-lymphomas should be analyzed separately [4, 5].

Recent studies also revealed that Hodgkin's disease was heterogeneous, and about 30% of morphologically defined Hodgkin's disease turned out to be T- or B-lymphoma based on immunophenotypic and immunogenotypic analyses. The cellular origin of Hodgkin's disease is still not clear [6]. Therefore, non-Hodgkin's lymphoma, which has been named on the basis of Hodgkin's disease, becomes inadequate in terminology. In addition, new disease entities such as ATL and immunoblastic lymphadenopathy (IBL)-like T-cell lymphoma have been established. Therefore, we propose that at least three different diseases, ATL, peripheral non-ATL T-lymphoma, and B-lymphoma, should be used instead of the all-inclusive non-Hodgkin's lymphoma. Here we summarize recent progress in research of peripheral T-cell lymphoma, including ATL, in Japan.

Recent progress in ATL research in Japan

1. Further epidemiological study on ATL in Japan

ATL is a unique T-cell malignancy with which human T-cell leukemia/lymphoma virus type I (HTLV-I) is

* This work was supported in part by Grants-in-Aid for Cancer Research (2S-1) and for Comprehensive 10-year Strategy for Cancer Control from the Ministry of Health and Welfare.

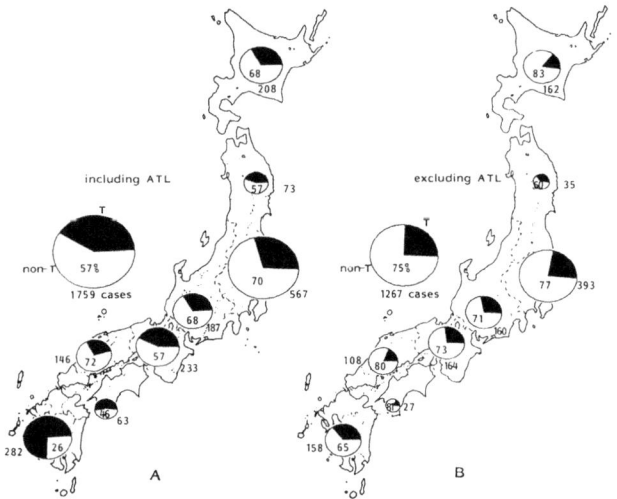

Fig. 1. Geographical distribution of birth places of patients with T- and B-lymphomas. (A) Distribution of 1759 patients including ATL. The number in circle indicates percentage of non-T-lymphoma. The number outside circle indicates number of cases. (B) Distribution of 1267 patients excluding ATL. Data were obtained from the 4th nation-wide survey of ATL [9].

closely associated [7, 8]. ATL occurs in adult HTLV-I carriers. The incidence of ATL was calculated to be 0.6 per 1 000 adult HTLV-I carriers (>20 years of age) from strict epidemiological surveys at specific places in ATL-endemic areas. From a nationwide survey of ATL [9], a total of 697 new cases of ATL can be counted every year in Japan. Approximately 80% of ATL patients were from southern Japan (Kyushu, Kii, and South Shikoku), and 10% were from northern Japan (Hokkaido and Tohoku) as shown in Figure 1. The ratio between T- and B-lymphomas in Kyushu was remarkably high (2.85) compared to that in other districts (0.52). When ATL cases were excluded from the cases of non-Hodgkin's lymphomas, the ratio between non-ATL T-lymphoma (peripheral T-lymphoma not associated with HTLV-I) and B-lymphoma was not very different by district in Japan. It was 0.55 in the Kyushu district and 0.31 in other districts.

2. HTLV-I-negative ATL

ATL is believed to be caused by HTLV-I [7, 8]. However, we found that 11 patients with ATL have typical clinicohematological, morphological, and immunophenotypic features, but no antibody to HTLV-I as well as no provirus integration [10–12]. The clinicohematological features of HTLV-I-negative ATL were the same as HTLV-I-positive ATL. From the clinical features, 7 patients were diagnosed as acute type, 2 as chronic type, and 2 others as lymphoma type of ATL according to the classification of subtypes of ATL [13]. Survival from the time of diagnosis was usually short (1–13+ months) except for 1 patient with chronic ATL (34 months).

Leukemia cells were positive for CD3 and CD4 and negative for CD8 in most patients. In karyotype anal-

ysis of HTLV-I-negative patients with ATL, we found the same very complicated chromosome constitutions as those found in HTLV-I-associated ATL [14, 15] such as trisomy for chromosomes 3, 7 or 7q, and 21, monosomy for chromosomes X, Y, 13, 14, and 17, rearrangements involving 6q21, 10p11–13, and 14q11 [16]. These results suggest that HTLV-I was not involved in leukemogenesis of HTLV-I-negative ATL and that there may be common factor(s) other than HTLV-I in the process of leukemogenesis in both HTLV-I-positive and -negative ATLs.

3. Multistep leukemogenesis model of ATL

HTLV-I can immortalize human T cells. However, the virus alone cannot explain the development of ATL because of the presence of a long latency period between HTLV-I infection and the disease manifestation as well as a very low occurrence rate of ATL among carriers of the virus. Recent studies have demonstrated that HTLV-I-pX (tax_1/rex_1) gene product, tax_1 (also called $p40^X$, X-lor, or pX protein), is responsible for activation of cellular genes, such as those for interleukin-2 (IL-2) or interleukin-2 receptor (IL-2R) in some T-cell lines [17]. Expression of tax_1/rex_1 mRNA was detectable in peripheral blood mononuclear cells from patients with ATL and healthy HTLV-I carriers by using reserved transcription of spliced mRNA of HTLV-I provirus followed by the polymerase chain reaction [18]. Viral antigens may be expressed only in 10^{-5} to 10^{-6} cells in circulating peripheral blood mononuclear cells. These facts indicate that HTLV-I may immortalize infected T cells via the autocrine circuit consisting of IL-2 and IL-2R.

This autocrine circuit may be responsible for polyclonal proliferation of HTLV-I-infected T cells in healthy carriers [19]. However, monoclonality of leukemic cells in ATL cannot be explained by the autocrine model. This line of thought is also supported by the occurrence of a few ATL cases that are apparently unassociated with HTLV-I. In addition, monoclonal integration of HTLV-I proviral DNA has been detected in peripheral blood lymphocytes of about 40% of anti-HTLV-I seropositive patients with strongyloidiasis [20]. White blood cell count and an absolute lymphocyte count are within the normal range in these patients. These facts indicate that specific immune stimulations to T cells may cause monoclonal proliferation of certain normal T cells. Then the monoclonal proliferation of the HTLV-I-infected T cells may continue as long as the specific immune stimulations such as the infestation of *Strongyloides stercoralis* continue. However, the monoclonal proliferation of HTLV-I-infected T cells in this situation is benign and does not indicate a malignant state.

Analysis of the age-dependent occurrence of anti-HTLV-I-seropositive ATL is of interest in considering its leukemogenesis. It was analyzed for 357 cases collected during nationwide surveys that were carried out

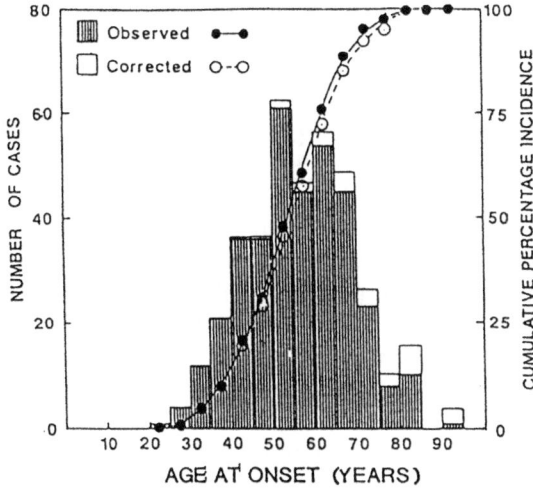
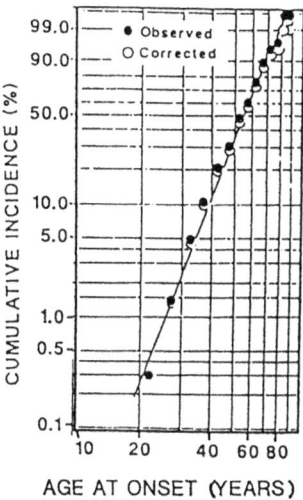

A   B

Fig. 2. The distribution of the age at disease onset of ATL patients. (A) The original ages were categorized into five-year ranks. The observed (shaded bar) and corrected (white bar) numbers of patients in each rank are shown. The corrected number in each rank was obtained by standardization by the accumulated death rate for each age rank according to data from the national population survey in Japan conducted in 1985. The cumulative percentages of ATL occurrence, both observed (●) and corrected (○), are shown by curves. (B) Weibull plots of the cumulative percentage of ATL occurrence by age. Lines were obtained for the observed (●), and the corrected (○). The ordinate indicates log [log $1/(1 - f(t))$] and the abscissa, log t.

From these analysis, onset age distribution of ATL patients can be described by a Weibull distribution model. The density function is as follows; $f(t) = a/b \cdot t^{a-1} \cdot \exp(-t^a/b)$, where t is the age (yr). a and b are 5.03 and $8.00x^{-8}$ for all cases. The figures were reproduced with permission of authors and publisher from the paper described by Okamoto et al. (Jpn J Cancer Res 1989; 80: 191–5.)

between 1982 and 1985 in Japan [1, 21]. It was assumed that patients were infected with HTLV-I during infancy and that the age at onset of ATL could be regarded as the incubation period of the disease. As shown in Figure 2, ATL development started from the age of 24 years, peaked at 50–54 years, and then decreased. Cumulative percentage incidence of these ATL patients can be simply described by a Weibull model of the typical tear-off type [22]. These results suggest that ATL leukemogenesis may be the result of accumulation of numerous critical events, most likely somatic mutations within HTLV-I-immortalized T cells. Parameters' values for the density functions of the Weibull model ('a' as shape parameter and 'b' as scale parameter) to describe the onset of ATL were as follows; $a = 5.03$, $b = 8.0 \times 10^{-8}$. The putative number of independent leukemogenic mutations involved in ATL is estimated to be approximately five (represented as parameter 'a') from the analysis [22]. Although HTLV-I infection plays a primary role as an initiator in the pathogenesis of ATL, it may be only a prerequisite for accumulation of later events and may not be the direct cause of the disease unless HTLV-I is subsequently shown to possess a mutagenic potential in T cells. Thus, the increase in number of HTLV-I-infected T cells may imply the increase in incidence of malignant transformation of the HTLV-I-infected T cells in vivo. The rarity of HTLV-I-negative ATL may be explained mainly by the later events and suggests that ATL could occur without HTLV-I infection if the T-cell population of a particular differentiation lineage were to be immortalized by another less common mechanism.

It is considered that the rates of ATL-prone somatic mutations are very low and/or that quite a large number of HTLV-I-immortalized cells are required for ATL development within the normal human life span. The presence of HTLV-I-negative ATL suggests that unknown cellular oncogenes closely related to the transformation of inducer/helper T cells may exist, although we are unable to speculate further on the nature of the target genes for the mutations involved in ATL leukemogenesis.

Immunoblastic lymphadenopathy (IBL)-like T-cell lymphoma

A group of systemic lymphoproliferative disorders have been described under the heading of angioimmunoblastic lymphadenopathy with dysproteinemia (AILD) and IBL. In spite of fatal outcome in most cases, AILD and IBL were considered as nonneoplastic lymphoproliferative disorders (possibly abnormal hyperimmune B-cell disorders) and as a prelymphoma state of immunoblastic sarcoma. Some reports documented the high incidence of malignant lymphoma in patients with AILD and IBL.

In 1979, we reported that IBL or AILD was a peripheral T-cell lymphoma on the basis of surface marker analysis and cytological and histopathological findings, and proposed a new disease entity, 'IBL-like T-cell lymphoma,' as a variant of peripheral T-cell lymphoma [23]. The most important findings were summarized in three following points: Firstly, atypical large lymphoid cells were observed in the aspiration cytology smear of swollen lymph nodes and these cells were cytologically considered to be lymphoma cells. Secondly, these atypical large lymphoid cells could form rosettes with sheep erythrocytes, namely E-rosettes, indicating that these cells were of a T-cell nature. Thirdly, the important diagnostic histological finding of IBL-like T-cell lymphoma was focal or sheetlike neoplastic proliferation of atypical lymphoid cells consisting of immunoblasts and so-called 'pale-cells' in the background of histologic features indistinguishable from those of AILD or IBL [23–26].

Further study revealed that immunogenotypic analysis was important to show clonal proliferation of T cells in these cases evidenced by rearrangement of the T-cell receptor beta-chain gene and germ-line configuration of the immunoglobulin heavy chain gene [24]. Then most AILD/IBL turned out to be IBL-like T-cell lymphoma.

IBL-like T-cell lymphoma may be divided into two groups on the basis of surface marker analysis: the CD4-positive group and the CD8-positive group [24, 27]. However, there were no significant differences in clinical manifestations, histologic findings and survivals between the both groups [24]. Further studies are necessary to clarify the differences between the CD4-positive group and the CD8-positive group.

Present state of treatment of peripheral T-cell lymphoma in Japan

Despite recent progress in combination chemotherapy, the prognosis of patients with ATL is still poor [3, 4]. A randomized study of T-lymphomas [3, 4] revealed that complete response (CR) was achieved in only about 28% of patients with ATL treated with doxorubicin (Adriamycin)-containing first-generation combination chemotherapy [4]. Interestingly, CR and four-year survival rates were significantly associated with clinical diagnosis, but not with pathology; the CR rate was 28% for ATL versus 63% for non-ATL T-lymphoma, and the four-year survival rate was only 8% for ATL versus 46% for non-ATL T-lymphoma.

The primary reason for the poor CR rates is the poor condition of patients, evidenced by advanced performance status (PS), hypercalcemia, high levels of lactate dehydrogenase (LDH), large tumor burden, hyperleukocytosis, and infectious complications due to their immunodeficient state [28]. In this context, both special supportive therapy and effective anticancer drugs should be explored for ATL patients to improve treatment outcome.

Prognostic factors of peripheral T-lymphomas

1. Major prognostic factors of patients with ATL

Because of the diversity in clinical courses of patients with ATL [13], major prognostic factors should be identified to find patients with varying risks of death. In the third and fourth nationwide surveys of ATL conducted from 1984 to 1987 [9, 21], detailed clinical data of 854 patients with anti-HTLV-I antibody-positive ATL, newly diagnosed from 1983 to 1987, were obtained from 175 institutions. All subtypes of HTLV-I-associated ATL were included in this study.

Thirty-six pretreatment characteristics were analyzed [28]. There were 466 males and 388 females with a mean age of 57.1 years. Of the total, 269 were still alive with a median follow-up of 14 months from diagnosis, while 585 were dead with a median survival time (MST) of 6 months. MST was 10 months, and projected two- and four-year survival rates of all patients were 28% and 12%, respectively. As shown in Table 1, a Cox proportional hazards model analysis revealed that five factors – advanced PS, high LDH value, age $\geq$40 years, increased number of total involved lesions (TIL), and hypercalcemia – were negatively associated with survival (P < 0.01). The first four factors (PS, LDH, number of TIL, and age) were selected to construct a model to identify patients at low and high risk for shortened survival. The fifth factor, corrected calcium level, was not used to identify low-risk patients, because no patient with hypercalcemia was found among low-risk patients. Seventy-two combinations of the four factors were produced, and the estimated ratio of the hazard rate for death was calculated from a Cox model in each combination. One hundred seventy-eight patients with a hazard ratio of less than 0.5 were classified as a low-risk group, and 646 with hazard ratio of 0.5 or more were placed in a high-risk group [28].

Major prognostic factors of patients at high risk were found to be four factors: PS, LDH, age and corrected calcium level [28]. Then, the four factors, including hypercalcemia instead of number of TIL, were used to identify patients with the most aggressive type of

Table 1. Cox proportional hazards model analysis of survival.

Prognostic factor	No. of patients	Univariate	Multivariate (807 cases)[a]		
		P	Beta	P	Risk ratio
Age	854	0.0001	0.7475	0.0000	2.1
PS	832	0.0000	0.4059	0.0000	3.4
No. TIL	854	0.0000	0.2849	0.0016	1.8
Corrected Ca	820	0.0000	0.4151	0.0000	1.5
LDH	836	0.0000	0.3531	0.0000	2.0

TIL, total involved lesions.
[a] Statistically significant factors were selected at P < 0.01 by stepwise method of a Cox proportional hazards model.

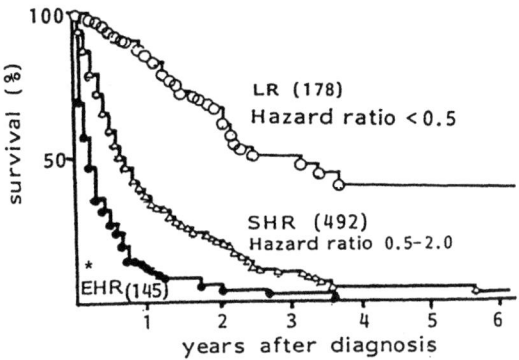

Fig. 3. Survival curves of patients with ATL at low risk, those at standard high risk (SHR) and those at extremely high risk (EHR).

Low-risk group, hazard ratio <0.5; High-risk group, hazard ratio ⩾0.5; SHR, patients having a hazard ratio of 0.5⩽ and <2.0. EHR, patients having a hazard ratio of ⩾2.0. Number in parentheses indicates number of patients.

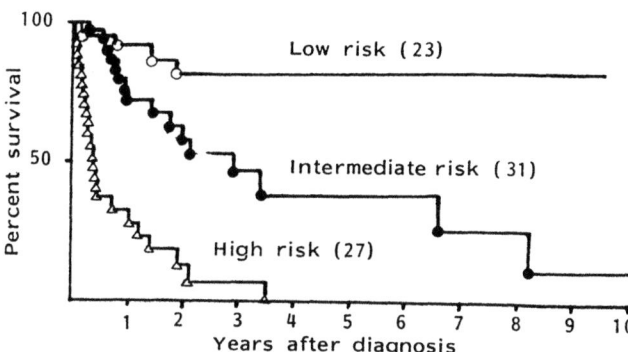

Fig. 4. Survival curves of patients with non-ATLT-lymphoma at low risk, those at intermediate risk and those at high risk. Number in parentheses indicates number of patients.

ATL. According to the estimated hazard ratio calculated for each combination of the four factors, patients at high risk were further classified into two subgroups, patients at extremely high risk (EHR), having a hazard ratio of 2.0 or more, and those at standard high risk (SHR), having a hazard ratio of less than 2.0 [28]. Survival curves of patients at low risk, EHR and SHR are shown in Figure 3. MST and projected two- and four-year survival rates were 38 months, 66.3 and 41.2% for low risk, and 7 months, 17.2 and 3.2% for high risk, respectively. In patients at SHR and those at EHR, MST was 9 months and 3 months, projected one-year survival rate was 20.6 and 13.5%, and projected two-year survival rate was 4.5 and 0%, respectively, indicating that patients at EHR represented the most aggressive type of ATL. The risk classification of ATL is useful in determining treatment strategy at diagnosis.

2. Prognostic factors of peripheral non-ATL T-lymphoma

Ninety-two adult patients with peripheral T-cell lymphoma, including IBL-like T-lymphoma and excluding ATL, were treated between January 1975 and December 1985 in the National Cancer Center Hospital.

Thirty-seven pretreatment characteristics were analyzed in this study. There were 64 males and 28 females with a mean age of 52.3 years. Of the total, 40 were still alive with a median follow-up time of 33.8 months from initial therapy, while 52 were dead with an MST of 9.7 months. MST and projected two- and four-year survival rates of all patients were 21.1 months, 51.6 and 39.7%, respectively. As shown in Table 2, a Cox proportional hazards model analysis revealed that two factors, high LDH value and advanced stage were negatively associated with survival (P < 0.01). The two factors were used to construct a model to identify patients at low, intermediate, and high risk. Eight combinations of the patients were produced, and the estimated ratio of the hazard rate for death was calculated

from a Cox model in each combination. Patients with a hazard ratio <0.4 were classified as a low-risk group, those with a hazard ratio of 0.4–1.9 as an intermediate risk group, and those with a hazard ratio ⩾2.0 as a high-risk group. The survival curves of the three risk groups are shown in Figure 4. For the low-risk group, MST was not reached, and projected two- and four-year survival rates were both 80.4%. MST and two- and four-year survival rates were 34.7 months and 62.3 and 38.4 for intermediate risk, and 4.4 months and 12.4 and 0% for high risk, respectively.

Conclusion

It is of interest to note that major prognostic factors were different among ATL, non-ATL T-lymphoma, and B-lymphoma, and that pathology was not a prognostic factor for T-cell diseases while it was the most important one for B-lymphoma. Because of the difference in cellular origin, clinical features, prognostic factors, treatment outcome, chromosomal aberrations, and etiology, at least three diseases, ATL, peripheral non-ATL T-lymphoma, and B-lymphoma, should be defined instead of the all-inclusive term non-Hodgkin's lymphoma, and each disease should be analyzed separately. Otherwise, the future of lymphoma research will not be promising.

Table 2. Major prognostic factors of peripheral non-ATLT-lymphoma.

Prognostic factors	Number of patients	Univariate	Multivariate[a]		Risk ratio
		P value	P value	beta	
LDH (N/H)	81(44/37)	0.0000	0.0029	0.5059	2.9
Stage (I/II/ III/IV	92(27/11/ 22/32)	0.0011	0.0002	0.7109	12.3

[a] Statistically significant factors were selected by stepwise method of a Cox proportional hazards model.
N, normal; H, high.

162

References

1. The T- and B-cell Malignancy Study Group, Statistical Analyses of Clinico-Pathological, Virological and Epidemiological Data on Lymphoid Malignancies with Special Reference to Adult T-Cell Leukemia/Lymphoma: A Report of the Second Nationwide Study of Japan. Jpn J Clin Oncol 1985; 15: 517–35.

2. Kadin ME, Berard CW, Nanba K et al. Lymphoproliferative diseases in Japan and western countries. Human Pathology 1983; 14: 745–7.

3. Shimoyama M, Ota K, Kikuchi M et al. For the Lymphoma study group (1981–1983), Chemotherapeutic results and prognostic factors of patients with advanced non-Hodgkin's lymphoma treated with VEPA or VEPA-M. J Clin Oncol 1988; 6: 128–41.

4. Shimoyama M, Ota K, Kikuchi M et al. For the Lymphoma Study Group (1981–1983), Major prognostic factors of adult patients with advanced T-cell lymphoma/leukemia. J Clin Oncol 1988; 6: 1088–97.

5. Shimoyama M, Ota K, Kikuchi M et al. For The Lymphoma Study Group (1981–1983), Major prognostic factors of adult patients with advanced B-cell lymphoma treated with vincristine, cyclophosphamide, prednisone and doxorubicin (VEPA) or VEPA plus methotrexate (VEPA-M). Jpn J Clin Oncol 1988; 18: 113–24.

6. Agnarsson BA, Kadin ME. The immunophenotype of Reed-Sternberg cells. A study of 50 cases of Hodgkin's disease using Fixed Frozen Tissues. Cancer 1989; 63: 2083–7.

7. Hinuma Y, Nagata K, Hanaoka M et al. Adult T cell leukemia: Antigen in an ATL cell line and detection of antibodies to the antigen in human sera. Proc Natl Acad Sci USA 1981: 78: 6476–80.

8. Yoshida M, Seiki M, Yamaguchi K et al. Monoclonal integration of human T-cell leukemia provirus in all primary tumors of adult T-cell leukemia suggests causative role of human T-cell leukemia virus in the disease. Proc Natl Acad Sci USA 1984; 81: 2534–7.

9. Tajima K. The T- and B-cell malignancy Study Group, and Co-authors, The fourth nationwide study on adult T-cell leukemia/lymphoma (ATL) in Japan: Estimates of risk for ATL and its geographical and clinical features. Int J Cancer 1990; 45: 237–43.

10. Shimoyama M, Minato K, Tobinai K et al. Anti-ATLA (antibody to adult T-cell leukemia-lymphoma virus-associated antigen)-negative adult T-cell leukemia-lymphoma. Jpn J Clin Oncol 1983; 13: 245–56.

11. Shimoyama M, Kagami Y, Shimotohno K et al. Adult T-cell leukemia/lymphoma not associated with human T-cell leukemia virus type I (HTLV-I). Proc Natl Acad Sci USA 1986; 83: 4524–8.

12. Shimoyama M. Human T-cell leukemia virus type I (HTLV-I) negative adult T-cell leukemia-lymphoma. Hematology Reviews 1990; 3: 211–22.

13. Shimoyama M. Adult T-cell leukemia-lymphoma and its clinical subtypes from the viewpoints of viral etiology. Vogt PK, Ed, Springer-Verlag Berlin Heidelberg, Current Topics in Microbiology and Immunology 1985; 115: 113–25.

14. ATL Karyotype Review Committee 1985, Kamada N, Shimoyama M, Sakurai M et al. Relation between chromosome aberrations and clinical features in 78 cases of adult T cell leukemia. Proc Jpn Cancer Ass 1986; 45: 733.

15. The Fifth International Workshop on Chromosomes in Leukemia-Lymphoma, Correlation of chromosome abnormalities with histologic and immunologic characteristics in non-Hodgkin's lymphoma and adult T cell leukemia-lymphoma. Blood 1987; 70: 1554–64.

16. Shimoyama M, Abe T, Miyamoto K et al. Chromosome aberrations and clinical features of adult T cell leukemia-lymphoma not associated with human T cell leukemia virus type I. Blood 1987; 69: 984–9.

17. Inoue J, Seiki M, Taniguchi T et al. Induction of interleukin 2 receptor gene expression by p40^X encoded by human T-cell leukemia virus type 1. EMBO J 1986; 5: 2883–8.

18. Kinoshita T, Shimoyama M, Tobinai K et al. Detection of mRNA for the tax_1/rex_1 gene of human T-cell leukemia virus type I in fresh peripheral blood mononuclear cells of adult T-cell leukemia patients and viral carriers by using the polymerase chain reaction. Proc Natl Acad Sci USA 1989; 86: 5620–4.

19. Yamaguchi K, Kiyokawa T, Nakada K et al. Polyclonal integration of HTLV-I proviral DNA in lymphocytes from HTLV-I seropositive individuals: an intermediate state between the healthy carrier state and smoldering ATL. Br J Haematol 1988; 68: 169–74.

20. Nakada K, Yamaguchi K, Furugen S et al. Monoclonal integration of HTLV-I proviral DNA in patients with strongyloidiasis. Int J Cancer 1987; 40: 145–8.

21. The T- and B-cell Malignancy Study Group, The third nationwide study on adult T-cell leukemia/lymphoma (ATL) in Japan: Characteristic patterns of HLA antigen and HTLV-I infection in ATL patients and their relatives. Int J Cancer 1988; 41: 505–12.

22. Okamoto T, Ohno Y, Tsugane S et al. Multi-step carcinogenesis model for adult T-cell leukemia. Jpn J Cancer Res 1989; 80: 191–5.

23. Shimoyama M, Minato K, Saito H et al. Immunoblastic lymphadenopathy (IBL)-like T-cell lymphoma. Jpn J Clin Oncol 1979; 9: 347–56.

24. Tobinai K, Minato K, Ohtsu T et al. Clinicopathologic, Immunophenotypic and Immunogenotypic Analyses of Immunoblastic Lymphadenopathy-Like T-Cell Lymphoma. Blood 1988; 72: 1000–6.

25. Watanabe S, Shimosato Y, Shimoyama M et al. Adult T-cell lymphoma with hypergammaglobulinemia. Cancer 1980; 46: 2472–83.

26. Watanabe S, Sato Y, Shimoyama M et al. Immunoblastic lymphadenopathy, angioimmunoblastic lymphadenopathy, and IBL-like T-cell lymphoma. A spectrum of T-cell neoplasia. Cancer 1986; 58: 2224–32.

27. Namikawa R, Suchi T, Ueda R et al. Phenotyping of proliferating lymphocytes in angioimmunoblastic lymphadenopathy and related lesions by the double immunoenzymatic staining technique. Am J Pathol 1987; 127: 279–87.

28. Shimoyama M, Takatsuki K, Araki K et al. Lymphoma Study Group (1984–1987), Major prognostic factors of patients with adult T-cell leukemia-lymphoma: A cooperative study. Leuk Res (in press).

Correspondence to:
Masanori Shimoyama, M. D.
Chief, Hematology-Oncology and Medical Oncology Division
National Cancer Center Hospital
5-1-1, Tsukiji, Chuo-ku, Tokyo 104, Japan

Annals of Oncology, Supplement 2 to Volume 2: 163–169, 1991.
© 1991 *Kluwer Academic Publishers*.

Original article ⸻

Peripheral T-cell lymphomas

Harald Stein, Dieter Dienemann, Friederike Dallenbach & Michael Kruschwitz
Institute of Pathology, Steglitz Medical Center, Free University of Berlin, Berlin, Germany

Summary. The development of T cells from stem (progenitor) cells to effector cells results from a two-wave process of proliferation and differentiation. The cells of the first differentiation wave are the precursor T cells, and those of the second differentiation wave are peripheral T cells. In the first differentiation wave, resting/circulating naive antigen-reactive T lymphocytes are produced which differ from each other in their antigen receptor-specificity. In the second differentiation wave, those T lymphocytes multiply whose antigen receptors have found the corresponding antigen. Thus three major forms of differentiation can be distinguished in the peripheral T cells: (1) resting/circulating naive antigen-reactive T cells, (2) activated T cells, and (3) effector T cells and memory T cells. In addition, there are at least three major organ-restricted sublines of peripheral T cells, i.e., nodal T cells, mucosa-associated T cells, and skin-associated T cells. Thanks to the availability of markers for most of the above-mentioned T-cell sublines and differentiation forms, all these cellular forms can be associated with certain lymphoma types, i.e., lymphomas of T-cell type can be divided into categories of precursor T-cell lymphomas and peripheral T-cell lymphomas. The peripheral T-cell lymphomas can be subdivided into those derived from lymph nodal, mucosal, and cutaneous T cells. The gut mucosal T-cell lymphomas are associated with enteropathy. The lymph node, mucosal, and cutaneous T-cell lymphomas can be further subdivided into those in which all tumor cells are similar to recirculating resting (nonactivated) T cells, those in which some of the tumor cells resemble activated T cells, and those in which all tumor cells resemble activated T cells. The second group includes pleomorphic T-cell lymphoma, Lennert's lymphoma, and angioimmunoblastic T-cell lymphoma, and the third group includes Ki-1$^+$ (CD30$^+$) anaplastic large-cell (ALC) lymphomas of T-cell type. The apparently constant association of Ki-1$^+$ T-ALC lymphoma with the breakpoint 5q35 underlines the justification of its classification as a separate entity.

The prerequisite for understanding peripheral T-cell lymphomas is the knowledge of the uniqueness of T cell differentiation. As demonstrated in Figure 1, three different types of differentiation pathways may be distinguished in the human body: Type I, the one-wave pathway of proliferation and differentiatiobn, results in the generation of terminally differentiated, nonproliferating effector cells from stem cells in a single wave of proliferation and differentiation. Examples of this differentiation pathway are granulopoiesis, erythropoiesis, and thrombopoiesis. In type II, the two-wave pathway of differentiation, the first wave of differentiation is associated with proliferation, and the second is not. This type is seen in the monocytic/macrophage system. In type III, the two-wave pathway of differentiation, both the first and the second waves of differentiation are associated with proliferation. This third type of differentiation is exclusive to the T and B cells of the lymphoid system.

The unique feature of T-cell development is two waves of proliferation and differentiation

In the first proliferation and differentiation wave,

T-cell-determined lymphoid stem cells (progenitor T cells) pass through an intermediate stage in the thymus to become what we call *precursor cells*, which then develop into *resting, naive antigen-reactive T lymphocytes* (Fig. 2). These T lymphocytes carry antigen receptors of varying specificity on their surface membrane. This means that the first proliferation and differentiation wave generates the 'diversity' of antigen receptors, which puts the organism in a position to produce lymphocytes with antigen receptors specific for the many millions of naturally occurring antigens. When an antigen-reactive T lymphocyte comes into contact with an antigen that fits its antigen determinant (*epitope*) in the recesses of the antigen receptor (*binding site*), i.e., binds to the antigen receptor, the lymphocyte reacts by forming blasts in a new, second wave of differentiation and proliferation. These antigen-induced proliferating blasts represent *activated T cells* or *blasts*, according to the definition of immunologists. The naive T lymphocytes with antigen receptors that do not react with the antigen determinants invading the organism remain in a resting phase, and are probably eliminated if they rest too long. The antigen-stimulated T blasts proliferate and transform into so-called *effector T cells*, or back into resting, antigen-reac-

Correlation between Proliferation and Differention

Lineage	Precursor Cell Pool	Mature competent cells	Activated/Effector Cells	Differen- tiation type
Granulocytic				I
Monocytic/ Macrophage				II
Lymphoid	Gene - R	Ag		III

= Proliferation

Fig. 1. The three main types of differentiation seen in the hemato-lymphoid system.

tive T cells. These previously activated, resting T lymphocytes are the carriers of the immunological memory. Thus the immunological memory comes about by a multiplication of antigen-specific lymphocytes. The regulatory mechanisms and course of the first proliferation and differentiation wave are thus fundamentally different from those of the second. The decisive difference is that the first wave is antigen independent and the second is antigen dependent. It therefore follows that the two differentiation and proliferation waves are controlled by different genes and divergent proliferation and differentiation inducers (i.e., accessory cells and cytokines). The second wave of proliferation and differentiation occurs in peripheral lymphoid tissue. Thus the resting, naive, antigen-reactive T cells and the activated T blasts, together with the memory T cells and effector T cells derived from them, comprise the *peripheral T cells.*

Peripheral T-cell lymphomas are the product of the antigen-reactive T cells and T cells of the second wave of T-cell proliferation and differentiation

The existence of the second wave of proliferation and differentiation in the T-cell lineage was ignored for a long time in schemes designed to relate T-cell lymphomas to normal differentiation [1, 2]. The availability of markers specific for activated lymphoid cells (i.e. interleukin-2 receptor [CD25] and Ki-1 [CD30]) has made it possible to prove that T-cell lymphomas derived from activated peripheral T cells are quite frequent [3, 4, 5]. Studies with these markers also revealed that the degree of differentiation of the lymphoma cells towards activated T cells varies greatly (Fig. 3). The spectrum ranges from small T-cell lymphomas, containing T cells of nonactivated stage, to medium-sized T-cell lymphomas and, more frequently, T-cell lymphomas consisting

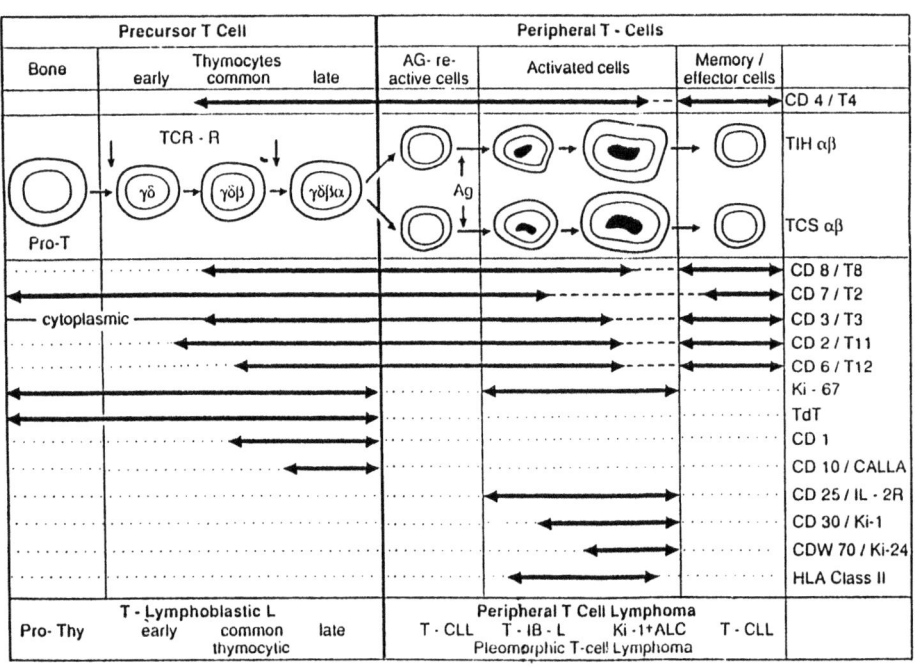

Fig. 2. Correlation between differentiation of T cells and expression of antigenic markers as well as allocation of T cell lymphomas to the physiologic T cell differentiation forms.

of a mixture of small, medium-sized, and large cells. In these tumors, only a portion of the tumor cells express activation antigens, indicating that the tumor cells are at various stages of differentiation between nonactivation and high activation. These tumors have been incorporated in Japanese classifications [6] and the updated Kiel classification [7] as pleomorphic T-cell lymphomas. Another type of T-cell lymphoma with activation markers is the anaplastic large-cell (ALC) lymphoma [3]. In this tumor type, all the tumor cells resemble highly activated T cells in terms of morphology and high expression of CD30.

Peripheral T-cell lymphomas of activated T cells can develop primarily or secondarily

The more T-cell lymphomas resemble highly activated T cells, the more often the tumors lack T-cell antigens [3, 8, 9]. This was one factor which delayed the discovery that the neoplastic cells in anaplastic large-cell tumors are often T-cell-derived. Furthermore, these tumors are frequently associated with intrasinusoidal dissemination, high content of macrophages and, in some instances, with erythrophagocytosis. These features were regarded in the past as being typical for macrophage tumors, and therefore the ALC lymphomas of T-cell type were classified in the past most frequently as malignant histiocytosis. It also happened that these cases were erroneously classified as anaplastic carcinomas or, less frequently, as malignant

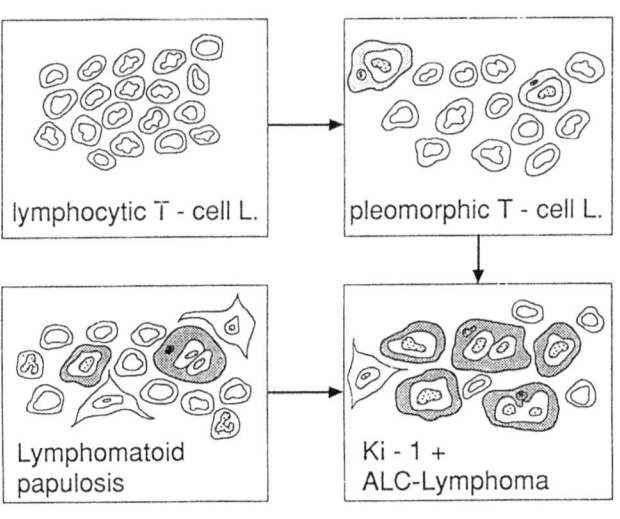

T - Cell ◯ ◎ ⊕   Makrophage △   Granulocyte �

Fig. 3. Schematic representation of the cellular composition seen most commonly in peripheral T cell lymphomas. Shaded areas represent expression of the lymphoid activation antigen CD30. The term 'pleomorphic', introduced by Japanese and European pathologists to define a peripheral T cell lymphoma category, is not correctly applied in this respect because the so-called pleomorphic T cell lymphomas do not only have highly irregular nuclei, but usually also show much variation in cell size (as outlined in the upper right).

melanomas because of the carcinoma-like intrasinusoidal spread. Many immunophenotypical and genotypical studies have confirmed that these tumors are of T-cell lineage and express activation markers, most constantly the CD30 molecule [3, 10, 11, 12, 13]. These studies also revealed that pleomorphic T-cell lymphomas and Ki-1$^+$ anaplastic large-cell (ALC) lymphomas of T-cell type (T-ALC) can develop both primarily and secondarily [14, 15, 16]. Most frequently, lymphocytic cutaneous T-cell lymphomas give rise to secondary pleomorphic T-cell lymphomas and T-ALC lymphomas. The secondary pleomorphic and anaplastic T-cell lymphomas appear to have a worse prognosis than the primary ones, indicating that the appearance of CD30 expression during the disease is a bad prognostic sign.

Primary Ki-1$^+$ ALC lymphomas of T-cell type represent a biological entity

Since lymphomas with the morphology of ALC lymphomas and CD30 expression are heterogenous in terms of antigen profile (Table 1), and thus in cellular origin, the justification of their distinction was repeatedly questioned. Prompted by the suggestion by Morgan *et al.* [17] that a chromosomal translocation involving a breakpoint at q35 in chromosome 5 was characteristic of malignant histiocytosis, Mason collected 17 malignant histiocytosis cases with this particular translocation and investigated them immunohistologically [18]. The result, shown in Table 2, is that all 17 cases with a breakpoint in the long arm of chromosome 5 at position q35 showed the features of Ki-1$^+$ ALC lymphomas. Bitter *et al.* [19] confirmed the exclusive association between Ki-1$^+$ ALC lymphoma and 5q35 translocation [19]. In five cases from Mason's collection, there was evidence based on antigen expression and/or genotypic studies that the neoplasm was of T-lymphoid derivation. It is highly likely that the 12 CD30$^+$ ALC lymphomas of null cell type could not be allocated to the T-cell lineage because of very limited phenotypical studies. Since the 5q35 breakpoint has not yet been observed as a constant genomic alteration in any other lymphoma type, including Hodgkin's disease, these findings by Mason *et al.* and Bitter *et al.* provide strong evidence that CD30$^+$ T-ALC lymphomas represent a biological entity. Genotypical investigations of three cases of CD30$^+$ ALC lymphomas of B-cell type (Dr. F. Cabanillas, Houston; personal communication) revealed a breakpoint on chromosome 6 involving the region on the long arm between 14 and 23. This shows that the B-ALC lymphoma differs not only in cellular origin, but also in genomic alteration from CD30$^+$ T-ALC lymphoma. Of course, further studies are needed to show how constant the latter genomic alterations are.

Table 1. Phenotype of 45 anaplastic large-cell lymphomas.

No. of cases	Ki-1 antigen	T-cell antigens	B-cell antigens	Macrophage antigens[a]	Interpretation
26	+	+	−	−	T-cell type
9	+	+	+	−	mixed T/B
7	+	−	+	−	B-cell type
3	+	−	−	−	O type

[a] Lysozyme, Ber-MAC3, KP1 (CD68).

Table 2. Translocation t(2; 5) (p23; q35) in 17 of 20 cases of Ki-1 (CD30)+ ALC lymphoma.

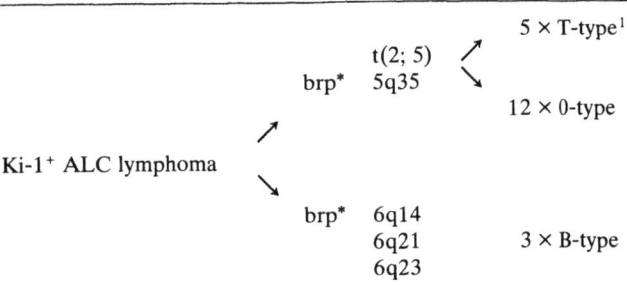

* brp = breakpoint.
[1] Data from Mason *et al.* (1989).
[2] Data from joint study with Dr. Cabanillas, Houston.

Table 3. Correlation between CD30 expression and morphologic features of T-cell lymphomas.

Cell type	Ki-1 (CD30)	Assumed cytokine release	Admixture of non-malignant cells	Morphologic type of lymphoma
Precursor T cells	−	→ −	none or little	T lymphoblastic L
Antigen-reactive T cells	−	→ −	none or little	lymphocytic TCL (T-CLL; CTCL)
Activated T cells	+	↗ little	little	pleomorphic TCL; ALC-type TCL
		↘ positive	extensive	Lennert's lymphoma; AILD-like TCL; macrophage-rich ALC type TCL; lymphomatoid papulosis

Table 4. Cytokine release by T cells.

Cell type	Cytokine relase
Precursor T cells	−
Quiescent antigen-reactive T cells	−
Activated T cells	+ or −

Peripheral T-cell lymphomas consisting of a mixture of neoplastic T cells and nonmalignant cells express activation markers

The presence of significant admixtures of nonneoplastic cells and neoplastic T cells is restricted to those lymphomas which contain at least some neoplastic T cells with features of activated cells (Table 3) [5]. This recalls the observation showing that only activated T cells are capable of releasing cytokines in large quantities (Table 4). In view of this, it is highly likely that the admixture of nonneoplastic cells, e.g., hyperplasia of venules and follicular dendritic cells in angioimmunoblastic-like T-cell lymphoma, the epithelioid macrophages in Lennert's lymphoma, and the many macrophages with or without erythrophagocytosis in Ki-1+ T-ALC lymphoma are the result of a production of certain types and mixtures of cytokines by the tumor cells. With the availability of cDNA probes specific for mRNA of cytokines, it should be possible to disprove or prove this concept in the near future using highly sensitive in situ hybridization techniques.

Intestinal T-cell lymphomas

There is more than 25 years' evidence based on selective gastrointestinal tract resistance to bacteria, viruses, parasites, toxins, and allergens and the homing of gut lymphocytes into the gut, that the gastrointestinal tract possesses its own unique T-cell population. This pointed to the possibility that there might be gut T-cell lymphomas that must be distinguished from nodal T-cell lymphomas. However, the lymphoma research community ignored this possibility for a long time. The simple reason for this appears to be that gut T-cell lymphomas were classified in the past as reticular cell sarcomas and, more recently, as true histiocytic malignancies. In 1937, Fairley and Mackiew were the first to emphasize the association between celiac disease and gut lymphomas [20]. These lymphomas were classified as reticular cell sarcomas or true histiocytic malignancies. In 1978, Isaacson and Wright reported immunohistological evidence based on staining of the tumor cells for α-1-antitrypsin, which seemed to confirm the histiocytic nature of these gut lymphomas [21]. However, with the availability of T-cell-specific monoclonal antibodies and the T-cell receptor β-chain gene probe, the T-cell nature of these malignancies could be demonstrated in a joint study with Isaacson's group [11]. With this finding, the discovery of intraepithelial lymphocytes as a novel T-cell type in 1978 became of interest once again [22]. The next important step in research progress was the generation of a monoclonal antibody designated HML-1 [23] that selectively reacts with a mucosa-lymphocyte antigen (MLA) that is expressed on all or nearly all intraepithelial T cells, but not with nodal T cells. The application of this antibody revealed strong reactivity of celiac disease-associated gut T-cell lymphomas with this antibody, whereas the nodal T-cell lymphomas were consistently negative [24, 25]. This strongly suggests that peripheral T-cell lymphomas can be derived either from nodal T cells or from intestinal T cells.

The mucosal (T) lymphocyte antigen (MLA)

The story of the discovery of the MLA molecule is in itself of interest, because this molecule was independently discovered three times by three different approaches. The French group searched for a mucosal tissue-restricted antigen. By immunizing with hairy cell leukemia cells, Poppema's group [26] obtained a monoclonal antibody (B-ly7) that, among B-cell lymphomas, is only reactive with hairy cell leukemia cells. In search of further activation-associated antigens, our group [27] succeeded in generating a monoclonal antibody (Ber-ACT8) that selectively reacts with activated CD8 cells. Further investigations revealed that all three monoclonal antibodies are directed against the same molecular target [27, 28]. Cross-blocking experiments showed that Ber-ACT8 and B-ly7 recognize the same or neighboring epitopes, whereas the HML-1 antibody reacts with a second epitope. Extended immunohistological studies in normal and diseased lymphoid tissue disclosed an identical reactivity of all three antibodies. The investigation of 60 T-cell lymphomas confirmed the results previously obtained with HML-1 and revealed two additional T-cell lymphomas expressing the molecule (Table 5). One of these was localized in the vocal cord and the other in the mesentery. The analysis of a large number of B-cell lymphomas confirmed that the MLA is absent from all B-cell lymphomas except the vast majority of hairy cell leukemia cells. These studies confirm that the MLA is well suited as a marker for reactive and malignant mucosa-restricted T cells as well as for hairy cell leukemia cells.

Skin-based peripheral T-cell lymphomas express a cutaneous lymphocyte antigen (CLA)

In order to investigate the possible relationship between gut T-cell lymphomas and cutaneous T-cell lymphomas, the analysis for the mucosa T cell-associated antigen was extended to the latter type of T-cell lymphomas [29]. The results, including the findings of other investigations, are provided in Table 6. They show that only a small number of T-cell lymphomas with a marked and diffuse infiltration of basal layers in the epidermis were positive, whereas all other cases, including those with so-called classical Pautrier's abscesses, were consistently negative. This speaks against there being a relationship between mucosal T cells and T cells with an affinity to skin. Very recently, evidence was provided that dermatotropic T cells constitute a unique tissue-restricted T-cell subtype. The evidence

Table 5. Mucosa lymphocyte antigen (MLA) expression in T-cell lymphomas and B-cell lymphomas as identified with the monoclonal antibodies HML-1 and Ber-ACT8[a]

Type of lymphoma	Total no. of cases	Site of biopsy or location	HML-1[+] cases	Ber-ACT8[+] cases
Precursor T-cell (lymphoblastic) lymphoma	5	Mediastinum	0	0[b]
Peripheral T-cell lymphomas				
pleomorphic	25	Lymph node	0	0
pleomorphic	9	Jejunum	9[c]	9
pleomorphic	1	Vocal cord	1	1
angioimmuno-blastic	5	Lymph node	0	0
T anaplastic large-cell (ALC)	5	Lymph node	0	0
T anaplastic	1	Mesentery	1	1
B-cell lymphomas	85		0	0
Hairy cell leukemia	20		18	18

[a] Data from Isaacson's and our own group.
[b] Identical results were obtained with B-ly7 in the cases tested.
[c] All cases were associated with celiac disease.

Table 6. Expression of the mucosa lymphocyte antigen (MLA) antigen in cutaneous T-cell lymphomas as identified with the monoclonal antibodies HML-1 and Ber-ACT8.

Pattern of epidermal infiltrate	No. of case	HML-1/Ber-ACT8	
		Epidermal infiltrate	Corium infiltrate
Dense in basal layers	6	+	−[a]
Dense to low in all layers	12	−	−
Pautrier abscesses	20	−	−

[a] Less than 15% weakly positive.

comes from the discovery by Picker et al. [30] of a new 200-kd molecule designated cutaneous lymphocyte antigen (CLA) that is recognized by the monoclonal antibody HECA-452. CLA is restricted in its occurrence to T cells in cutaneous chronic infiltrates and cutaneous T-cell lymphomas.

Classification of T-cell lymphomas in relation to stages of T-cell development as well as nodal and extranodal T-cell populations

The investigation of the expression of the mucosal T-cell antigen and the cutaneous T-cell antigen in peripheral T cells clearly showed that both populations represent nonoverlapping T-cell populations. With the discovery of these two antigens, at least three different

168

types of tissue-restricted T cells and neoplastic equivalents can be defined (Table 7).

According to expression or nonexpression of the corresponding molecules, all three tissue-restricted peripheral T-cell types can give rise to T-cell lymphomas. In light of these data, together with findings on the expression of precursor T-cell markers and activation markers, it appears reasonable to classify T-cell lymphomas as shown in Table 8.

Acknowledgement

This work was supported by the *Deutsche Krebshilfe, Mildred-Scheel-Stiftung*. The authors also thank Mr. B. Young for help preparing the text.

Table 7. Tissue-restricted T cells, their antigen profile and frequency, as well as their neoplastic counterparts.

	Tissue-restricted sublines	Frequency in peripheral blood	Group of peripheral T-cell lymphomas	Main observed subtypes	Incidence of subtype within within the main subgroup
Peripheral	mucosa T cells MLA[+a]	3%	intestinal TCL* (ITCL)	small-cell[1] pleomorphic[2] large-cell[3]	rare frequent frequent
	skin-associated T cells CLA[+b]	10–15%	cutaneous TCL (CTCL	small-cell[1c] pleomorphic[2c] large-cell[3**d]	frequent frequent rare (often terminal)
	nodal T cells MLA[-]/CLA[-]	80–90%	nodal TCL (NTCL)	small-cell[1] pleomorphic[2] large-cell[3**]	rare frequent frequent

* Usually associated with celiac disease; ** It is not yet clear how often the tissue-associated antigens are expressed on the T-cell lymphomas of large cell type.
[1] All tumor cells resemble non-activated CD30[-] T cells.
[2] A varying percentage, but not all of the tumor cells are large and express CD30 and/or CD25.

[3] All or nearly all tumor cells are large and express CD30.
[a] MLA = gut mucosa lymphocyte antigen.
[b] CLA = cutaneous lymphocyte antigen.
[c] The exact frequency of CLA expression is not yet determined.
[d] The expression of CLA is not yet analyzed.

Table 8. Classification of T-cell lymphomas in relation to stages of T-cell development as well as to nodal, cutaneous, and gut mucosal T-cell populations.

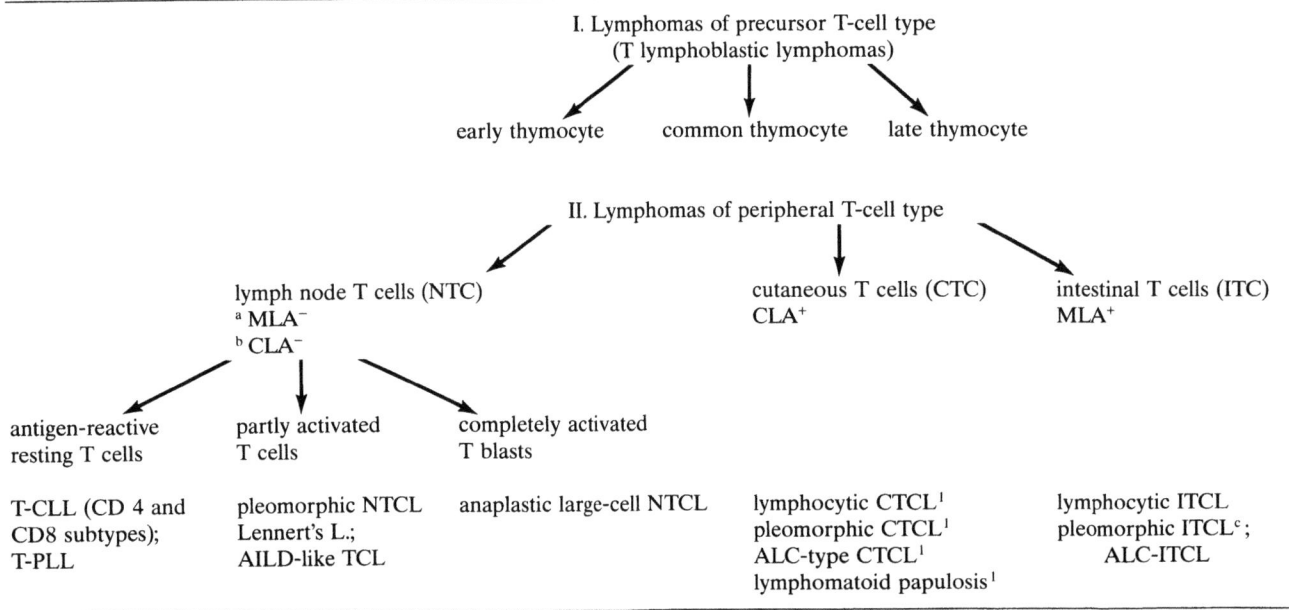

[a] MLA = gut mucosa lymphocyte antigen;
[b] CLA = cutaneous lymphocyte antigen;

[c] associated with celiac disease.
[1] The exact incidence of CLA remains to be determined.

References

1. Janossy G, Grant-Prentice H. T-cell subpopulations, monoclonal antibodies and their therapeutic applications. Clin Haematol 1982; 11: 631–660.
2. Foon KA. Todd RF 3d. Immunologic classification of leukemia and lymphoma. Blood 1986; 68: 1–31.
3. Stein H, Mason DY, Gerdes J, O'Conner N, Wainscoat J, Pallesen G, Gatter K, Falini B, Delsol G, Lemke H, Schwarting R, Lennert K. The expression of the Hodgkin's disease-associated antigen Ki-1 in reactive and neoplastic lymphoid tissue. – Evidence that Reed-Sternberg cells and histiocytic malignancies are derived from activated lymphoid cells. Blood 1985; 66: 848–858.
4. Stein H, Gerdes J. Phänotypische und genotypische Marker bei malignen Lymphomen. Ein Beitrag zum zellulären Ursprung des Morbus Hodgkin und der malignen Histiozytose sowie Implikationen für die Klassifikation der T-Zell und B-Zell-Lymphome. Verh. Dtsch. Ges. Path. 1986; 70: 127–151.
5. Stein H, Dallenbach F, Dienemann D. Differenzierungslinien physiologischer and maligner Zellen des lymphatischen Systems. Verh Dtsch Ges Pathol 1988; 72: 57–85.
6. Suchi T, Lennert K, Tu LY, Kikuchi M, Sato E, Stansfeld AG, Feller AC. Histopathology and immunohistochemistry of peripheral T-cell lymphomas: a proposal for their classification. J Clin Pathol 1987; 40: 995.
7. Stansfeld AG, Diebold J, Kapanci Y, Kelenyi G, Lennert K, Mioduszewska O, Noel H, Rilke F, Sundström C, van Unnik JAM, Wright DH. Updated Kiel Classification for lymphomas. Lancet 1988; i: 292–293.
8. Picker LJ, Weiss LM, Medeiros LJ, Wood GS, Warnke RA. Immunophenotypic criteria for the diagnosis of non-Hodgkin's lymphoma. Am J Pathol 1987; 128: 181–201.
9. Said JW, Shintaku IP, Parekh K, Pinkus GS. Specific phenotyping of T cell proliferations in formol-fixed paraffin-embedded tissues: Use of antibodies to the T cell receptor βF1. Am J Clin Pathol 1990; 93: 382–386.
10. Delsol G, Al Saati T, Gatter KC, Gerdes J, Schwarting R, Caveriviere P, Rigal-Huguet F, Robert A, Stein H, Mason DY. Coexpression of epithelial membrane antigen (EMA), Ki-1, and interleukin-2 receptor by anaplastic large cell lymphomas. Am J Pathol 1988; 130: 59–70.
11. Isaacson PG, Spencer J, Connolly CE, Pollock DJ, Stein H, O'Conner NTJ, Bevan DH, Kirkham N, Wainscoat JS, MaSON DY. Malignant histiocytosis of the intestine: A T cell lymphoma. Lancet 1985; ii: 688–691.
12. Weiss LM, Trela MJ, Cleary ML, Turner RR, Warnke RA, Sklar F. Frequent immunoglobulin and T cell receptor gene rearrangements in 'histiocytic' neoplasms. Am J Pathol 1985; 121: 369–373.
13. Beljaards RC, Meijer CJLM, Scheffer E, Toonstra J, van vloten WA, van der Putte SCJ, Geerts ML, Willemze R. Prognostic significance of CD30 (Ki-1/Ber-H2) expression in primary cutaneous large cell lymphomas of T origin: a clinicopathologic and immunohistochemical study in 20 patients. Am J Pathol 1989; 135: 1169–1178.
14. Engelhard M, von Schilling C, Diehl V, Pfreundschuh M, Brittinger G, Feller AC, Stein H, Zwingers T, Lennert K. Clinical analysis of Ki-1 lymphoma. Blut 1986; 53: 220 (abstract).
15. Engelhard M, von Schilling C, Diehl V, Pfreundschuh M, Brittinger G, Zwingers T, Feller AC, Stein H, Lennert K. CD30 (Ki-1)+ lymphoma: morphological and immunohistological characterization, identification of three subentities, and clinical analysis of 92 cases. Blood 1990; (submitted).
16. Kaudewitz P, Stein H, Dallenbach F, Eckert F, Bieber K, Burg G, Braun-Falco O. Primary and secondary Cuntaneous Ki-1+ (CD30+) Anaplastic Large Cell Lymphomas. Morphologic, Immunohistologic, and Clinical Characteristics. Am J Pathol 1989; 135: 359–367.
17. Morgan R, Hecht BK, Sandberg AA, Hecht F, Smith SD. Chromosome 5q35 breakpoint in malignant histiocytosis. N Eng J Med 1986; 314: 1322 (Letter).
18. Mason DY, Bastard C, Rimokh R, Dastugue N, Huret JL, Kristoffersson U, Magaud JP, Nezelof C, Tilly H, Vanier JP, Hemet J, Warnke R. CD30-positive large cell lymphomas (Ki-1 lymphoma) are associated with a chromosomal translocation involving 5q35. Brit J Haematol 1990; 74: 161–168.
19. Bitter MA, Franklin WA, Larson RA, McKeithan TW, Rubin CM, Le Beau MM, Stephens JK, Vardiman JW. Morphology in Ki-1 (CD30)-positive non-Hodgkin's lymphoma is correlated with clinical features and the presence of a unique chromosomal abnormality, t(2; 5) (p23; q35). Am J Surg Pathol 1990; 14: 305–316.
20. Fairley NH, Mackiew FP. Clinical and biochemical syndrome in lymphadenoma and allied diseases involving mesenteric lymph glands. Brit Med J 1937; 1: 375–380.
21. Isaacson PG, Wright DH. Malignant histiocytosis of the intestine: its relationship to malabsorption and ulcerative jejunitis. Hum Pathol 1978; 9: 661–677.
22. Guy-Grand D, Griscelli C, Vassali P. The mouse gut T lymphocyte, a noval type of T cell: Nature, origin, and traffic in mice in normal graft-versus-host conditions. J Exp Med 1978; 148: 1661–1677.
23. Cerf-Bensussan N, Jarry A, Brousse N, Lisowska-Grospierre B, Guy-Grand D, Griscelli C. A monoclonal antibody (HML-1) defining a novel membrane molecule present on human intestinal lymphocytes. Eur J Immunol 1987; 17: 1279–1285.
24. Spencer J, Cerf-Bensussan N, Jarry A, Brousse N, Guy-Grand D, Krajewski AS, Isaacson PG. Enteropathy-associated T cell lymphoma (malignant histiocytosis of the intestine) is recognized by monoclonal antibody (HML-1) that defines a membrane molecule on human mucosal lymphocytes. Am J Pathol 1988; 132: 1–5.
25. Stein H, Dienemann D, Sperling M, Zeitz M, Riecken EO. Identification of a T cell lymphoma category derived from intestinal mucosa-associated T cells. Lancet 1988; ii: 1053–1954.
26. Visser L, Shaw A, Slupsky J, Vos H, Poppema S. Monoclonal antibodies reactive with hairy cell leukemia. Blood 1989; 74: 320–325.
27. Kruschwitz M, Fritzsche G, Schwarting R, Micklem K, Mason DY, Falini B, Stein H. Ber-ACT8: A new monoclonal antibody defining a trimeric antigen associated with activated CD8 T cells, gut mucosa T cells, and hairy cell leukemia cells (submitted).
28. Schwarting R, Dienemann D, Kruschwitz M, Fritzsche G, Stein H. Specificities of monoclonal antibodies B-ly7 and HML-1 are identical. Blood 1990; 320.
29. Sperling M, Kaudewitz P, Braun-Falco O, Stein H. Reactivity of T cells in mycosis fungoides exhibiting marked epidermotropism with the monoclonal antibody HML-1 that defines a membrane molecule on human mucosal lymphocytes. 1989, Amer J Path 1989; 134: 955–960.
30. Picker LJ, Michie SA, Rott LS, Butcher EC. A unique phenotype of skin-associated lymphocytes in human: Preferential expression of the HECA-452 epitope by benign and malignant T cells at cutaneous sites. Am J Pathol 1990; 136: 1053–1068.

Correspondence to:
Prof. Dr. H. Stein
Institut für Pathologie
Klinikum Steglitz
Hindenburgdamm 30
D-1000 Berlin 45, Germany

Annals of Oncology, Supplement 2 to Volume 2: 171–176, 1991.
© 1991 *Kluwer Academic Publishers.*

Original article ────────────────────

The present status of therapy for patients with aggressive non-Hodgkin's lymphoma

Julie M. Vose & James O. Armitage
University of Nebraska Medical Center, Omaha, Nebraska, USA

Summary. The aggressive non-Hodgkin's lymphomas include some of the malignancies most frequently cured with chemotherapy. However, not all patients are cured, and the best treatment approach remains uncertain. The most common aggressive non-Hodgkin's lymphomas are diffuse large-cell lymphoma and immunoblastic lymphoma. Most recent studies suggest no useful difference between these two groups. When these lymphomas are localized at presentation they are highly curable. Earlier studies showed that radiotherapy alone had a high relapse rate. Chemotherapy alone has been found to have an excellent cure rate, but when followed by radiotherapy, the amount of chemotherapy can be reduced with the same good result. A number of chemotherapy regimens have been shown to cure approximately 50% of patients with disseminated large-cell lymphoma. It appears that a number of regimens including m-BACOD, MACOP-B, LNH-84, ProMACE-CytaBOM, CAP-BOP, COP-BLAM, F-MACHOP, and perhaps full-dose CHOP achieve similar results when prognostic factors are taken into account. Currently the most important area for therapeutic research (unless new drugs are found) is in identifying those patients likely to be cured with our present treatments and those patients for whom alternative therapies such as bone marrow transplantation need to be considered as part of the primary treatment. This is true not only for large-cell lymphoma but also for the less common aggressive non-Hodgkin's lymphomas such as lymphoblastic lymphoma, small noncleaved-cell lymphoma, and peripheral T-cell lymphoma.

Introduction

Over the past 15 years, the development of intensive combination chemotherapy has dramatically improved the treatment of aggressive non-Hodgkin's lymphoma (NHL). One of the first large series of patients with diffuse large-cell lymphoma, the most common type of aggressive NHL in which cure was documented, was reported in 1973 by De Vita *et al.* [1]. This series demonstrated that regimens originally designed for the treatment of Hodgkin's disease such as MOPP (mechlorethamine, vincristine, procarbazine, and prednisone) or C-MOPP (cyclophosphamide, vincristine, procarbazine, and prednisone) could produce long-term disease-free survival in over 30% of patients [1]. The next major development in the treatment of aggressive NHL was the addition of doxorubicin (Adriamycin) to produce regimens such as CHOP (cyclophosphamide, Adriamycin, vincristine, and prednisone) [2] or BACOP (bleomycin, Adriamycin, cyclophosphamide, vincristine, and prednisone) [3]. Further intensification with the addition of other chemotherapy agents such as methotrexate, etoposide, or cytarabine [4–6] or the use of infusional chemotherapy [7] have more recently been utilized to improve on the results of the first combinations. Because all patients are not equally likely to be cured with these

protocols, a detailed analysis of prognostic factors must be included in any comprison of treatment regimens.

Pathology

When comparing different treatments for aggressive NHL, it is important to be certain that similar patients were treated. There are a number of diffeent classification schemes utilized for NHL. The Rappaport classification [8] was introduced in the 1950s and has been used for many years by pathologists and clinicians alike; however, several other systems such as the Kiel [9] and Lukes-Collins [10] are utilized by different groups throughout the world. In 1982 an attempt to unify pathologic diagnoses for NHL was made by developing the Working Formulation [11]. This classification schema can be used in conjunction with the previous classifications for comparisons.

Although incorporation of the Working Formulation has clarified pathologic classification, there is still a high rate of discordance among the pathologists utilizing the Working Formulation. When the expert pathologists who originally developed the Working Formulation were tested for consistency of their diagnoses, the rate of reproducibility ranged from 53 to 93% [12]. Even so, histologic classification remains the basis for therapy. For the purposes of this manuscript, diffuse mixed, diffuse large-cell, and immunoblastic lymphomas will be considered together. Small non-cleaved-cell and lymphoblastic lymphomas (i.e., true 'high-grade' disorders) will be dealt with separately.

Subgroups of patients with special treatment considerations

1. Localized NHL

Approximately 30% of patients with aggressive NHL appear to have localized disease (stage I or minimal stage II) [11]. As might be expected, patients with localized, minimal disease have a much better outlook than patients with more extensive disease. Radiation therapy alone for localized disease has produced long-term survival rates ranging from 30 to 75% in various studies [13, 14]. The best results have been seen in patients with surgically staged, nonbulky, stage I disease.

In patients treated initially with radiotherapy, a number of studies have demonstrated a reduced frequency of relapse with adjuvant chemotherapy [15, 16]. Several investigators have more recently used an abbreviated course of chemotherapy preceding radiotherapy in patients with localized diffuse large-cell lymphoma. Patients treated with three cycles rather than six who then receive involved-field radiotherapy consistently demonstrate >80% long-term disease-free survival [17–18].

Some sites of localized extranodal lymphomas may dictate specific treatment approaches. For example, patients with sinus or epidural lymphoma are at a high risk for central nervous system (CNS) lymphoma and should be considered for CNS prophylaxis along with their primary therapy. Furthermore, lymphomas of the gastrointestinal tract are associated with lymphomas in the Waldeyer's ring (and vice versa) in approximately 20% of the cases. Most importantly, careful staging is needed to insure that apparently limited lymphomas are truly localized, allowing for the best results to be obtained with the least toxic therapy.

2. Elderly patients

Several studies have found that patients who are older than approximately 60 years of age have a worse prognosis when treated for large-cell lymphoma [19–22]. However, when studies are closely evaluated, the poorer prognosis of elderly patients is not always due to poorer tumor response. Elderly patients have been found to demonstrate poorer survival secondary to increased treatment-related toxicity [21], or as a result of other medical conditions not necessarily related to the lymphoma or its therapy [22]. While some older patients will not be candidates for intensive regimens,

otherwise healthy elderly patients should not lose their chance for cure.

3. HIV-associated lymphomas

Patients with the acquired immunodeficiency syndrome (AIDS) have been noted to be at increased risk for several neoplasms including aggressive NHL. Originally only primary CNS lymphomas in human immunodeficiency virus (HIV)-positive patients less than age 60 years were considered as diagnostic criteria for AIDS; however, in 1985 sufficient data was available to warrant the inclusion of systemic high-grade B-cell NHL as well [23]. Currently, NHLs occur in 5–10% of patients with AIDS.

The pathologic spectrum of these lymphomas is unusual when compared to the patient population. The majority of AIDS-associated NHLs are immunoblastic, or small non-cleaved lymphoma [24]. The clinical setting and management options are distinct in the AIDS-associated lymphomas as the underlying immunodeficiency makes intensive therapy difficult.

The survival of patients with AIDS-associated NHL is shortened in most clinical trials compared to the usual survival of patients with non-AIDS-associated NHL treated with similar protocols. In one of the initial analyses, the use of the CHOP variant regimens (cyclophosphamide, Adriamycin, vincristine, prednisone, with bleomycin and/or methotrexate) were evaluated [25]. Although an initial 53% of the patients obtained a complete remission, most remissions were of very short duration. Several other combination chemotherapy regimens including ProMACE-MOPP [26] and MACOP-B [27] have been evaluated and found to have similar results. Despite attempts at adequate therapy, the vast majority of patients with AIDS-associated primary CNS lymphomas have died within three months of diagnosis [28]. In order to improve the results of treatment for AIDS-related lymphomas, future trials may need to be designed combining reduced-dose chemotherapy with antiviral agents and/or immunoregulators.

4. High-grade NHLs

Lymphoblastic lymphoma
In 1975, Barcos and Lukes used the term *convoluted lymphocytic lymphoma* to describe this subgroup of predominantly young male patients who often presented with a large mediastinal mass and had rapid progression to disseminated lymphoma [29]. Nathwani *et al.* [30] subsequently recognized both convoluted and nonconvoluted cell types in these lymphomas and classified them as lymphoblastic lymphoma. Although the disease occasionally appears to be localized at diagnosis, it evolves rapidly to systemic involvement. Bone marrow involvement is present at diagnosis in approximately 30% of the cases; however, as the disease

progresses, as many as 80% of the patients eventually develop bone marrow and peripheral blood involvement [31].

The treatment of lymphoblastic lymphoma with chemotherapy regimens utilized for intermediate-grade NHL has demonstrated excellent initial results in most trials; however, the patients who present with high levels of lactate dehydrogenase (LDH), bone marrow involvement, or CNS involvement usually relapse and eventually die of progressive disease. Studies in pediatric patients have found that regimens developed for acute lymphoblastic lymphoma (ALL), such as the LSA2-L2 regimen, are more effective than regimens used for the treatment of other aggressive lymphomas. Wollner and colleagues found that patients treated with the LSA2-L2 protocol had a 76% two-year disease-free survival compared with a 26% two-year disease-free survival for patients treated with the COMP protocol [32].

Small non-cleaved NHL
This type of lymphoma also is more common in young patients, an age group similar to that of patients with lymphoblastic lymphoma. The clinical presentation is also similar, with most patients having rapidly progressive disease. In the United States and Europe these account for approximately 1–2% of all NHL.

Most therapeutic trials for the treatment of small noncleaved NHL have been carried out in the pediatric population, with few trials on adults available for analysis. Several multiagent chemotherapy regimens combined with CNs prophylaxis have been shown to achieve high remission rates and long-term disease-free survival. Protocols that were designed for ALL (e.g., LSA2-L2) seem to be inferior to protocols specific for the small noncleaved NHL. This was confirmed in a Children's Cancer Study Group (CCSG) trial in which patients with small noncleaved NHL had a much improved prognosis when treated with COMP (cyclophosphamide, vincristine [Oncovin], methotrexate, and prednisone) compared with those children treated with LSA2-L2 [32]. Most trials utilizing modern multiagent chemotherapy for childhood small noncleaved NHL report overall survival rates of approximately 50–75%. However, children and adults with poor prognostic features, including an unresected tumor bulk >10 cm, pretreatment LDH >500 IU/L, or involvement of the CNs or bone marrow, have a significantly worse prognosis with a projected relapse-free survival of 28% [33]. These and other studies have pointed out that patients who present with these poor prognostic characteristics need more intensive therapy.

Peripheral T-cell NHLs
Although this category remains somewhat controversial, many centers would also classify patients with high-stage peripheral T-cell NHL in the high-grade lymphoma category. Some earlier analyses have not found immunophenotype to be of prognostic significance

[34, 35]; however, several recent studies with uniformly treated patients have found this to be the case [36, 37]. An analysis of 110 uniformly treated patients at our institution found that stage IV B-cell NHL patients had a higher complete remission rate than their stage IV T-cell NHL counterparts (67% versus 0%; P = 0.002), as well as a much improved overall survival at three years (44% versus 0%; P = 0.002) [37]. Based on this recent information, some institutions are now utilizing early autologous bone marrow transplantation in this high-risk patient population.

Choosing a chemotherapy regimen for the treatment of aggressive non-Hodgkin lymphomas

Since the recognition several years ago that aggressive NHL could be cured by combination chemotherapy, many new approaches have been evaluated. There have been a large number of regimens developed and studied in clinical trials. In evaluating the results of these regimens, it is important to remember that the initial results may be modified with time. For example, CHOP, as utilized in the SWOG experience, had an initial complete response rate of 67% with a projected relapse-free survival of 70% at two years and a median overall survival of 22 months [38]. However, a decade later, the complete-remission rate was reported as 53%, with a relapse-free survival of 50% and an overall survival of 30% [39]. Also, because newer regimens are often tested on patient populations that are likely to withstand the side effects, when the regimen is later evaluated on a general lymphoma population the results are often modified.

A large number of prognostic factors have been identified to be predictive of outcome with therapy for aggressive NHL. For example, bulky tumor [40], age [22, 41], stage [42], site of involvement [43], and systemic symptoms [44] have all been identified as important prognostic characteristics in various trials. It may be unreasonable to compare trials in which prognostic variables such as age vary widely.

A multitude of regimens have not been developed to improve on the original results with CHOP. Most of the recently developed second- and third-generation regimens have added new agents and used the principle of dose intensification. High-dose methotrexate with leucovorin rescue was added to the standard BACOP group of drugs to form the M-BACOD regimen. This regimen was reported to achieve a 72% complete-remission rate with 44% of all patients disease-free at five years [45]. However, because the high-dose methotrexate was costly, required alkalization of the urine with large-volume hydration, and demonstrated a high mucositis rate, a lower dose of methotrexate with leucovorin rescue was substituted to form the m-BACOD program [46]. This program produced a 61% complete-remission rate with 40% of all patients disease-free at a median follow-up of 3.3 years, and less severe mucositis when compared to M-BACOD. Another regimen using these agents is the MACOP-B regimen, originally developed in Vancouver [47]. This intensive regimen, which is delivered over 12 weeks, was originally reported to achieve an 84% complete-remission rate and an overall actuarial survival of 64% in 125 patients, with a median follow-up time of 18 months. This treatment was also moderately toxic with a 10% incidence of sepsis and frequent mucositis. When these regimens have been evaluated at other institutions with different patient populations, the results have been variable. For example, m-BACOD was evaluated by the Eastern Cooperative Oncology Group and Cancer and Leukemia Group B and found to have a 54% complete-remission rate [48], not dissimilar to the original 61% complete-remission rate. When the MACOP-B regimen was evaluated in a Southwest Oncology Group pilot study it produced only a 50% complete-remission rate [49].

Another intensive regimen evaluated for the treatment of aggressive NHL was the ProMACE series developed at the National Cancer Institute. This regimen was originally given as alternating with MOPP, based on the Goldie-Coldman hypothesis [50]. The original series produced a 76% complete-remission rate [51]. Another similar regimen, ProMACE-Cyta-BOM, utilizing other active agents was reported to produce complete-remission rate of 79% [52]. These regimens also produced a moderate amount of toxicity, with a toxic-death rate of 4–10%. It remains to be seen if these results can be duplicated in cooperative-trial settings. Another intricate regimen, the LNH-80 regimen [53] has been extensively evaluated in Europe and also found to have encouraging results. A few programs have also evaluated the effect of using infusional bleomycin and vincristine along with the other standard agents in an attempt to decrease the toxicity. The COP-BLAM III and CAP-BOP III series are examples of such regimens; however, the results are still preliminary.

In order to adequately compare these advanced regimens for the treatment of aggressive NHL, randomized trials in similar ptient populations must be conducted. The Southwest Oncology Group activated such a randomized study comparing CHOP with m-BACOD, MACOP-B, and ProMACE-CytaBOM in 1986. This study will take many patients and years to complete; however, it may aid oncologists in the selection of the most appropriate protocol for the treatment of aggressive NHL, or, alternatively, none of the regimens may be found to be superior to the others.

Special circumstances, such as lymphoblastic lymphoma or small non-cleaved NHL, may require a treatment strategy that is specifically designed for that patient population. Furthermore, patients that are at high risk for relapse, such as stage IV peripheral T-cell lymphomas or poor-risk lymphoblastic and small non-cleaved cell NHL, may require further intensification after initial chemotherapy.

Salvage therapy

Once patients relapse after receving an effective, first-line chemotherapy regimen for aggressive NHL, the results with conventional salvage chemotherapy regimens have been disappointing. Many such regimens have been designed utilizing both established agents as well as investigational agents. One of the largest series, reported from M. D. Anderson Cancer Center, utilized methyl-gag, ifosfamide, methotrexate, and etoposide (MIME). The investigators reported treating 123 patients with relapsed NHL with this regimen [54]. Although the complete-response rate was approximately 30%, only 20% of those complete responders were long-term, disease-free survivors. These results would be consistent with a potential cure rate of only 6% of the original population. Another ifosfamide-containing salvage regimen that has been evaluated is the IMVP-16 regimen. Along with ifosfamide, this regimen utilizes methotrexate and etoposide. Five of 41 patients (12%) treated with this regimen achieved a complete remission [55]. At the time of publication, four of the five patients remained in complete remission.

Another popular salvage regimen recently has been the DHAP regimen (dexamethasone, cytarabine, and cisplatin). The original evaluation of this regimen reported on results in 83 patients with relapsed NHL [56]. Although 28 of these patients achieved a complete remission, only 8 patients were alive in complete remission after an 11-month median follow-up. Several other regimens using these and other agents have been utilized in patients with relapsed aggressive NHL with similar results [57–59].

Because of these very discouraging results with conventional salvage chemotherapy, the use of high-dose chemoradiotherapy with autologous bone marrow transplantation (ABMT) has become increasingly utilized as a method to overcome drug resistance. Philip et al. [60] demonstrated that it is possible to predict outcome with ABMT based on the responsiveness of the tumor to salvage chemotherapy administered at traditional doses. Of patients who had never been in complete remission with conventional chemotherapy, 9 of 34 (26%) achieved a complete remission with ABMT; however, none of these patients were long-term disease-free survivors. Ten of the 22 patients (45%) who had been in complete remission but had become resistant to chemotherapy achieved complete remission, but only 14% of these patients achieved long-term disease-free survival. Forty of the 44 patients (91%) who had relapsed from a complete remission and still had chemotherapy-sensitive disease had a complete response to ABMT. The most important observation from this analysis was the fact that 36% of these chemosensitive patients were long-term disease-free survivors [60]. Although no randomized trials have as yet been completed, it would appear that ABMT offers an improved outcome over conventional salvage chemotherapy for patients with relapsed aggressive NHL.

Optimal treatment strategy

Patients with aggressive NHL can be successfully treated with any one of a number of front-line chemotherapy regimens. However, special attention should be paid to characteristics, such as stage, histologic subtype, or immunophenotype, that may direct the therapy toward the use of protocols containing specific drugs or intensification approaches. Unfortunately, the relative efficacy of the many regimens developed for the treatment of aggressive NHL remains unknown. In order to answer these important questions, patients should be encouraged to participate in clinical trials. Once it has been established that cure canot be achieved with front-line chemotherapy, eligible patients should receive high-dose therapy with ABMT to optimize chances for long-term disease-free survival.

References

1. DeVita VT, Chabner B, Hubbard SP et al. Advanced diffuse histiocytic lymphoma, a potentially curable disease. Lancet 1973; 1: 248–250.
2. McKelvey EM, Gottlieb JA, Wilson HE et al. Hydroxyldaunomycin (Adriamycin) combination chemotherapy in malignant lymphoma. Cancer 1976; 38: 1484–1493.
3. Skarin AT, Rosenthal DS, Maloney WC et al. Combination chemotherapy of advanced non-Hodgkin's lymphoma with bleomycin, Adriamycin, cyclophosphamide, vincristine, and prednisone (BACOP). Blood 1977; 49: 759–770.
4. Longo DL, DeVita Jr, Duffey P et al. Randomized trial of ProMACE-MOPP v. ProMACE-CytaBOM in Stage II–IV aggressive non-Hodgkin's lymphoma. Proc Am Soc Clin Oncol 1987; 6: 206.
5. Klimo P, Connors JM. Updated clinical experience with MACOP-B. Semin Hematol 1987; 24: 26–34.
6. Coiffier B, Bryon PA, Berger F et al. Intensive and sequential combination chemotherapy for aggressive malignant lymphomas (protocol LNH-80). J Clin Oncol 1986; 4: 147–153.
7. Boyd DB, Coleman M, Papish SW et al. COPBLAM III: Infusional combination chemotherapy for diffuse large-cell lymphoma. J Clin Oncol 1988; 6: 425–433.
8. Rappaport H. Tumors of the hematopoietic system in Atlas of Tumor Pathology, section 3, Fasicle 8, Washington DC, UA Armed Forces Institute of Pathology, 1966.
9. Lennert K, Mohri N, Stein H et al. The histopathology of malignant lymphoma. Br J Haematol 1975; 31: 193–203.
10. Lukes RJ, Collins RD. Immunologic characterization of human malignant lymphomas. Cancer 1974; 34: 1488–1503.
11. National Cancer Institute sponsored study of classification of non-Hodgkin's lymphomas. Summary and description of a Working Formulation for clinical usage. The non-Hodgkin's lymphoma Pathologic classification Project. Cancer 1982; 49: 2112–2135.
12. NCI Non-Hodgkin's Classification Project Writing Committee. Classification of non-Hodgkin's lymphomas. Reproducibility of major classification systes. Cancer 1985; 55: 91–95.
13. Levitt SH, Lee CR, Bloomfield CP et al. The role of radiation therapy in the treatment of early stage large cell lymphoma. Hematol Oncol 1985; 3: 33–37.
14. Vokes EE, Ultman JE, Golomb HM et al. Long-term survival of patients with localized diffuse histiocytic lymphoma. J Clin Oncol 1985; 3: 1309–1317.
15. Nisson NI, Ersbol J, Hansen HS et al. A randomized study of radiotherapy versus radiotherapy plus chemotherapy in Stage I–II non-Hodgkin's lymphomas. Cancer 1983; 52: 1–8.
16. Carde P, Burgers IMV, van Glabbekem M et al. Combined radiotherapy-chemotherapy for early stage non-Hodgkin's lymphoma. Radiotherapy Oncology 1984; 2: 301–304.
17. Miller TP, Jones SE. Initial chemotherapy for clinically localized lymphoma of unfavorable histology. Blood 1983; 62: 413–418.
18. Connors JM, Klimo P, Fairey RN et al. Brief chemotherapy and involved field radiation therapy for limited stage, histologically aggressive lymphoma. Ann Intern Med 1987; 107: 25–30.
19. Jagannath S, Valasquez WS, Tucker SL et al. Stage IV diffuse large cell lymphoma: a long-term analysis. J Clin Oncol 1985; 3: 39–45.
20. Dixon DO, Neilan B, Jones JE et al. Effect of ages on therapeutic outcome in advanced diffuse histiocytic lymphoma: The Southwest Oncology Group experience. J Clin Oncol 1986; 4: 295–305.
21. Tirelli U, Zagonel V, Serraino J et al. Non-Hodgkin lymphomas in 137 patients ages 70 or older: A Retrospective European Organization for Research and Treatment of Cancer Lymphoma Group Study. J Clin Oncol 1988; 6: 1708–1713.
22. Vose JM, Armitage JO, Weisenburger DD et al. The importance of age in survival of patients treated with chemotherapy for aggressive non-Hodgkin's lymphoma. J Clin Oncol 1988; 6: 1838–1844.
23. Ross RK, Dworsky RL, Paganini-Hill A et al. Non-Hodgkin's lymphoma in never married men in Los Angeles. Br J Cancer 1985; 52: 785–787.
24. Levine AM, Gill PS. AIDS related malignant lymphoma: Clinical presentation and treatment approaches. Oncology 1987; 1: 41–46.
25. Gill PS, Levine AM, Kraib M et al. AIDS-related malignant lymphoma: results of progressive treatment trials. J Clin Oncol 1987; 5: 1322–1328.
26. Knowles DM, Chamulak GA, Subar M et al. Lymphoid neoplasia associated with the acquired immunodeficiency syndrome (AIDS). Ann Intern Med 1988; 108: 744–753.
27. Barmudez MA, Grant KM, Rodvien R et al. Non-Hodgkin's lymphoma in a population with or at risk for acquired immunodeficiency syndrome: Indications for intensive chemotherapy. Am J Med 1989; 86: 71–76.
28. So YT, Beckstead JHY, Davis PL. Primary central nervous system lymphoma in acquired immunodeficiency syndrome: A clinical and pathological study. Ann Neurol 1986; 20: 566–572.
29. Barcos MP, Lukes RJ. Malignant lymnphoma of convoluted lymphocytes – A new entity of possible T-cell type. In: Sinus LF, Godden JO (eds). Conflicts in childhood cancer. An evaluation of current management, Vol. 4, New York Liss, p 147, 1975.
30. Nathwani BN, Kim H, Rappaport H. Malignant lymphoma, lymphoblastic. Cancer 1976; 38: 964–983.
31. Levine AM, Forman SJ, Meyer PR et al. Successful therapy of convoluted T-lymphoblastic lymphoma in adults. Blood 1983; 61: 92–98.
32. Wollner N, Wachtel AE, Exelby PR et al. Improved prognosis in children with intra-abdominal non-Hodgkin's lymphoma following LSA$_2$-L$_2$ protocol chemotherapy. Cancer 1980; 45: 3034–3039.

33. Bernstein JI, Coleman N, Strickelr JG et al. Combined modality therapy for adults with small non-cleaved cell lymphoma (Burkitt's and non-Burkitt's type). J Clin Oncol 1986; 4: 847–858.

34. Horning SJ, Weiss CL, Crabtree CG et al. Clinical and phenotypic diversity of T-cell lymphomas. Blood 1986; 67: 1578–1582.

35. Simoyama M, Ota K, Kikuchi M et al. Major prognostic factors of adult patients with advanced T-cell lymphoma/leukemia. J Clin Oncol 1988; 6: 1088–1097.

36. Coiffier B, Berger F, Byron P-A et al. T-cell lymphomas; Immunologic, histologic, clinical and therapeutic analysis of 63 cases. J Clin Oncol 1988; 6: 1584–1589.

37. Armitage JO, Vose JM, Linder J et al. Clinical significance of immunophenotype in diffuse aggressive non-Hodgkin's lymphoma. J Clin Oncol 1989; 7: 1783–1790.

38. McKelveny EM, Gottlieb JA, Wilson HE et al. Hydroxyldaunomycin (Adriamycin) combiantion chemotherapy in malignant lymphoma. Cancer 1976; 38: 1484–1493.

39. Coltman CA, Jr., Dahlberg S, Jones SE et al. CHOP is curative in thirty percent of patients with large cell lymphoma: A twelve-year Southwest Oncology Group follow-up. Proc Am Soc Clin Oncol 1986 (abstr); 5: 197.

40. Fisher RI, DeVita VT, Johnson BL et al. Prognostic factors for advanced diffuse histiocytic lymphoma following treatment with combination chemotherapy. Am J Med 1977; 63: 177–182.

41. Dixon DO, Neilan B, Jones JE et al. Effect of age on therapeutic outcome in advanced diffuse histiocytic lymphoma: The Southwest Oncology Group experience. J Clin Oncol 1986; 4: 295–305.

42. Todd MB, Portlock CS, Farber LR et al. Prognostic indicators in diffuse large-cell histiocytic lymphoma. Int J Radiat Oncol Biol Phys 1986; 12: 593–601.

43. Armitage JO, Dick FR, Corder MP et al. Predicting therapeutic outcome in patients with diffuse histiocytic lymphoma treated with cyclophosphamide, Adriamycin, vincristine, and prednisone (CHOP). Cancer 1982; 50: 1695–1702.

44. Jagannath S, Valasquez WS, Tucker SL et al. Tumor burden assessment and its implication for a prognostic model in advanced diffuse large cell lymphoma. J Clin Oncol 1986; 4: 859–865.

45. Skarin AT, Conellos GP, Rosenthal DS et al. Improved prognosis of diffuse histiocytic and undifferentiated lymphoma by use of high-dose methotrexate alternating with standard agents (M-BACOD). J Clin Oncol 1983; 1: 91–98.

46. Canellos GP, Skarin AT, Klatt MM et al. The m-BACOD combination chemotherapy regimen in the treatment of diffuse large-cell lymphoma. Semin Hematol 1987; 24: 2–7.

47. Klimo P, Connors JM. MACOP-B chemotherapy for the treatment of advanced diffuse large-cell lymphoma. Ann Intern Med 1985; 102: 596–602.

48. Gordon LI, Harrington D, Glick JH et al. Randomized Phase III comparison of CHOP versus m-BACOD in diffuse large cell and diffuse mixed lymphoma: Equivalent complete remission and time to treatment failure but greater toxicity with m-BACOD. Proc Am Soc Clin Oncol 1989 (Abstr); 8: 255.

49. Miller TP, Dana BW, Weick JK et al. Southwest Oncology Group Clinical trials for intermediate and high-grade non-Hodgkin's lymphoma. Semin. Hematol 1988; 25: 17–22.

50. Goldie JH, Coldman AJ, Gudauskas GA. Rationale for the use of alternating non-cross resistant chemotherapy. Cancer Treat Rep 1982; 66: 439–449.

51. Longo D, DeVita VT Jr, Duffey P et al. Randomized trial of ProMACE-MOPP (Day 1, D8) PM vs. ProMACE-CytaBOM (PC) in Stage II–IV aggressive Non-Hodgkin's lymphoma. Proc Am Soc Clin Oncol 1987 (Abstr); 6: 206.

52. Browne MJ, Hubbard SM, Longo DL et al. Excess prevalence of pneumocytis carinii pneumonia in patients treated for lymphoma with combination chemotherapy. Ann Intern Med 1986; 104: 338–344.

53. Coiffier B, Bryon PA, French M et al. Intensive chemotherapy in aggressive lymphomas: Updated results of LNH-80 Protocol and Prognostic Factors affecting response and survival. Blood 1987; 70: 1394–1399.

54. Cabanillas F, Hagemeister FB, McLaughlin P et al. Results of MIME regimen for recurrent or refractory lymphoma. J Clin Oncol 1987; 5: 407–412.

55. Hagberg H, Cavallin-Stahl E, Lind J. Ifosfamide and etoposide as salvage therapy for non-Hodgkin's lymphoma. Scand J Haematol 1986; 36: 61–64.

56. Velasquez WS, Cabanillas F, Salvador P et al. Effective salvage therapy for lymphoma with cisplatin in combination with high-dose Ara-C and dexamethasone (DHAP). Blood 1988- 71: 117–122.

57. O'Donnell MR, Forman SJ, Levine AM et al. Cytarabine, cisplatin and etoposide chemotherapy for refractory non-Hodgkin's lymphoma. Cancer Treat Rep 1987; 71: 187–189.

58. Warrell RP, Coonley CJ, Straus DJ et al. Treatment of patients with advanced malignant lymphoma using gallium nitrate administered as a sevenday continuous infusion. Cancer 1983; 51: 1982–1987.

59. Helms SR, Oblon DJ, Braylan RC et al. Etoposide, carmustine, bleomycin and methotrexate with leucovorin rescue as retreatment for unfavorable non-Hodgkin's lymphoma. Cancer Treat Rep 1985; 69: 783–786.

60. Philip T, Armitage JO, Spitzer G et al. High-dose therapy and autologous bone marrow transplantation after failure of conventional chemotherapy in adults with intermediate-grade or high-grade non-Hodgkin's lymphoma. N Engl J Med 1987; 316: 1493–1498.

Request for reprints:
Dr. Julie M. Vose
600 S. 42nd Street
Section of Hematology/Oncology
Department of Internal Medicine
University of Nebraska Medical Center
Omaha, Nebraska 68198, USA

Annals of Oncology, Supplement 2 to Volume 2: 177–180, 1991.
© 1991 *Kluwer Academic Publishers.*

Original article

Prospective multicenter trial for the response-adapted treatment of high-grade malignant non-Hodgkin's lymphomas: Updated results of the COP-BLAM/IMVP-16 protocol with randomized adjuvant radiotherapy*

M. Engelhard, P. Meusers, G. Brittinger, N. Brack, W. Dornoff, W. Enne, W. Gassmann,
H. Gerhartz, M. Hallek, J. Heise, W. Hettchen, D. Huhn, K. Kabelitz, R. Kuse, E. Lengfelder,
F. Ludwig, I. Meuthen, H. Radtke, C. Schadeck, C. Schöber, E. Schumacher, W. Siegert,
H.-J. Staiger, E. Terhardt, E. Thiel, M. Thomas, T. Wagner, M. G. Willems, W. Wilmanns,
T. Zwingers, H. Stein, M. Tiemann & K. Lennert
Department of Hematology, University of Essen, Hufelandstr. 55, D-4300 Essen, Germany

Summary. In a prospective multicenter trial the efficiency of the response-adapted COP-BLAM/IMVP-16 protocol to induce complete remissions (CR) in high-grade malignant non-Hodgkin's lymphomas as well as the prognostic relevance of adjuvant radiotherapy were investigated. From 1986–1989, 548 patients (median age 56 years) with stage II–IV (Ann Arbor) disease were treated with five cycles of COP-BLAM followed by two cycles of IMVP-16. If only a partial remission was obtained at the time of first restaging (RS) after three cycles (delayed response), treatment was switched to IMVP-16 (two to five courses) immediately. Patients achieving CR by the second RS after chemotherapy were randomized to adjuvant radiotherapy or observation. Responses to chemotherapy were 63% CR in patients completing the second RS (N = 350) or 72% if patients achieving late CR by consolidating radiotherapy are added; responses were 58% or 65% if all deaths prior to the second RS are included (N = 50). Overall and relapse-free survival were 71% and 68% at one year and 63% and 61% at two years. Multivariate risk factor analysis proved the early (by first RS) CR response to possess predominant prognostic relevance for survival. A significant advantage of adjuvant radiotherapy over no further treatment for duration of CR is not yet discernible. These results emphasize the importance of a rapidly achieved CR, thus contributing to the design of future trials.

Key words: non-Hodgkin lymphoma, randomized trial, response-adapted strategy

Introduction

Since it became evident that high-grade malignant non-Hodgkin's lymphomas (NHL) can be cured, even in cases of advanced disease, by appropriate chemotherapy, efforts were made to improve response rates, and thereby survival, by modifications of treatment protocols [1]. The accumulating international experience with several therapeutic regimens later revealed that the chance of cure depends not only on the pattern of initial disease extent and activity but on the subsequent dynamics of initial response [2]. Recent treatment approaches have therefore focused on exposing the tumor to more cytotoxic drugs in shorter intervals at higher dosages, thus increasing the dose intensity [3]. In accordance with these considerations, the present study was designed to evaluate the remission-inducing efficiency of the response-adapted sequential application of two non-cross-resistant multicomponent regi-

mens, namely COP-BLAM (cyclophosphamide, vincristine, prednisone, bleomycin, doxorubicin [Adriamycin], and procarbazine) [4] and IMVP-16 (ifosfamide, methotrexate, and etoposide) [5]. Additionally, the prognostic relevance of adjuvant radiotherapy for the stabilization of complete remissions was investigated.

Patient characteristics

Previously untreated patients aged 15–75 years presenting with a diagnosis of high-grade malignant non-Hodgkin's lymphoma according to the Kiel classification in stage II–IV disease (Ann Arbor classification) were eligible for the study. Immunohistochemical analysis is not yet completed. Histological evaluations were performed at and/or confirmed by the Kiel Lymph Node Registry (K. Lennert) or the Institute for Pathology, Freie Universität Berlin (H. Stein). Initial

* Supported by the BMFT, Germany.

clinical stage was assessed by a complete staging examination including all modern endoscopic and imaging techniques as well as bone marrow cytology and histology. These investigations were repeated at the restaging evaluations (RS) with particular attention to all areas of initial lymphoma involvement.

Study design

The study was performed as a prospective multicenter randomized trial according to the following design [6]: Initial chemotherapy consisted of a sequential application of the COP-BLAM (as in reference 4 but without dose escalation) and the IMVP-16 [5] regimens. Clinical response was evaluated by the first RS after three cycles of COP-BLAM. Patients attaining complete response (CR) continued therapy with two consolidating courses of COP-BLAM (total of five cycles) followed by two cycles of IMVP-16, while patients achieving only partial response (PR) were switched immediately to IMVP-16 (two to five cycles). All patients in complete remission after chemotherapy (second RS) were then randomized to adjuvant involved-field or main bulk radiotherapy (40 Gy) or treatment-free observation, excluding those with initial bulky disease ($\geqslant 10$ cm) for whom radiotherapy was recommended. Clinical response was defined in the usual categories of CR or PR as previously described [6]. Survival probabilities [7], significance of observed differences [8], and multivariate analysis of prognostic factors [9] were calculated according to standard procedures.

Results

From 1986 to 1989, 548 qualified patients were recruited to the study from 82 participating centers. Patient characteristics including initial parameters of disease and incidence of lymphoma entities and stages are summarized in Tables 1 and 2. By the date of analysis (March 1, 1990) 488 patients had completed phase 1 of chemotherapy and the first RS, including 19 early deaths; 381 had reached the second RS or died in the interval (N = 31, Table 3). In 10 patients in CR, therapy-related deaths resulted predominantly from pulmonary complications. Of all patients achieving CR, 110 qualified and gave informed consent for randomization to adjuvant radiotherapy versus treatment-free observation, of whom 74 have been followed for $\geqslant 3$ months and have thus become evaluable. Median observation time for all patients from the date of diagnosis is 12 (range 1–50) months; those having already completed chemotherapy were followed for 11 (range 2–30) months after the second RS. Response to chemotherapy is delineated in Table 3 rendering an overall CR rate of 58–65%. The precise rate depends on the point of reference, with only minor, nonsignificant differences between the histological entities (data

Table 1. Incidence of initial parameters.

Qualified patients	n = 548	
Sex	m : w = 1.2	
Median age (range)	56 (17–75) years	
age	>50 yr	65%
	>65 yr	25%
B-symptoms		51%
Extranodal manifestation		56%
Bone marrow involvement		12%
LDH	>240 U/L	49%
Karnofsky index	<70%	25%
Bulky disease	$\geqslant 10$ cm	19%
Total serum protein	<60 g/L	9%

Table 2. Incidence of histologic subtypes and stages.

NHL subtype	Stage			Sum	
	II	III	IV	n	(%)
Centroblastic	98	76	126	300	(55)
Immunoblastic	28	21	37	86	(16)
Lymphoblastic + Burkitt	5	3	13	21	(4)
Unclass. high-grade	43	13	44	100	(18)
Large cell anaplastic (Ki1 lymphoma)	15	11	15	41	(7)
Total	189	124	235	548	
(%)	(34)	(23)	(43)		

Table 3. Evaluation of remission rate.

	n	Deaths in CR/total	Rate of CR	
			RS	Including all deaths
Therapy phase 1	548	4/19		
Restaging 1	469		47%	46%
Therapy phase 2	410	6/31		
Restaging 2	350		63%	58%
Follow-up period[a]	312		72%	65%

[a] Late CR induced after partial response at second RS by additional radio- (n = 22/29) or chemotherapy (n = 7/29).
CR: Complete remission.
RS: Restaging evaluation.

not shown). Of 180 patients obtaining only a PR by the first RS and being followed until the second RS or death, 49 were submitted to the IMVP-16 protocol immediately, while in 131 cases of minimal residual disease the standard protocol (two cycles of COP-BLAM, two cycles IMVP-16) was continued. In patients switched early to IMVP-16, 37% CR were achieved as compared to 42% in those switched late with similar probabilities for overall and relapse-free survival in both groups (data not shown). Relapses occurred early in 5% of all patients between the first and second RS and late in 23% at a median of 6 (range 2–28) months after completion of chemotherapy. Of all relapses, 21% became evident in sites of initial disease, 52% developed as a combination of local recurrence and new manifestations, and 27% occurred only in new locations (e.g., central nervous system or bone marrow). Salvage chemotherapy regimens (including autologous bone marrow rescue in five cases) induced second remissions in 14% of the patients treated, 48% died rapidly of progression or toxic side effects (N = 6) and the rest are currently undergoing salvage treatment. Overall and relapse-free survival of all patients (Fig. 1) were 73 and 68%, respectively, at one year and 64% and 61%, respectively, at two years with the median not yet reached. Moderate, though nonsignificant differences of overall survival were seen in the comparison of lymphoma entities (Fig. 2) and even less significant differences between patients randomized to radiotherapy as opposed to no further treatment (Fig. 3). Relapse-free survivals in each of these subsets of patients were quite similar. Results of a multivariate analysis of factors previously identified as relevant for prognosis are listed in Table 4 according to their importance for the short-range (first RS) and long-term

Table 4.

Priority of relevance	Prognostic factors significantly relevant with respect to	
	Dynamic of response (CR after 3 cycles)	Overall survival probability
1.	− B-symptoms − tumor size >5 cm Ø − serum LDH >240 U/L	+ CR after 3 cycles − Karnofsky <70% − increasing age
2.	− extranodal manifestation	+ CR after 7 cycles − serum LDH >240 U/L − B-symptoms

+: Favorable; −: Unfavorable; CR: complete response.

(overall survival) prognosis. Parameters related to the extent or biological activity of the disease significantly influence the probability of an early CR after three cycles of therapy. This rapid CR is the most important prognostic determinant for overall survival.

Discussion

Since the introduction of anthracyclines into the therapeutic program significantly increased the response rates and thereby improved survival of patients with

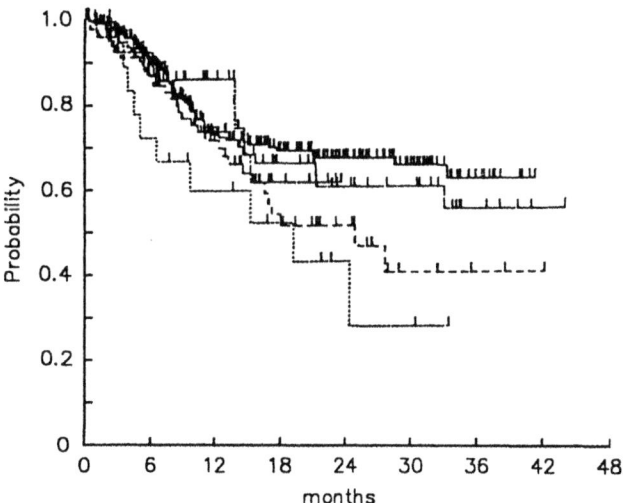

Fig. 2. Overall survival probability of all patients according to histological lymphoma entity (Kiel classification).

————	centroblastic	N = 300
- - - - -	immunoblastic	N = 86
··············	lymphoblastic + Burkitt	N = 21
− − − −	unclassifiable high grade	N = 100
−·−·−·−	large cell anaplastic (Ki-1)	N 41
		P > 0.05

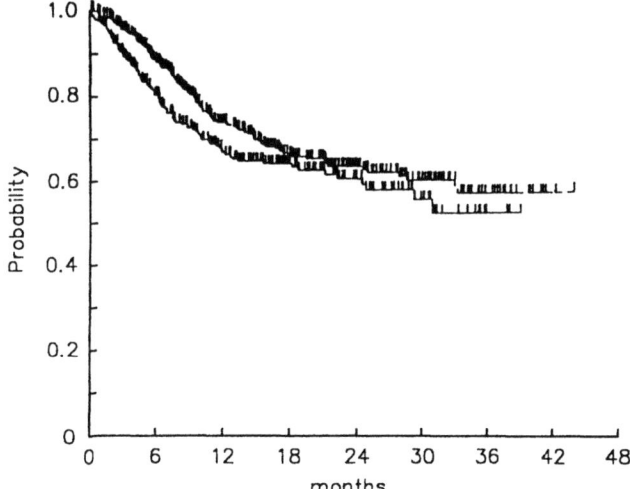

Fig. 1. Survival probability of all patients treated by COP-BLAM/IMVP-16 with relapse free survival calculated from earliest verification of CR (first or second RS) and regardless of whether chemotherapy has already been completed.

- - - - -	overall survival (upper curve)	N = 548
————	relapse-free survival (lower curve)	N = 349

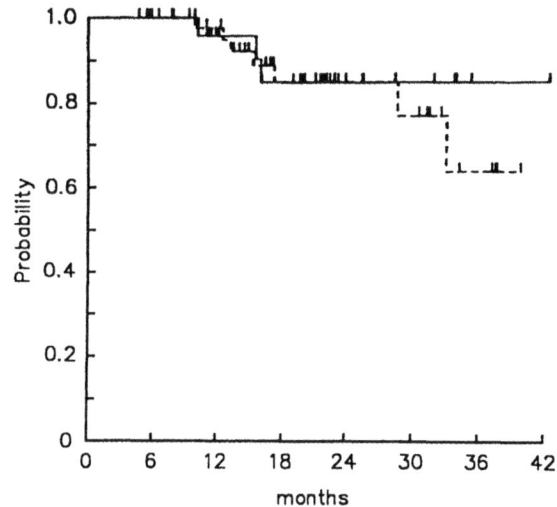

Fig. 3. Overall survival probability of patients randomized to adjuvant radiotherapy versus treatment-free observation after CR obtained by chemotherapy

————	randomized	N = 74
————	radiotherapy no	N = 44
- - - - -	radiotherapy yes	N = 30
		P > 0.05

high-grade malignant NHL, numerous protocols have been developed with the intention of further improving the treatment results. The more recent strategies ('third-generation' protocols) are characterized by six- to nine-drug combinations applied in intricate modifications of dosage and schedule and thus by an increased dose intensity [1, 3], as compared to the early cyclic regimens. Although these strategies have succeeded in raising the CR rates, their impact on survival still remains to be supported by long-term observations.

The protocol presented here was designed to encompass cytotoxic drugs active both in the induction and salvage treatment of lymphoma and included in two already established regimens [10]. The study thus allowed a multicenter clinical setting presumed to represent treatment conditions realistically achievable outside of strictly experimental environments. According to this concept, all patients qualified by age, histology, and stage of disease were eligible for this study and were evaluated regardless of whether factors indicative of high risk (e.g., low performance status, bulky disease) were present or of whether they died early in the treatment phase. Because of these considerations, the overall CR rates obtained (Table 3) can be favorably compared to other contemporary multicenter trials, are reminiscent of those achieved earlier by the CHOP regimen worldwide (including a pilot trial of the same study group) but differ from those reported in some recent limited institution studies [1].

One aim of the study was to assess the efficacy of a response-adapted strategy by introducing the transition to the second regimen early in patients reaching only a partial response by the first RS performed after three cycles. More than one third of these delayed responders (whose state is known to be associated with a high risk) later achieved CR. These CRs proved to be as stable as those obtained in the group switched later to the second regimen, although the latter group, by definition, represented a prognostically more favorable subset of patients. While the delayed responders thus seem to profit from the early exposure to a new regimen, it remains to be shown whether this approach of early salvage can be improved by different dosages or combinations of drugs, possibly warranting the early application of bone marrow ablative therapy followed by (autologous) marrow rescue.

While the data assembled thus far in the chemotherapy phase of this study already permit an estimation of its CR-inducing potential, including the separate analysis of different subsets of patients (e.g., immunohistological subtypes, particular manifestation sites), evidence for the prognostic relevance of adjuvant involved-field radiotherapy as opposed to no further treatment remains quite vague. Preliminary results seem to indicate that radiotherapy applied after successful completion of chemotherapy may not significantly contribute to the stabilization of CR and may thus be irrelevant for cure. A definitive evaluation of this crucial issue still demands the long-term observation of all patients randomized accordingly. However, as the multivariate analysis indicates (Table 4), a number of factors can already be shown to have significant effects on long-term prognosis. Among the factors associated with the tumor initially (e.g., systemic activity, site or extent of disease) as well as age and the performance status of the patient, the tumor-related parameters prove to exert significant adverse influence on the rapid achievement of complete response as established by the first RS evaluation. If the end point for this type of analysis is overall survival, an early CR – along with a reduced performance status and increasing age – emerges as the most relevant prognostic factor. The combined evidence of this study thus supports the concept of the ultimate importance of therapeutic success early in the treatment period of high-grade malignant NHL as already implied in the conclusions from separate studies [2]. Taking the only moderate toxicity of the protocol presented here into account, it seems promising to intensify the initial phase of therapy with the aim of increasing rapid complete response rates, as is currently being investigated in a pilot trial by this study group.

References

1. Yi PI, Coleman M, Saltz L et al. Chemotherapy for large cell lymphoma: A status update. Semin Oncol 1990; 17: 60–73.
2. Armitage JO, Weisenberger DD, Hutchins M et al. Chemotherapy for diffuse large-cell lymphoma – Rapidly responding patients have more durable remissions. J Clin Oncol 1986; 4: 160–164.
3. DeVita VT Jr, Hubbard SM, Young RC. The role of chemotherapy in diffuse aggressive lymphomas. Semin Hematol 1988; 25: 2–10.
4. Laurence J, Coleman M, Allen SL et al. Combination chemotherapy of advanced diffuse histiocytic lymphoma with the six-drug COP-BLAM regimen. Ann Intern Med 1982; 97: 190–195.
5. Cabanillas F, Hagemeister FB, Bodey GB et al. IMVP-16: an effective regimen for patients with lymphoma who have relapsed after initial combination chemotherapy. Blood 1982; 60: 693–697.
6. Gerhartz HH, Thiel E, Brittinger G et al. German-Austrian multicenter trial for aggressive non-Hodgkin lymphomas: COP-BLAM/IMVP-16 chemotherapy with randomized adjuvant radiotherapy. Blut 1988; 56: 139–142.
7. Kaplan EL, Meier P. Non-parametric estimation from incomplete observations. J Am Statist Assoc 1958; 53: 457–481.
8. Mantel N. Evaluation of survival data and two new rank order statistics arising in its consideration. Cancer Chemother Rep 1966; 50: 163–170.
9. Cox DR. Regression models and life tables. J Roy Statist Soc 1972; 34 (series B): 187–220.
10. Coleman M, Armitage JO, Gaynor M et al. The COP-BLAM programs: Evolving chemotherapy concepts in large cell lymphoma. Semin Hematol 1988; 25, No 2, Suppl 2: 23–33.

Correspondence to:
Dr. Marianne Engelhard
Department of Hematology
University of Essen
Hufelandstr. 55
D-4300 Essen, Germany

Annals of Oncology, Supplement 2 to Volume 2: 181–185, 1991.
© 1991 Kluwer Academic Publishers.

Original article

Autologous bone marrow transplantation for advanced stage adult lymphoblastic lymphoma in first complete remission
Report of the Non-Hodgkin's Lymphoma Cooperative Study Group (NHLCSG)

G. Santini,[1] P. Coser,[2] T. Chisesi,[3] A. Porcellini,[4] R. Sertoli,[5] A. Contu,[6] O. Vinante,[7] A. M. Congiu,[1] A. M. Carella,[1] T. D'Amico,[1] D. Pierluigi,[1] E. Rossi,[1] D. Scarpati[8] & V. Rizzoli[9]

[1] Division of Hematology, Ospedale S. Martino, Genoa; [2] Division of Hematology, Ospedale Civile, Bolzano; [3] Division of Hematology, Ospedale Civile, Vicenza; [4] Division of Hematology, Ospedale Civile, Cremona; [5] National Cancer Institute, Genoa; [6] Division of Oncology, Ospedale Civile, Sassari; [7] Division of Oncology, Ospedale Civile Noale; [8] Institute of Radiology, Genoa; [9] Institute of Hematology, Parma, Italy

Summary. Thirty-six successive adult patients with lymphoblastic lymphoma entered a study of sequential chemotherapy consisting of an intensive LSA2-L2-type protocol to induce first complete remission. Eighteen patients in first CR (median age 22 years, range 15–51), underwent autologous bone marrow transplantation after receiving a conditioning regimen consisting of cyclophosphamide and total body irradiation. Of these 18 patients, 2 were in stage III and 16 in stage IV; 15 showed mediastinal and 9 bone marrow involvement at diagnosis. The transplant procedure was well tolerated and no treatment-induced deaths occurred. At this time, 14 out of 18 patients are alive and well between 1 and 60 months post transplant (median follow-up time 46 months) with an actuarial disease-free survival of 74%. This phase II study suggests that high-dose chemo-radiotherapy followed by autologous bone marrow transplantation may improve long-term disease-free survival in advanced stage adult lymphoblastic lymphoma.

Introduction

Lymphoblastic lymphoma (LBL) is a distinct subgroup of high-grade malignant non-Hodgkin's lymphomas (NHL) [1], often characterized by a mediastinal mass in addition to peripheral adenopathies, rapidly involving bone marrow and peripheral blood [2].

Sequential multiagent chemotherapy has improved the prognosis of the disease. The first encouraging results were attained in children [3–5] while only recently has progress been made in adults [6–9]. However, because of the high relapse rate, long-term survival in adults with advanced stage disease is still unsatisfactory [7–9].

In a small number of studies, patients with high-grade malignant NHL in complete remission (CR) following conventional chemotherapy were treated with high-dose chemotherapy and chemoradiotherapy followed by allogeneic bone marrow transplant (BMT) or autologous bone marrow transplantation (ABMT). When results in LBL patients were analyzed separately, bone marrow transplant appeared to prolong survival and disease-free survival (DFS) in poor prognosis patients, when performed in CR [10–15]. Recently, more homogeneous studies have reported very encouraging results in the same group of patients [16, 17]. In order to confirm the real impact of ABMT in LBL,

our pilot study [16] has been extended to a larger number of adult, advanced-stage patients in first CR after a sequential LSA2-L2-type regimen.

Materials and methods

Patients and treatment

Thirty-six patients with lymphoblastic lymphoma classified according to the 'Working Formulation' [1] were studied between January 1985 and April 1990.

During this period all new patients seen at the cooperating centers were entered in the prospective study. The eligibility criteria were as follows: (1) age ≥15 years; (2) lymph node biopsy confirming LBL diagnosis, and phenotype if possible; (3) advanced stage (II with mediastinal bulky disease >15 cm, III, or IV); and (4) less than 25% blasts in the bone marrow and less than 10% circulating blasts. Immune membrane markers were determined using a panel of monoclonal antibodies [18]. Informed consent was requested from every patient.

Pretreatment tests included chest x-ray, chest computerized tomography (CT), abdominal ultrasound and/or CT scan. Two posterior iliac crest bone biopsies were carried out on all patients, as were bone marrow aspiration and a lumbar puncture for chemical and cytological examination of the liquor. Cytological or pathological tests on accessible sites were conducted in all cases. Involvement of the pericardium, kidney, liver, and spleen was based on clinical criteria alone. The stage of the disease, according to the Ann Arbor classification [19], was determined just before ABMT.

In order to obtain a CR, patients were treated with a sequential regimen derived from LSA2-L2 [3], including an induction-consolidation therapy of 64 days duration, which is similar to the same phases of the original protocol. The schedule and doses of the eight drugs are reported in Table 1.

Once a CR was confirmed by restaging, patients entered the second treatment step consisting of a conditioning regimen of high-dose radio-chemotherapy followed by autologous bone marrow rescue.

All patients received cyclophosphamide (CY) 60 mg/kg on days -4 and -3, total body irradiation (TBI) 10 Gy on day -1, and bone marrow infusion on day 0. The TBI was given in a single dose, from a ^{60}Co source at a rate of ~4 cGy/min. The patients were adequately hydrated and received Mesna (to prevent hemorrhagic cystitis), as well as fuoresemide and antiemetic drugs.

Bone marrow collection and purging

Bone marrow was collected as described elsewhere [20]. In 9 patients who presented with partially infiltrated marrow at diagnosis, the harvested marrows were purged with a dose of Maphosphamide (ASTA-Z 7557) able to spare 5% of normal granulocyte-macrophage colony-forming units (GM-CFU), as reported by Gorin et al. [21]. In our patients a median dose of 80 μg/2 × 10^7 cells was used (range 50-100) (Table 3).

The marrows were placed in 5-mL plastic tubes (2.5 mL of marrow and 2.5 mL dimethyl sulfoxide [DMSO] 20% in medium) and then cryopreserved and stored in

Table 1. Induction/Consolidation Protocol.

	Dose (m^2)		Days of treatment
Induction			
Vincristine	1.4	mg I.V.	1, 8, 15, 22, 29
Adriamycin	30	mg I.V.	8, 15, 22
Cyclophosphamide	750	mg I.V.	15, 22, 29
L-Asparaginase	10.000	U I.V.	8-14
Prednisone	40	mg P.O.	1-29
Methotrexate	10	mg I.T.	3, 10, 17, 24
Consolidation			
Daunomycin	50	mg I.V.	43, 46, 49
Cytosine arabinoside	200	mg I.V.	43-49
Methotrexate^b	400	mg I.V.	64

^{a} Continuous infusion;
^{b} I.V. MTX 1/4 dose push, 3/4 dose in 4 hours. Leucovorin rescue 15 mg/P.O. every 6 hours for 6 doses, beginning 24 hours after the end of the MTX infusion.

the vapor phase of a liquid nitrogen freezer [13]. The bone marrow aspirates contained a median of 2.0 × 10^8/kg nucleated cells (range 1.0-3.5 × 10^8/kg) and, in unpurged marrows, a median of 1.5 × 10^4/kg GM-CFU (range 1.1-4.2 × 10^4/kg).

Clinical report

All patients were isolated after transplant and fitted with a Hickman catheter.

The patients received intestinal tract decontamination therapy (colistin, neomycin, and amphotericin B), while an empirical antibiotic regimen (an aminoglycoside and a cephalosporin) was administered intravenously if bouts of fever associated with granulocytopenia occurred. Patients showing clinical evidence of herpes simplex virus were treated with acyclovir. Patients also received parenteral hyperalimentation, and platelet transfusions from individual donors were given when platelet counts fell below 20 × 10^9/L. Leukocyte-free erythrocyte concentrates were administered when hemoglobin dropped below 10 g/dL. All allogeneic cells were irradiated (20 Gy).

Statistical methods

The DFS curve was estimated by the Kaplan and Meier method [22]. The statistical analysis was performed in April 1990.

Results

Patients and tumor responses

One patient died early of sepsis and hemorrhage; of the 35 evaluable patients, 24 achieved CR (69%), 6 attained partial remission (PR) (17%), and 5 were nonresponders (NR) (14%). In spite of salvage therapy, only 2 PR patients are still alive, while all the other PR and NR patients died of progressive disease at 7, 11, 16, and 20 and 3, 3, 8, 9, and 14 months from diagnosis, respectively.

Twenty-four patients in CR were registered for ABMT. One, who had persistent hypoplastic bone marrow four months after induction-consolidation, was registered for allotransplant and is now alive and well 34 months after the procedure (41 months after diagnosis). Three refused transplant and underwent maintenance therapy for two years. The treatment consisted of weekly therapy rotating six drugs (vincristine, doxorubicin [Adriamycin], cyclophosphamide, methotrexpatients, 2 relapsed at 10 and 22 months from CR and died at 19 and 28 months from diagnosis, respectively. The third is alive and well at 57 months from CR and 59 from diagnosis. Two patients are now scheduled, and 18 have already undergone ABMT. This latter group consisted of 12 males and 6 females, median age 21 years (range 15-43). Two were stage III, and 16 were stage IV; 4 presented with B symptoms (fever, weight loss), 15 with mediastinal (83%) and 9 with bone marrow involvement (50%). Six of the latter showed blasts in the peripheral blood. There was spleen involvement in 7 cases, pleura and liver in 4, kidney in 3, and isolated gut, muscle, pericardium, bone, or lung involvement in 5 individuals.

Of these 18 patients, 16 were included in the study upon diagnosis, while 2 entered the study after receiving six cycles of CHOP [23] at another institution and achieving a PR (Table 2). The immunological phenotype of these patients is reported in Table 3.

The results of the ABMT procedure are summarized in Table 4. All patients were in first CR when transplanted. The median time between attainment of CR and ABMT was 2 months (range 1–19). Only the first patient was transplanted 19 months after CR and after 18 months of maintenance chemotherapy.

Currently 14 of the 18 patients are in continuous complete remission (CCR); the median follow-up time is 46 months (range 1–60) with an actuarial DFS probability of 74% (Fig. 1). Of the 9 patients who presented at diagnosis with bone marrow involvement, 4 died at 3, 5, 5 and 9 months post transplant of leukemic relapse without lymph node involvement (Table 4).

Table 2. Patients' characteristics.

Patient no.	Sex/age (ys)	Histology/(in. stage, symptoms)		Med involv +/−	BM involv +/−	ExtraN involv	Previous therapy	Status at induction/consolidation
1	F/18	LBL-NC	(IV, B)	+	−	1, 2	−	diagnosis
2	F/31	LBL-C	(IV, A)	+	+	−	−	diagnosis
3	M/27	LBL-NC	(IV, A)	+	+	3	−	diagnosis
4	F/43	LBL-NC	(III, A)	+	−	−	6 × CHOP	PR
5	M/16	LBL-NC	(IV, A)	−	+	3	6 × CHOP	PR
6	F/36	LBL-C	(IV-B)	+	−	1	−	diagnosis
7	M/17	LBL-NC	(IV-A)	+	−	4	−	diagnosis
8	M/26	LBL-C	(IV, A)	+	−	5	−	diagnosis
9	M/18	LBL-NC	(IV, A)	+	+	3	−	diagnosis
10	M/15	LBL-C	(IV, A)	+	+	−	−	diagnosis
11	F/38	LBL-NC	(IV, B)	+	+	1, 6	−	diagnosis
12	F/16	LBL-C	(IV, A)	+	+	3	−	diagnosis
13	M/15	LBL-C	(IV, A)	+	+	3	−	diagnosis
14	M/15	LBL-NC	(IV, A)	+	+	1, 2, 3	−	diagnosis
15	M/24	LBL-C	(IV, A)	+	−	9	−	diagnosis
16	M/18	LBL-NC	(IV, A)	+	−	2, 4, 8	−	diagnosis
17	M/30	LBL-NC	(IV, B)	−	−	2, 3, 4, 7	−	diagnosis
18	M/27	LBL-C	(III, A)	−	−	−	−	diagnosis

In. stage: initial stage; Med involv: mediastinal involvement; BM involv: bone marrow involvement; ExtraN involv: extranodal involvement; LBL: lymphoblastic lymphoma; NC: non convoluted; C: convoluted; 1: pleura; 2: liver; 3: spleen; 4: kidney; 5: muscle; 6: pericardium; 7: gut; 8: skin; 9: lung; CHOP: cyclophosphamide, Adriamycin, oncovin prednisone; PR: partial response.

Table 3. Immunologic characterization of LBL.

Cases	OKT3	OKT4	OKT6	OKT8	OKT9	OKT10	OKT11	Ia	CALLA	B1	C-Ig	S-Ig	Immunotype
1	−	−	−	−	++	+	+	+	−	−	−	−	T
2	++	++	−	++	−	++	Nd	+	+	−	−	−	T
3	−	−	−	−	+	+	−	++	++	++	++	−	Pre-B
4	Nd	Nd	Nd	Nd	Nd	Nd	Nd	Nd	Nd	Nd	Nd	Nd	Nd
5	−	−	−	−	−	−	−	++	++	−	−	−	Non T/B
6	++	+	−	++	−	−	++	−	−	−	Nd	Nd	T
7	++	−	−	−	++	−	++	−	−	−	Nd	Nd	T
8	++	+	+	+	−	++	++	−	−	−	Nd	Nd	T
9	++	−	−	+	+	−	++	−	−	−	Nd	Nd	T
10	++	++	++	−	++	Nd	++	−	+	−	−	−	T
11	−	−	−	−	−	−	−	++	++	−	−	−	Non T/B
12	−	−	+	−	+	++	−	−	−	−	Nd	Nd	T
13	++	−	+	−	++	++	Nd	−	−	−	Nd	Nd	T
14	+	Nd	++	Nd	++	++	Nd	−	−	−	−	−	T
15	++	+	Nd	+	+	Nd	Nd	−	−	Nd	Nd	Nd	T
16	−	Nd	−	Nd	−	+	−	++	++	++	−	−	Pre-B
17	++	++	−	++	+	−	−	−	−	−	Nd	Nd	T
18	−	−	−	−	−	Nd	Nd	++	++	+	−	−	Pre-B

Antibody staining was scored as: −, 0 to 10%; +, 11 to 50%; ++, 51 to 100%. Nd: not determined; LBL: lymphoblastic lymphoma; Non T/B: non-T, non-B.

Table 4. Results of cytoreductive therapy and ABMT in first CR LBL.

Case no.	Time from CR to ABMT	Purging (μg/2 × 10⁷ cells)	Duration of CCR (mos. from ABMT)	Cause of death (mos. from ABMT)
1	19[a]	–	60+	–
2	3	70	58+	–
3	2	100	56+	–
4	1	–	52+	–
5	2	50	2	leuk. rel. (3)
6	4	–	52+	–
7	2	–	48+	–
8	1	–	47+	–
9	2	90	45+	–
10	1	70	3	leuk. rel. (5)
11	3	100	41+	–
12	2	80	7	leuk. rel. (9)
13	4	80	4	leuk. rel. (5)
14	2	60	21+	–
15	3	–	11+	–
16	1	–	5+	–
17	2	–	1+	–
18	3	–	1+	–

[a] Transplanted after 18 months of maintenance chemotherapy.
CCR: continuous complete remission; leuk. rel.: leukaemic relapse.

Toxicity

All patients had pancytopenia (leukocyte nadir <0.1 × 10⁹/L). Marrow engraftment occurred in all. In the 9 patients who had no initial bone marrow involvement, the median time to self-sustaining granulocyte recovery (>0.5 × 10⁹/L) was 13 days (range 12–15), while the median time for platelet recovery (>20 × 10⁹/L) was 22 days (range 15–53). In the other 9 patients, whose marrow had been purged, recovery was delayed, with granulocyte recovery (>0.5 × 10⁹/L) on day 18 (range 12–83) and platelet recovery (>20 × 10⁹/L) on day 35 (range 25–105).

All patients suffered from nausea and vomiting (grade 3), and most had diarrhea (grade 2). Grade 2–3 mucositis was observed in all patients. For these reasons all patients required parenteral hyperalimentation. Abnormal liver function was observed in 6 patients (grade 1–2), but the elevation of liver enzymes was very transient. Only 1 patient developed severe liver and kidney toxicity (grade 3), but again the episode was short-lived. All patients required antibiotic therapy and transfusions during the aplastic phase. Eight cases of bacterial sepsis occurred (grade 1–3), but all responded to parenteral antibacterial therapy. Five patients developed herpes simplex labialis, requiring acyclovir.

Discussion

The experience gained in the treatment of children shifted the therapeutic approach toward a sequential chemotherapy borrowed from protocols that had proved so successful in the therapy of ALL [3–5]. The

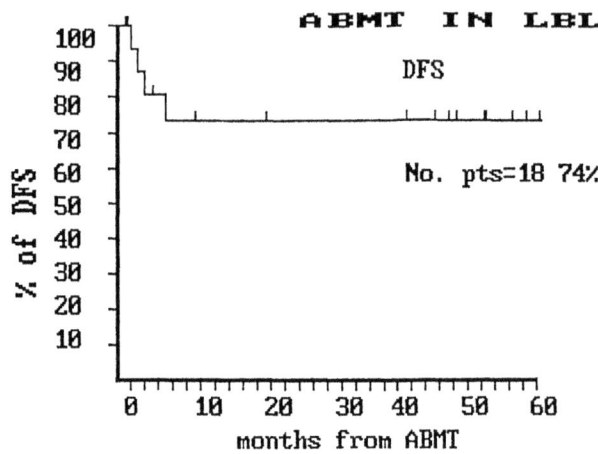

Fig. 1. Probability of DFS for 18 LBL patients in first CR following an autograft.

employment of these treatments in adult patients yielded similar results [6–9].

However, even if overall results are very good, survival and DFS are markedly influenced by a series of prognostic factors such as age [8], advanced stage of the disease and bone marrow involvement [7, 9] with a three-year DFS of approximately 20%. Most of the relapses occur while on treatment; discrediting the value of a prolonged aggressive maintenance chemotherapy.

The failure of conventional treatment to influence the outcome of these high-risk patients prompted the use of high-dose radiotherapy and/or chemotherapy followed by bone marrow rescue. A small number of studies on the use of allogeneic BMT for the treatment of LBL in adults has shown that it is possible to improve the prognosis for patients with HLA-compatible siblings [10–12]. However, this option is limited by the availability of a suitable donor.

ABMT is an increasingly safe procedure with a larger applicability, but few data, based on very limited series, are available on ABMT in LBL in CR [13–15]. Results seem encouraging; when ABMT data on patients autografted in first CR are scrutinized to sort out LBL cases, the seven-year DFS of these patients is 65% [15]. Recent results of the NHLCSG and the French group in advanced-stage patients lend support to this approach [16, 17].

Our study was designed to compress the sequential induction-consolidation therapy into 64 days and to avoid any subsequent maintenance therapy after attaining a CR. We planned to eradicate possible minimal residual disease with megachemo-radiotherapy followed by ABMT.

This approach seems particularly suitable for high-risk LBL patients, such as those entered into our study, who present with one or more of those risk factors linked with poor survival, such as age, advanced stage, and bone marrow involvement at diagnosis.

In line with reports from other investigators, the sequential treatment adopted in our protocol proved efficacious; 24 of 35 evaluable patients attained CR (69%) [6, 8, 9].

Three CR patients refused to proceed to ABMT, 1 underwent allogeneic BMT, 2 are on the waiting list, and 18 underwent ABMT in first CR. Of these 18 patients, 14 are currently in CCR, off therapy, 1–60 months (median 46 months) after ABMT (Table 4), with a five-year DFS probability of 74% (Fig. 1). Four patients died of leukemic relapse three, five, five, and nine months after transplant; all 4 cases presented with bone marrow involvement.

The overall toxicity of the ABMT procedure was acceptable. The mild toxicity was probably related to the good clinical condition of the patients at the time of the procedure and probably also to the fact that none of them had received prior mediastinal radiation therapy.

This study is not able to confirm whether it is necessary to purge the bone marrow with maphosphamide [24–26], but initial bone marrow involvement appears to be an unfavorable prognostic factor.

Because of the limited size of our study, we do not feel entitled to draw definite conclusions. However, considering the strong likelihood of failure with conventional therapy, the results obtained in these high-risk patients suggest that ABMT in first CR is able to improve long-term DFS with acceptable toxicity.

In addition, in comparison with the very prolonged treatment period reported in the literature, the short overall duration of treatment, including induction-consolidation phases followed by ABMT, represents a definite improvement in terms of quality of life.

References

1. Rosenberg SA, Berard CW, Brown BW et al. National Cancer Institute sponsored study of classification of non-Hodgkin's lymphomas: summary and description of a working formulation for clinical usage. Cancer 1982; 49: 2112–2135.
2. Nathwani BN, Diamond LW, Winberg CD et al. Lymphoblastic lymphoma: a clinicopathologic study of 95 patients. Cancer 1981; 48: 2347–2357.
3. Wollner N, Burchenal JH, Leiberman PH et al. Non-Hodgkin's lymphoma in children: a comparative study of two modalities of therapy. Cancer 1976; 37: 123–134.
4. Weistein HJ, Vande ZB, Jaffe N et al. Improved prognosis for patients with mediastinal lymphoblastic lymphoma. Blood 1979; 53: 683–694.
5. Anderson JR, Wilson JF, Jenkin DT et al. Childhood non-Hodgkin's lymphoma: the results of a randomized therapeutic trial comparing a 4-drug regimen (COMP) with a 10-drug regimen (LSA2-L2). Brit J Haematol 1983; 308: 559–565.
6. Levine AM, Forman SJ, Meyer PR et al. Successful therapy of convoluted T-lymphoblastic lymphoma in the adult. Blood 1983; 61: 92–98.
7. Mazza P, Bertini M, Macchi S et al. Lymphoblastic lymphoma in adolescents and adults. Clinical, pathological and prognostic evaluation. Eur J Cancer Clin Oncol 1986; 22: 1503–1510.
8. Slater DE, Mertelsmann R, Koziner B et al. Lymphoblastic lymphoma in adults. J Clin Oncol 1986; 4: 57–67.
9. Coleman CN, Picozzi VJ, Cox RS et al. Treatment of lymphoblastic lymphoma in adults. J Clin Oncol 1986; 4: 1628–1637.
10. Ernst P, Maraninchi D, Jacobsen N et al. Marrow transplantation for non-Hodgkin's lymphoma: a multi-centre study from the European Co-operative Bone Marrow Transplant Group. Bone Marrow Transplant 1986; 1: 81–86.
11. Phillips GL, Herzig RH, Lazarus HM et al. High-dose chemotherapy, fractionated total-body irradiation, and allogeneic marrow transplantation for malignant lymphoma. J Clin Oncol 1986; 4: 480–488.
12. Nademanee AP, Forman SJ, Schmidt GM et al. Allogeneic bone marrow transplantation for high risk non-Hodgkin's lymphoma during first complete remission. Blut 1987; 55: 11–18.
13. Verdonck LF, Dekker ML, Kempen ML et al. Intensive cytotoxic therapy followed by autologous bone marrow transplantation for non-Hodgkin's lymphoma of high-grade malignancy. Blood 1985; 65: 984–989.
14. Braine HG, Santos GW, Kaizer H et al. Treatment of poor prognosis non-Hodgkin's lymphoma using cyclophosphamide and total body irradiation regimens with autologous bone marrow rescue. Bone Marrow Transplant 1987; 2: 7–14.
15. Goldstone AH, Singer CRJ, Gribben JG et al. Fifth report of EBMTG experience of ABMT in malignant lymphoma. Proc. XIVth Ann. Meet. Eur. Coop. Group for Bone Marrow Transplantation. Bone Marrow Transplant 1988; 3 (suppl 1): 33–36.
16. Santini G, Coser P, Chisesi T et al. Autologous bone marrow transplantation for advanced stage adult lymphoblastic lymphoma in first complete remission. A pilot study of the non-Hodgkin's lymphoma Co-operative Study Group (NHLCSG). Bone Marrow Transplant 1989; 4: 399–404.
17. Milpied N, Ifrah N, Kuentz M et al. Bone marrow transplantation for adult poor prognosis lymphoblastic lymphoma in first complete remission. Br J Haematol 1989; 73: 82–87.
18. Weiss LM, Bindl JM, Picozzi VJ et al. Lymphoblastic lymphoma: an immunophenotype study of 26 cases with comparison to T cell acute lymphoblastic leukemia. Blood 1986; 67: 474–478.
19. Carbone PP, Kaplan HS, Musshoff K et al. Report of the committee on Hodgkin's disease staging. Cancer Res 1971; 31: 1860–1861.
20. Thomas ED, Storb R. Technique for human marrow grafting. Blood 1970; 36: 507–515.
21. Gorin NC, Douay L, Laporte JP et al. Autologous bone marrow transplantation using marrow incubated with ASTA Z 7557 in adult acute leukemia. Blood 1986; 67: 1367–1376.
22. Kaplan EL, Meier P. Non-parametric estimation from incomplete observations. J Am Stat Assoc 1958; 53: 457–481.
23. McKelvey EM, Gottlieb JA, Wilson HE et al. Hydroxyldaunomycin (Adriamycin) combination chemotherapy in malignant lymphoma. Cancer 1976; 38: 1484–1493.
24. Yager AM, Kaiser H, Santos GW et al. Autologous bone marrow transplantation in patients with acute non lymphocytic leukemia, using ex vivo marrow treatment with 4-hydroperoxy-cyclophosphamide. N Eng J Med 1986; 315: 141–146.
25. Gorin NC, Aegerter P, Auvert B for the EBMTG. Autologous bone marrow transplantation (ABMT) for acute leukemia in remission: fifth European survey. Evidence in favour of marrow purging. Influence of pretransplant intervals. Bone Marrow Transplant 1988; 3 (suppl 1): 39–41.
26. Rizzoli V, Mangoni L, Aglietta M et al. Italian Study Group, Hematology Unit – Parma University. Autologous bone marrow transplantation in acute leukemia using maphosphamide treated marrow. Exp Hematol 1988; 16: 543 (abstract).

Correspondence to:
Dr. Gino Santini
Division of Hematology
Ospedali Civili Genova
Viale Benedetto XV, 10
16132, Genova, Italy

Annals of Oncology, Supplement 2 to Volume 2: 187–190, 1991.
© 1991 *Kluwer Academic Publishers.*

Original article ————————————————————

Radioimmunotherapy of B-cell lymphoma

Janet F. Eary
University of Washington Medical Center, Division of Nuclear Medicine, Department of Radiology, Seattle, Washington, USA

Summary. Radioimmunotherapy has evolved from an attractive concept to implementation in clinical trials for evaluation of toxicity and efficacy. Non-Hodgkin's lymphoma is a useful setting for evaluation of this novel form of therapy. Groups investigating radioimmunotherapy for non-Hodgkin's lymphoma are implementing single high doses and multiple smaller doses of beta emitters I-131 and Y-90 attached to antibodies. All groups giving multiple small doses observe partial responses to treatment with variable hematopoietic toxicity. Single very high doses have yielded complete responses with hematologic toxicity requiring reinfusion of stored bone marrow. A review of radioimmunotherapy trials for non-Hodgkin's lymphoma with a discussion of pertinent related issues is presented.

Key words: lymphoma, radioimmunotherapy, radioisotopes, radiolabeled antibody

Since the modern concept of radioimmunotherapy was envisioned in the early 1970s, clinical studies began as trials to use antibodies attached to radioisotopes for imaging sites of metastatic disease. Eventually as these techniques became familiar, clinical trials evolved to utilize radiolabeled antibodies at high specific activities in attempts to treat malignancy. While most of these trials are in their early phases of evaluation of toxicity and efficacy, several requirements for successful radioimmunotherapy are evolving. Selection of isotope for radioimmunotherapy has settled primarily on the use of beta emitters because of their long particle range in tissue and because of concerns over heterogeneity of antibody binding within the tumor. Beta-emitting isotopes are readily available, and many can be used with stable attachments to radiolabeled antibodies (Table 1). It has also become apparent that antibodies and their fragments, which have increased residence time in tumor, are more efficacious in selectively radiating the tumor as target compared to normal organs. This, in combination with focal tumor uptake, are the requirements for successful treatment of malignant disease. At this time the goals of most groups performing radioimmunotherapy trials are those of increasing uptake and residence time of radiolabeled antibodies in tumor sites, while increasing clearance of background radioactivity from normal organs, particularly the radiosensitive bone marrow.

Lymphoma is an ideal malignancy for treatment with radiolabeled antibodies because of its exquisite sensitivity to radiation. It is a disseminated disease, with well-characterized surface antigens, and numerous antibodies are available that have excellent binding characteristics for diseased and normal lymphocytes. In addition, compared to solid tumors, it has a number of other favorable characteristics. Most lymphomas have adequate vascularization for delivery of radiolabeled antibody to the interior of tumor; they have high levels of antigens on cells, with high numbers of cells bearing antigen; and they do not develop necrotic hypoxic centers that commonly affect solid tumors. Patients can be selected with a wide variety of states of disease progression, and often are not in a state of critical compromise when experimental therapy can be administered. In addition, lymphoma has a long history of well-established effective clinical regimens for comparison to the toxicity and efficacy of new radioimmunotherapy trials.

In this discussion, a review of major radioimmunotherapy trials for lymphoma will be presented with emphasis on description of therapeutic protocols and approaches. A review of current toxicity and efficacy data will be presented, with a focus on the work performed at the University of Washington Medical

Table 1. Isotopes considered for radioimmunotherapy.

Isotope	Emission	Half-life	Photons
I-131	0.34 MeV β (13%) 0.61 MeV β (86%)	8.1 d	364 keV (82%)
Y-90	2.29 MeV β (100%)	6.4 hr.	none
Re-186	0.93 MeV β (22%) 1.07 MeV β (70%)	90.6 hr.	137 keV (9.2%)
Re-188	1.97 MeV β (24%) 2.13 MeV β (74%)	6.9 hr.	155 keV (15%)

188

Center in conjunction with the Fred Hutchinson Cancer Research Center.

Review of clinical data

Construction of a radioimmunotherapy trial for lymphoma takes into consideration issues that are faced by investigators attempting to treat carcinomas as well. One major consideration is dosing schedule. Should a large single dose be administered, or several smaller doses over a long period of time? Radioisotopes with desirable physical characteristics must be chosen as therapeutic agents, with attention paid to ability to gather biodistribution data using trace-labeled antibody doses for therapy planning. In addition, investigators must decide if bone marrow toxic doses will be administered, and whether there will be institutional plans for bone marrow storage and rescue if necessary. And finally, estimates of internal radiation absorbed dose to tumors and normal organs are imperative for comparison of data to standard radiation therapy techniques in oncology. A review of the protocols and results of several groups engaged in clinical trials of radioimmunotherapy of lymphoma is presented (Table 2).

Investigators at the University of Washington, in conjunction with the Fred Hutchinson Cancer Research Center, have established a well-defined protocol for evaluation of treatment of patients with non-Hodgkin's B-cell lymphoma (Table 3). Patients admitted onto the protocol must have bone marrow containing less than 15% tumor, for storage and possible reinfusion after treatment. They must also have evaluable disease, and life expectancy greater than one month. Other laboratory parameters must be

Table 2. Radioimmunotherapy of non-Hodgkin's lymphoma.

Group	Radio-isotope	Dose	No. of patients	Results
University of Washington/ Fred Hutchinson Cancer Research Center	I-131	Single 250–630 mCi	7	6CR/1PR
University of California, Davis	I-131	Divided 20–60 mCi	23	23PR
Center for Molecular Medicine and Immunology	I-131	Divided 30 + 20 mCi	6	4PR
University of California, San Diego	Y-90	10 mCi	1	PR
University of Michigan	I-131	25–149 mCi	5	3PR

Table 3. University of Washington/Fred Hutchinson Cancer Research Center Lymphoma study design.

1. Cryopreserve bone marrow
2. Dosimetry studies (0.5, 2.5, 10.0 mg/kg antibody)
3. Therapeutic infusion
   a) estimated to deliver 1500 cGy to normal organs
   b) radiation dose escalation 175 cGy increments/3 pts
   c) hospitalize until body radioactivity level is <30 mCi
   d) follow daily CBC as outpatient
4. Autologous bone marrow transplant if indicated

normal, without the presence of human anti-mouse antibody from previous antibody exposures. Patients receive up to three trace-labeled doses of anti-B-cell antibody, in an escalating dose protocol, for evaluation of optimal biodistribution for treatment. Biodistribution that is favorable for treatment includes dosimetry estimates that demonstrate that tumor receives greater radiation dose per millicurie administered than any normal organ excluding bone marrow [1]. If patients meet these criteria from any one of the trace-labeled radioactivity doses, then they are entered into the treatment aspect of the protocol. Treatment is based on rads delivered to the highest normal organ, and is currently at 1675 rads to the highest normal organ (excluding bone marrow). These involve administrations of single high specific activity radiolabeled antibody doses of 300–700 mCi. At current dose levels, patients require reinfusion of stored bone marrow because of severe hematologic toxicity. At present, 7 patients have been treated, with 6 of the 7 experiencing complete response of disease for 6–12+ months. The remaining patient had a partial remission [2]. Radiation doses estimated to be delivered to tumor range from 850 to 4200 rads, and no normal organ (nonmarrow) toxicity has been observed. In addition, a number of observations were made about the patient groups as a whole. Patients with smaller tumor burden were more likely to achieve favorable biodistribution with the pan-B-cell antibodies, and those patients also had longer clearance time of the antibody, which enabled tumor antibody residence time to equal that of the physical half-life of the isotope. The tumor uptake, expressed as percent of the injected dose per gram, did not vary significantly from one patient to the next; however, the deciding factors between treatment and leaving the protocol were residence of radioactivity in tumor and speed of clearance of radioactivity from normal organs. This group continues on a dose-escalation protocol, with reinfusion of stored bone marrow when peripheral blood counts reach a nadir post treatment. Since toxicities have been minimal and there have been no problems with bone marrow engraftment, the group believes that normal organ toxicity will be at a significantly higher internal radiation absorbed dose.

The group at the University of California, Davis, treats patients with non-Hodgkin's lymphoma using I-131 labeled Lym-1 antibody [3, 4]. Their treatment protocol is designed to avoid life-threatening bone marrow toxicity by administering several smaller radio-labeled antibody doses. Patients receive 20–60 mCi at a time at two- to six-week intervals. Patients who continue on the protocol can receive cumulative doses of I-131 as great as 300 mCi. Most of the 23 patients have experienced a partial response. Toxicities observed from treatment have been minor. Several patients had transient thrombocytopenia, but toxicities most commonly encountered were fever, chills, and hives, all related to the time of infusion of the antibody dose. Dosimetry estimates were 2–50 rads/mCi to tumor whole body 0.3–0.5 rads/mCi for the whole body, and 0.5–1.2 rads/mCi for bone marrow. Evaluation of toxicity and efficacy of this treatment protocol is still ongoing.

I-131 is also the radioisotope used for radioimmunotherapy trials for lymphoma at the Center for Molecular Medicine and Immunology/University of New Jersey [5]. Their experimental therapy protocol involves use of the anti-lymphoma antibody EPB-2. Six patients who were heavily pretreated with other therapeutic modalities received 30 mCi I-131 EPB-2 followed by 20 mCi EPB-2 one week later. Of 5 patients evaluable for response, 3 had partial responses. In this particular patient group, significant myelotoxicity was considered to be dose-limiting. This trial is also currently ongoing.

Similar to the University of Washington group, the investigators at the University of Michigan use the MB-1 antibody (anti-CD37) attached to I-131 as the therapeutic agent [6]. Theirs is also a dose-escalation study designed to avoid bone marrow transplantation. To date, 5 patients who failed standard treatment have been treated. Initial single doses ranged from 25 to 149 mCi I-131. One patient who received an intermediate dose (67 mCi) received a second dose of 110 mCi five weeks later. In this group, significant hematopoietic toxicity was not observed; 3 of 5 patients had partial tumor responses. The group plans to continue this treatment protocol and to select patients who are less heavily pretreated and have a smaller tumor burden at the outset of treatment.

The group at the University of California, San Diego, is exploring the uses of patient-specific anti-idiotype antibodies chelated to the pure beta emitter, Y-90 [7]. Circulating idiotype was removed from circulation by administration of unlabeled anti-idiotype antibody. This was followed by examination of biodistribution of the labeled antibody by imaging an In-111 labeled form of the antibody. After these preliminary studies, the patient received 10 mCi Y-90 anti-idiotype antibody. On subsequent lymph node biopsy, antibody deposition was documented in the tumor. The patient demonstrated partial regression of disease.

As evidenced by the brief discussions of the projects presented above, current radioimmunotherapy trials for non-Hodgkin's lymphoma involve the use of beta-emitting radioisotopes as the therapeutic agents. I-131

is in wide use because of the fact that it is readily available at high specific activity in labeling-grade form. It also uses standardized well-described labeling procedures that attach the radiolabel covalently to the protein [8]. Another advantage it has is that there is, in addition to the beta particle, a gamma photon that can be imaged with standard nuclear medicine techniques. This allows for observation of the biodistribution of the radiolabeled antibody for estimation of internal radiation absorbed dose for normal organs and tumor sites. In contrast, radiometals such as Y-90, and Re-186 (Table 1) are attached to proteins by binding to a chelate that is attached to the protein. These have the advantage of higher beta-particle energies. Y-90, however, has no gamma photon to enable observation of biodistribution of the antibody in the patient. In this case, some investigators make biodistribution observations with In-111 substitutes in the chelate for Y-90. When adequate biodistribution for treatment is observed by imaging with a gamma camera, then the antibody radiometal chelate is switched to Y-90 [7]. Underlying this procedure is the assumption that the two radiometal chelates behave in the same way in the patient. Early radiometal chelates had problems associated with stability and translocation of the radiometal from the protein to nonspecific sites in the body. However, new and more stable chelates are being designed and put into use for radiolabeled antibodies [9]. Another potential advantage of the pure beta-emitting isotopes is radiation safety. Without high-energy penetrating gamma photons, there is little exposure risk for hospital and radiochemistry personnel.

Another issue that is apparent from the review of clinical trials concerns the type of dose scheduling for administration of the therapeutic radiolabeled antibody. The group at the University of Washington, which has the most experience with bone marrow transplantation, believes that a single high therapeutic dose (requiring bone marrow transplantation) has a more effective tumor cell kill, with less sublethal damage that can be repaired. Other groups mentioned in this review seek to treat the tumor repeatedly, giving a more constant dose rate to effect cell kill. Using multiple doses has the risk of inducing patients to form human anti-mouse antibodies (HAMA). Most groups observe that a sizable proportion of their patients who have received repeated doses of mouse-derived antibody form HAMA [10, 11]. This may have the effect of altering biodistribution of the antibody in the patient by forming complexes with the infused antibody that localize in nontumor sites such as the liver. The presence of HAMA also predisposes some patients to having anaphylactoid reactions on subsequent antibody administrations.

Associated with these issues are questions related to the validity of internal absorbed radiation dose estimates for the radiolabeled antibody therapeutic dose. Estimation of radiation internal absorbed dose is difficult compared to radiation oncology techniques [1].

The radioisotope is distributed throughout the body with specific uptakes and retention times that are different from site to site. In contrast, the dose delivered to tissues in standard radiation therapy is very accurately modeled and calibrated. At present, the dosimetry estimations for radioimmunotherapy doses are compared to rads delivered to tumor and normal organs in standard radiation therapy. Radiation delivered by a radioisotope resident at the tumor site for as long as the half-life of the radioisotope (hopefully) delivers a 'hyperfractionated' dose at an extremely low dose rate. Only by observing the biologic effects of doses delivered at these dose rates in animal models and in patients on experimental trials will we be able to determine the relative biological effects of radiation doses delivered to tissues in this manner and be able to compare them to toxicity data in standard radiation therapy.

In summary, radioimmunotherapy trials for treatment of non-Hodgkin's lymphoma are showing promising results. This disease is an ideal setting for radioimmunotherapy because of well-documented radiation sensitivity, the abundant information available on the nature of tumor and normal lymphocyte markers, and the presence of tumors that provide good perfusion and access to intravenously administered agents. Patients in these trials have had good responses to treatment without nonmarrow toxicity. Marrow toxicity in high-dose protocols is easily overcome with bone marrow reinfusion [1]. Issues regarding radioisotopic effectiveness and radiolabeled antibody dose scheduling, toxicity, and biodistribution are being addressed. Because of these important biologic aspects, non-Hodgkin's lymphoma is the setting in which radioimmunotherapy techniques can be evaluated and refined to their fullest potential.

References

1. Eary JF, Press OW, Badger CC, Durack L, Richter KY, Krohn KA, Fisher D, Porter B, Williams D, Martin P, Appelbaum FR, Levy R, Brown S, Miller R, Nelp W, Bernstein ID. Imaging and treatment of B-cell lymphoma. J Nucl Med 1990; 31: 1257–1268.
2. Press OW, Eary JF, Badger CC, Martin PJ, Appelbaum FR, Levy R, Miller R, Brown S, Nelp W, Krohn K, Fisher D, DeSantes K, Porter B, Kidd P, Thomas ED, Bernstein ID. Treatment of refractory non-Hodgkin's lymphoma with radiolabeled MB-1 (Anti-CD37) antibody. J Clin Onc 1989; 7: (8) 1027–1038.
3. DeNardo GL, DeNardo SJ, O'Grady LF, Lewis JP, Mills SL, Macey DJ, Epstein AL. Treatment of chronic lymphocytic leukemia (CLL) with I-131 LYM-1. J Nucl Med 1989; 30: (5) 827–828.
4. DeNardo SJ, DeNardo GL, Macey DJ, Mills SL, O'Grady LF, McGahan JP, Epstien AL. Successful radioimmunotherapy in patients with lymphoma: results of dose fractionation of I-131 LYM-1 MoAb. J Nucle Med 1988; 29:(5) 847.
5. Sharkey RM, Horowitz JA, Stein R, Belisle EH, Hansen HJ, Pinsky CM, Hall TC, Goldenberg DM. Tumor targeting and radioimmunotherapy (RAIT) of B-cell lymphoma with a new monoclonal antibody (MAb), EPB-2. Antibody Immunoconjugates, and Radiopharmaceuticals 1990; 3: (1) 53.
6. Kaminski MS, Fig L, Del Rosario R, Miller R, Buchsbaum D, Mudgett E, Wahl RL. Radioimmunotherapy of advanced B-cell lymphoma with none bone marrow ablative doses of 131-I MB-1 antibody. Antibody Immunoconjugates, and Radiopharmaceuticals 1990; 3: (1) 58.
7. Halpern S, Parker BA, Vassos A, Frincke J, Amox D, Miller R, Green MR, Royston I. 90 Yttrium (90Y) anti-idiotype monoclonal antibody therapy of non-Hodgkin's lymphoma. J Nucl Med 1989; 30: (5) 778.
8. Eary JF, Krohn KA, Kishore RA, Nelp WB. Radiochemistry of halogenated antibodies. In: Zalutsky MR (ed). Antibodies in Radiodiagnosis and Therapy. Boca Raton, Florida, CRC Press; 1989; 83–102.
9. Deshpande SV, De Nardo SJ, Kukis DL, Moi MM, McCall MJ, DeNardo GL, Meares CF. Yttrium-90 labeled monoclonal antibody for therapy: Labeling by a new macrocyclic bifunctional chelating agent. J Nucl Med 1990; 31: 473–479.
10. Kalades PM, Khazaeli MB, Hazzard E, Vanderbegt DL, LoBuglio AF, Gilman SC. Detection of human anti-murine antibody (HAMA) following infusion of onciscint CR103. Comparison of Elisa with a double antigen radiometric assay. Antibody Immunoconjugates, and Radiopharmaceuticals 1990; 3: (1) 54.
11. Zimmer AM, Kuzel T, Duda RB, Webber DI, Spies WG, Gilyon K, Samuelson E, Spies SM, Rosen ST. Radioimmunotherapy retreatment of patients with HAMA: effect of cold antibody titration on the pharmacokinetics of radiolabeled antibodies. Antibody Immunoconjugates, and Radiopharmaceuticals. 1990; 3: (1) 53.

Correspondence to:
Janet F. Eary, M.D.
Assistant Professor, Radiology & Pathology
Division of Nuclear Medicine, RC-70
University of Washington Medical Center
1959 N.E. Pacific
Seattle, WA 98195, USA

Annals of Oncology, Supplement 2 to Volume 2: 191–200, 1991.
© 1991 *Kluwer Academic Publishers.*

Original article _____

The occurrence of opportunistic non-Hodgkin's lymphomas in the setting of infection with the human immunodeficiency virus

James M. Pluda, Robert Yarchoan & Samuel Broder
The Clinical Oncology Program, National Cancer Institute, Bethesda, MD 20892, USA

Summary. The incidence of non-Hodgkin's lymphoma (NHL) has increased by over 50% in the United States since 1973. There is epidemiologic evidence that some of this increase is the result of AIDS-related lymphoma and that this component is increasing. Prolonged survival in the setting of a variety of immunodeficiency states is associated with an increased incidence of NHL. The development of antiretroviral therapy and improved therapy for the complications of AIDS has resulted in prolonged survival of patients with AIDS. As these patients survive longer with profound immunodeficiency, they have an increased cumulative risk of developing NHL. This may result in even more AIDS-related NHL in the future than predicted from current epidemiological studies. An increased understanding of the pathogenesis of AIDS-related NHL may lead to means of preventing their occurrence. Also, therapies that may prevent immunodeficiency from developing in HIV-infected patients may reduce the likelihood of NHL developing. Current efforts at treating these lymphomas are aimed at preventing the myelosuppression and immunosuppression associated with current regimens, lymphoma relapses within the central nervous system, and the opportunistic infections associated with treatment of these tumors. Ultimately, the best means of preventing the development of these lymphomas is by preventing infection with HIV.

Key words: AIDS, immunosuppression, lymphoma, pathogenesis, survival, therapy

Introduction

Acquired immunodeficiency syndrome (AIDS), a disorder caused by infection with the human immunodeficiency virus (HIV), was first recognized in 1981 as a new illness occurring in individuals in certain high-risk groups [1–4]. Soon after the recognition of AIDS and its related syndrome as new disorders, a clustering of high-grade non-Hodgkin's lymphoma (NHL) was noted in these same risk groups infected with HIV. Many of these lymphomas occurred with unusual sites of presentation [5–13]. In 1985, the Centers for Disease Control (CDC) expanded the case definition for AIDS to include certain high-grade NHL as an AIDS-defining illness in particular settings [14]. Epidemiologically, there is evidence that the incidence of HIV-associated NHL continues to rise, and at present, these tumors now comprise approximately 3% of all new AIDS-defining illnesses reported to the CDC [15–17]. AIDS has added a new dimension to the problem of NHL, and it is likely to be a major factor in lymphoma incidence and mortality in the coming decade.

The lymphomas most frequently seen in the setting of HIV infection are large-cell immunoblastic (LC-IBL) or small-noncleaved-cell lymphomas (SNCCL) of the B-cell type. The frequency of the small noncleaved category of lymphoma is remarkable because this subtype is rather rare in the United States, accounting for

only 5% of all NHLs [18]. The majority of these lymphomas present in extranodal sites, particularly the central nervous system (CNS).

Primary CNS disease occurs in approximately one fourth of patients who present with NHL antemortem, and an additional percentage have secondary involvement of the CNS [7, 11, 13]. The response of these tumors to standard chemotherapeutic regimens is poorer than that seen when similar tumors occur in non-HIV-infected patients. Overall, AIDS-associated lymphoma patients have a relatively short survival. Fatal opportunistic infections are a frequent complication during treatment [9, 11, 13, 19].

Immunodeficiency and NHL

It is not surprising that NHL develops in patients with immunosuppression caused by infection with HIV. There is a large body of evidence derived from experience with other immunodeficient patients that NHLs occur at a significantly increased rate in the setting of immunosuppression. In patients with primary immunodeficiency disorders, NHLs account for more than 50% of all tumors seen [20, 21]. The Wiskott-Aldrich syndrome (WAS) is an excellent example; WAS is an X-linked recessive disorder characterized by the presence of immunodeficiency, eczema, and thrombocytopenia. The risk of such patients developing a malignancy is 126 times that of unaffected individuals. Overall, the risk of developing a malignancy is 2% per year of life for the first 25 years of life [22]. Nearly 75% of the malignancies seen with this disorder are lymphoreticular in origin, and high-grade B-cell lymphomas predominate [22–24]. Interestingly, these lymphomas tend to occur in extranodal sites, especially the CNS; this is very similar to the presentation of NHL seen in the setting of HIV infection [22, 24]. As supportive therapies for the complications associated with WAS improve and patients live longer, it appears that their risk of developing a NHL is increasing as well [22, 24]. Other primary immunodeficiency disorders that are associated with a substantial increase in the incidence of lymphoproliferative malignancies include severe combined immunodeficiency, ataxia-telangiectasia, and common variable hypogammaglobulinemia [20].

Malignancies in the setting of secondary immunosuppression, particularly iatrogenic, have also been well documented. Patients receiving immunosuppressive therapy following organ transplants are at particular risk, with approximately 5–7% of these patients developing malignancies; more than one third of these tumors are NHL [25]. As noted with other immunodeficiency states, there is a high incidence of primary CNS involvement. Thirty-six percent of transplant patients developing NHL have disease limited to the brain at the time of diagnosis [25]. Interestingly, Kaposi's sarcoma (KS), a rare tumor in the general population but one of the first identified AIDS-defining illnesses, may also occur in as many as 3% of all patients receiving organ transplants [26]. Thus, the two most common tumors seen in the setting of AIDS are also seen with significantly increased frequency in the setting of iatrogenic immunosuppression.

Although the cause of immunosuppression varies between the primary immunodeficiency disorders and transplantation patients, the underlying immune system defects predisposing to the development of lymphoma are similar [27]. Immunosuppression may allow for abnormalities in B-cell proliferation and development resulting in unregulated expansion of B-cell populations. This may, in turn, allow for errors to occur resulting in oncogenic-virus activation, or other cellular events leading ultimately to malignant transformation. The underlying immunosuppression may also result in a failure of immunosurveillance, thus allowing newly developed malignant cells to replicate and establish themselves as tumors. It would appear that whatever the basis of a patient's immunodeficiency state, the common pathway of immune dysregulation may ultimately lead to the development of a malignant lymphoma.

NHL in the general population

The Surveillance, Epidemiology, and End Results (SEER) Program database of the National Cancer Institute (NCI) has been collecting information on the occurrence of cancer in a population base representing 9% of the United States population since 1973. Information from that database shows that the incidence of NHL has increased by more than 50% from 1973 to 1987 (the last year for which final figures are available [28]. The factors contributing to this rise are unknown. This increase began before the epidemic of HIV infection and appears to be largely caused by factors other than HIV, but the recent development of AIDS-related NHL will amplify this trend. Several populations have been shown to be at a relatively high risk of developing NHL, and perhaps an understanding of the pathogenesis of AIDS-related lymphomas will shed light on the pathogenesis of lymphomas in the general population and vice versa.

There have been numerous reports of increased development of NHL in persons with occupational exposure to certain chemicals. A brief discussion of some of these may be useful. Several epidemiologic studies have demonstrated an association between the use of phenoxy acid herbicides like 2,4-dichlorophenoxyacetic acid (2,4-D) and NHL in farmers and forestry workers [29–34]. In some of these studies, the risk appeared to follow a dose-response relationship, being directly related to the number of acres sprayed with 2,4-D and to the duration and frequency of exposure [32, 34]. Development of NHL has also been associated with exposure to chlorophenols, compounds commonly employed in the shoe or leather industry as well as the forestry and wood-products industry. Persons with a significant exposure to these compounds have an increased risk of developing NHL [29, 30]. Also, cabinet makers and carpenters, whose occupation exposes them to creosote (a wood preservative), solvents, and wood dust, develop NHL at a rate greater than that in the general public [35, 36]. Painters exposed to various solvents, and chemical manufacturing workers with exposure to alkyl sulfates and organic solvents, have also been reported to develop NHL more frequently [35, 37, 38].

Pathogenesis of occupation-related NHL

The mechanism(s) involved in increasing the incidence of NHL in persons exposed to various chemical agents is currently not known. It is easiest to hypothesize a causal relationship in persons exposed to phenoxy acids. These compounds might conceivably act by directly inducing a somatic mutation leading to neoplastic transformation. Alternatively, exposure may lead to immunosuppression which, as previously noted, may lead to development of an NHL in its own right. Nevertheless, 2,4-D, the agent most frequently used by subjects in epidemiologic studies, has not been shown to induce lymphoid tumors or to be significantly immunosuppressive in animals [34, 39–41]. The pesticide may have been contaminated by smaller quantities of toxic isomers or other chemicals, such as dioxin, a compound known to cause suppression of cell-mediated immunity and thymic involution in animals [42, 43]. Alternatively, a combined effect of several chemicals may be most likely to induce NHL.

The possibility of a role for zoonotic viruses in the development of certain hematological malignancies, including NHL, has been raised because of epidemiologic studies suggesting an increase of these forms of tumors in farmers raising chickens or cows and in persons involved in the food-processing industry [33, 44–48]. Both bovine leukemia virus (a C-type RNA virus infecting cattle) and the virus causing Marek's disease (a herpesvirus) have been suggested as possible etiologic agents. To date, no serologic or other direct evidence has been found linking these viruses to human tumors. However, there is evidence that viruses can cause tumors without serological evidence of viral infection [49]. Alternatively, it is possible that these viruses may be oncogenic only in conjunction with some other factors [50]. Thus, although the evidence for zoonotic infection playing a role in the development of lymphomas is weak, this possibility cannot be dismissed and may warrant further research.

Survival of HIV-infected patients

There is recent evidence that patients with AIDS are experiencing a significant improvement in their survival as a result of the development of AZT and other therapeutic advances. The median survival of patients diagnosed with AIDS reported to the San Francisco Department of Health has increased from 10.8 months for those diagnosed in 1985 to 15.6 months for those diagnosed in 1987 [51]. This improvement has been particularly striking for patients presenting with *Pneumocystis carinii* pneumonia (PCP). In these patients the median survival during the same period has increased from 10.5 to 17.9 months [51]. Although improved methods of diagnosis, treatment, and prophylaxis for PCP may have contributed to this phenomenon [52–56], there is evidence that the use of AZT has resulted in prolonged survival over and above any effect of PCP prophylaxis [51, 57, 58]. In New York State, only 30% of patients diagnosed with AIDS in 1984 were alive at 18 months, whereas 60% diagnosed with AIDS in 1987 survived for 18 months [59]. The main therapeutic advance made in this time period was the development and wide availability of AZT. In agreement with these figures, we have observed that the median survival of AIDS patients receiving AZT-containing therapies was 20.8 months from the time of their AIDS-defining illness (Fig. 1). Thus, with the advent of clinical advances in the treatment of HIV infection, patients with this disease are experiencing a prolongation of their survival, resulting in a growing population of patients with severe immunosuppression who are living for longer periods of time.

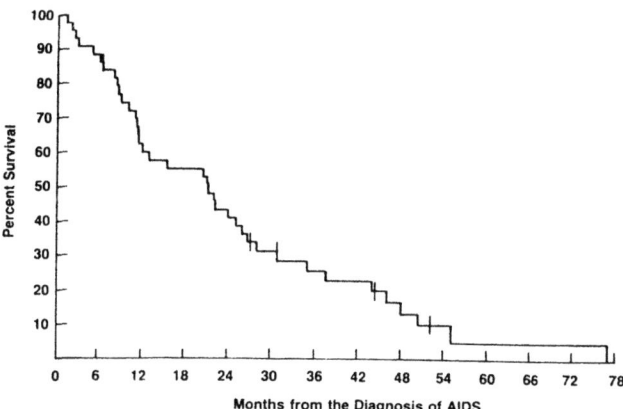

Fig. 1. Kaplan-Meier plot of the survival of 43 patients with AIDS receiving long-term dideoxynucleoside therapy entered into three phase I studies in the Clinical Oncology Program of the National Cancer Institute from 1985 to 1987. Survival was determined from the time of diagnosis of their AIDS-defining illness. Each tick mark represents a patient alive at the time of analysis.

Clinical aspects of NHL in patients with AIDS

As with the primary immunodeficiency disorders, prolonged survival of patients with AIDS and severe immunosuppression may lead to an increased incidence of NHL developing as an 'opportunistic' neoplasm. Recently, our group at the NCI published a study of the development of NHL in 55 patients with AIDS or severe AIDS-related complex (ARC) enrolled on their first three AZT-containing phase I studies from 1985 to 1987 [60]. These cases demonstrate several interesting clinical factors associated with AIDS-related lymphomas. All of these tumors were high-grade lymphomas with extranodal presentations. All but one were B-cell type, and this patient subsequently developed a second distinct B-cell lymphoma. Two patients developed new or enlarging brain lesions in the setting of previously diagnosed toxoplasmosis. However, brain biopsies of these lesions revealed NHL. A high index of suspicion and the aggressive utilization of invasive biopsy techniques may be necessary to differentiate between other AIDS-related diseases and the presence of a new NHL. It is therefore probable that some of these tumors, particularly those arising in the CNS, may be missed, resulting in an underreporting of the overall incidence of these tumors in the general population. Another patient receiving treatment with a steroid-containing regimen demonstrated that, as previously reported [61, 62], the use of steroids to treat NHL in patients with KS may result in dramatic flares of their KS. Thus, consideration should be given to the exclusion of steroids from chemotherapeutic regimens for NHL administered to patients with HIV infection, particularly in the presence of KS.

The treatment of AIDS-related NHL has been disappointing, with a decreased rate and durability of complete responses compared to patients without AIDS, and an increased incidence of opportunistic in-

194

fections [7, 9, 11, 13, 19]. The patients in our study were no different, having a median survival of 7 months for those patients presenting with visceral disease, and 1.8 months for patients presenting with primary CNS disease [60]. Thus, improved, less immunosuppressive therapeutic strategies in conjunction with prophylaxis for opportunistic infections are needed for the treatment of AIDS-associated lymphomas, and this will be an important area of future research.

Prolonged survival and the development of NHL in patients with AIDS

As previously reported, the patients who developed lymphoma in our cohort had AIDS for a median of 22.5 months and had fewer than 50 T4 cells/mm³ for a median of 15.3 months prior to the development of lymphoma [60]. Thus, these patients had survived in a state of profound immunodeficiency for a substantially longer period than would have been expected prior to the development of antiretroviral therapy. The possibility that AZT may play a direct role in the development of these tumors should be considered. AZT can act as a mutagen, and vaginal malignancies have been seen in mice and rats receiving lifelong high-dose AZT [63, 64]. However, we feel that this is a much less likely cause for the occurrence of the lymphomas than is the prolongation of patient survival in the setting of profound immunodeficiency, since the lymphomas that were seen were very typical of those arising in the setting of HIV infection and other immunodeficiency states [60].

Based on the most recent data available, the estimated probability of developing an NHL after three years of antiretroviral therapy among the 55 patients in our cohort is 31.1% (95% confidence interval 15.8–52.2%) [J. M. Pluda, R. Yanchoan, S. Broder, unpublished data]. Overall, they have an 8% chance of developing lymphoma per year of follow-up [60]. We believe that these lymphomas arising in the setting of prolonged survival with severe immunosuppression at a substantially increased rate represented an 'opportunistic' disease process and as such may be referred to as opportunistic neoplasms. Extrapolating from the SEER database, one can predict that by 1992 there will be an excess of 3800 cases of NHL in males aged 20 to 49 above that predicted by the incidence of NHL prior to the AIDS epidemic (Fig. 2). It is felt that these excess cases will be due largely to AIDS-related lymphomas. Ongoing research may eventually project significantly more cases of AIDS-related NHL developing by 1992 (M. H. Gail, personal communication). Using the incidence of NHL observed in our patient population, we predicted that nearly 5000 of the cases of AIDS reported in 1989 with an AIDS-defining illness other than NHL will develop an NHL at some time during their illness [60]. Thus, each of these analyses predicts that AIDS-related opportunistic NHL will become a

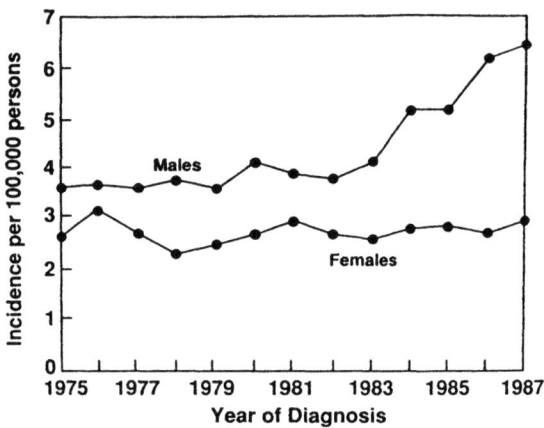

Fig. 2. Plot of data from the Surveillance, Epidemiology, and End Results Program of the National Cancer Institute on the incidence of non-Hodgkin's lymphoma developing in males and females of all races ages 20–49 years from 1975 to 1987.

significant component of the NHL diagnosed in the very near future.

One must interpret the information and projections mentioned above cautiously. There is a paucity of information on the temporal development of NHL in other cohorts of patients with AIDS or severe ARC, particularly since the development of effective antiretroviral therapy. It is possible that because of the screening process in our clinics (patients were selected as being clinically stable without any active opportunistic infections or malignancies), the NCI patients may not be entirely representative of the general AIDS or ARC population. Nevertheless, the estimated probability of an NHL developing in 24.3% of patients at 30 months and 31.1% of patients on antiretroviral therapy for 36 months is striking. It would appear from these data that the development of an opportunistic NHL may be an important limiting factor in the survival of patients treated with currently available modalities.

Pathogenesis of AIDS-related NHL

Although the exact pathogenesis of AIDS-related NHL is unknown, many interrelated factors have been postulated to be involved. Patients with AIDS or ARC have been found to have polyclonal B-cell proliferative lymph node expansion [65–67]. This polyclonal expansion may be induced by several factors. Infection with HIV may induce polyclonal B-cell activation through mitogenic or antigenic stimulation, or via an HIV-induced T-cell-dependent B-cell activation mechanism [68–70]. Also, patients with HIV infection have increased numbers of circulating B cells infected with Epstein-Barr virus (EBV), which may in part be a result of their profound immunodeficiency and defective T-cell regulation of EBV infection [70, 71]. However, direct EBV infection has not been documented in the majority of tumors, and there is some evidence that infection of tumor cells may occur after transformation [65, 72–75]. The molecular events resulting in B-cell activation in patients with HIV infection bear further study.

While the exact mechanism of the polyclonal B-cell proliferation is unknown, this expansion of dividing cells may provide a milieu for transforming events to occur. These crucial events have been fully elucidated, but there is evidence in many cases of AIDS-related Burkitt's lymphoma (BL) that a c-*myc* oncogenic rearrangement similar to that seen in both endemic and sporadic BL, involving the juxtaposition of the c-*myc* oncogene (on chromosome 8) and an immunoglobulin gene (kappa light chain on chromosome 2, lambda light chain on chromosome 22, or immunoglobulin heavy chain on chromosome 14), with the (8:14) translocation being seen most frequently [65, 73, 74, 76–79]. Even though the tumors arise within the setting a polyclonal B-cell expansion, no significant evidence exists to indicate that the tumors themselves are polyclonal. Pelicci and colleagues have found that the tumors are monoclonal and have a single c-*myc* rearrangement [65].

The means by which these translocations are able to result in the development of BL are uncertain. It has been argued that the c-*myc*/immunoglobulin translocation occurs in B cells that are actively dividing either during the normal course of B-cell development or because of EBV transformation, but that the tumorigenic effects are only expressed later when the cell undergoes a phenotypic switch from the proliferating blast to the resting cell, even though the cell is unable to stop dividing because of c-*myc* activation [80]. In addition, c-*myc* activation may result in phenotypic features that allow a BL cell to escape immune surveillance by cytotoxic T cells: (1) the absence or low expression of certain class I major histocompatibility complex antigens, (2) the insufficient expression of adhesion molecules required for the effector-target cell interactions, or (3) the downregulation of most of the EBV-coded antigens expressed in EBV-transformed normal cells [80]. These selection advantages are greatly magnified in HIV-infected patients who already have profound defects in T-cell immunity and increased numbers of circulating EBV-infected cells, as mentioned above. Thus the selection advantages conferred by the c-*myc* oncogene translocation and activation associated with BL, in conjunction with the immunological defects present in HIV-infected patients and a more 'permissive' immunologic environment, may allow for the significantly increased development of this uncommon tumor.

It is also conceivable that other oncogenic viruses that have not as yet been identified play an important role in the transformation to the malignant state. There is a recent suggestion from epidemiologic studies of homosexual men who have KS but who lack HIV infection, that another sexually transmitted virus may be responsible for the ultimate malignant transformation of the KS spindle cell and that the disease takes on its aggressive nature in the setting of HIV-induced immunosuppression [81, 82]. It is similarly possible that an unidentified coinfecting virus may play a significant role in the development of AIDS-related NHL in an analogous manner.

The exact pathogenic mechanisms involved in the development of AIDS-related NHL are unclear, and more research is needed. If some of the various factors involved in this malignant transformation can be elucidated, it may be possible to interfere with the cellular events responsible for the malignant phenotype or to prevent cellular transformation altogether. For example, McManaway and colleagues recently reported that an antisense oligodeoxynucleotide constructed against an abnormal, tumor-specific c-*myc* messenger RNA transcript from a Burkitt's lymphoma cell line inhibited in vitro growth of this cell line but not the growth of normal cells [83]. Thus, novel approaches to the prevention and treatment of the development of AIDS-related NHL may be possible in the future based upon a better understanding of the molecular events resulting in the occurrence of these tumors. Also, preventing the decrease in T4 cells and the defects in T-cell function may be important in providing a more 'restrictive' immunologic environment in which these lymphomas may not develop.

Other retrovirus-associated lymphoproliferative disorders

Other pathogenic human retroviruses, in addition to HIV, are associated with the development of lymphoma and other hematologic malignancies. For example, hairy cell leukemia (HCL) is an uncommon B-cell neoplasm characterized by the presence of pancytopenia, splenomegaly, and the circulating leukemic cells with 'hairy' cytoplasmic projections from which the disease derives its name. An atypical form of HCL has been described in which the leukemic cell is of T-cell origin [84], and a retrovirus, human T-cell lymphotropic virus type II (HTLV-II), has been found in association with this T-cell form of HCL in two patients [85, 86].

Infection with another retrovirus, human T cell lymphotropic virus type I (HTLV-I), is associated with a hematologic disorder known as adult T-cell leukemia/lymphoma (ATLL) [87, 88]. This disorder is usually an aggressive hematological malignancy, with circulating leukemia cells, skin involvement, lymphadenopathy, and hypercalcemia being common clinical features. The malignant cells are most frequently T-helper (T4+ and CD4+) lymphocytes expressing the interleukin-2 (IL-2) receptor on their surface. Opportunistic infections secondary to the immunosuppression induced by infection with this virus are a profound source of morbidity and mortality in this population [89, 90]. Recently, Tanaka and colleagues demonstrated that the *tax* gene product of HTLV-I, a transcriptional transactivator, has transforming and tumorigenic activities, acting as a viral oncogene without a cellular homolog

[91]. This transforming activity of *tax* may play an important role in leukemogenesis of ATLL. Currently, no defined antitumor regimens have been consistently able to achieve durable complete remissions in this disease, although the therapeutic uses of anti-IL-2 receptor antibodies [92] are an exciting and promising new area of ongoing research.

Interestingly, there is evidence that HTLV-I may also play a role in the development of B-cell hematologic malignancies. Mann and colleagues recently reported that chronic lymphocytic leukemia (CLL) B cells taken from two patients infected with HTLV-I had surface immunoglobulin directed against HTLV-I antigens [93]. They speculated that infection with HTLV-I may have played an indirect role in B-cell leukemogenesis by providing an antigenic stimulus as well as altering T-cell regulatory processes leading to immunosuppression, thus resulting in a B-cell malignancy.

Implications of coinfection with HIV and HTLV-I

Coinfection with HIV and HTLV-I is becoming an increasingly important problem. Both viruses are spread in a similar manner and occur together in certain risk groups. A study of homosexual men in Trinidad revealed that 40% were HIV positive, and 15% of these had serological evidence of coinfection with HTLV-I [94]. Among intravenous drug abusers (IVDAs) in New York City, a similar 41% were found to be seropositive for HIV with 34% of these also being seropositive for HTLV-I or -II [95]. It has been estimated that between 5% and 33% of all IVDAs in the United States are infected with HIV (an estimated 61 000–398 000 persons) [96], and this number may be growing. Based on these figures, there may be as many as 135 000 IVDAs coinfected with HIV and either HTLV-I or -II in the United States at present.

The implications of simultaneous HIV and HTLV-I infection are not entirely known as yet. However, there is in vitro evidence that HTLV-I can enhance production of HIV from HIV-infected peripheral blood leukocytes. Zack and colleagues have observed that HIV-infected T cells produced large quantities of HIV after stimulation with noninfectious HTLV-I virions [97]. They felt that this was probably due to mitogenic stimulation of HIV-infected T cells. In patients coinfected with both viruses, it is possible that an HTLV-I infected cell actively producing virus could result in the activation of other T cells infected with HIV. Alternatively, cells coinfected with HIV and HTLV-I can have an explosive burst of HIV production because of cross-transactivation of HIV by the HTLV-I *rex* protein [98]. Therefore, patients infected with both viruses could produce more HIV than patients not infected with HTLV-I. This may have important implications in the rate of development of HIV-associated illnesses in this population of coinfected patients.

Infection with both HIV and HTLV-I may be involved in inducing unusual tumors and proliferative disorders. For example, there is a report of a lymphoproliferative disease involving HTLV-I-infected T8 lymphocytes in a patient coinfected with HIV and HTLV-I [99]. Therefore, the simultaneous infection of patients with these viruses might lead not only to acceleration of the development of lymphoid neoplasias but to the occurrence of new or previously rare forms of neoplasia.

Implications of anti-HIV therapies for lymphomagenesis

One can project that as the AIDS epidemic matures, there will be an increased incidence in the number of AIDS-related lymphomas. These cases will be a challenge to physicians and the health care delivery system alike. However, developments in the therapy of HIV infection and associated immunosuppression may affect these projections in various ways. One unknown factor is the effect of early intervention with AZT or other therapies. There is evidence that the administration of AZT to patients with asymptomatic or mildly symptomatic HIV disease and T4 cells between 200 and $500/mm^3$ can delay the progression of HIV disease [100, 101]. Conceivably, such therapy may also lower the incidence of lymphomas by preventing or delaying the occurrence of the severe immunodeficiency in HIV-infected patients. However, information on the long-term follow-up of patients treated with AZT at an early stage of disease is not known at present, and it is unclear how this issue will sort itself out. Newer antiretroviral therapies may be developed that offer improved HIV control and thus more effectively delay or prevent the severe immunosuppression associated with the development of lymphomas.

There is preliminary evidence in patients with primary immunodeficiency disorders that immune reconstitution may prevent the development of lymphomas. Neudorf and colleagues retrospectively analyzed the incidence of malignancy in patients with WAS and severe combined immunodeficiency (SCID) who were successfully immunoconstituted by bone marrow transplantation [102]. Of the 15 patients with WAS and the 48 with SCID receiving bone marrow transplants, no patient developed a malignancy. Although Neudorf and colleagues did not perform a case-controlled analysis, the lack of tumors in these patients appeared to be substantially different from patients not undergoing bone marrow transplantation. Thus it would appear that immunoreconstitution may prevent the occurrence of NHL in this population of patients with severe immunodeficiency. Long-term follow-up of these patients is necessary to ascertain whether the bone marrow transplantation truly prevents or simply delays the development of NHL.

While suppression of viral replication in HIV-infected patients may allow a partial reconstitution of the immune system, there appears to be some limitation to the ability of the immune system in patients with advanced AIDS to reconstitute itself. We do not understand the reasons for this, but the phenomenon may be related to thymic damage caused either directly by HIV or by opportunistic infections. Newer therapeutic approaches that not only prevent HIV infection of previously uninfected cells but destroy chronically infected cells throughout the body, including relative sanctuary sites like the brain and central nervous system, may prove more effective in allowing the immune system to reconstitute itself. For example, combinations of therapies that are cytocidal to HIV-infected cells [103, 104], with adequate anti-HIV prophylactic treatment, immune stimulation, and bone marrow transplantation, may someday prove effective in suppressing HIV in infected patients and reconstituting their immune system. This area of research warrants further investigation.

The most effective means of preventing HIV-related lymphomas is of course to prevent the initial infection with HIV. This represents substantial public health challenges to educate the population about the ways that HIV infection is contracted and about the avoidance of behavior that could lead to infection. In addition, work continues on ways to develop a vaccine that, when administered to persons at high risk, would adequately immunize them and thus prevent infection from occurring should they become exposed to the virus.

Chemotherapy of AIDS-related lymphomas

As previously mentioned, the response of AIDS-associated NHL to standard chemotherapeutic regimens is substantially poorer than that seen in non-AIDS-related lymphomas. In general, complete responses occur in approximately 50% of patients and these responses tend to be of relatively short duration with relapses in the central nervous system a frequent occurrence [9, 11, 13, 19]. AIDS-associated NHL patients also develop opportunistic infections at a very high rate, and their overall survival is substantially less than that seen in NHL occurring in the general population. In addition, these patients tolerate more aggressive chemotherapeutic regimens poorly, with even worse survival than in other patients receiving such treatment [8, 19]. The single most consistent prognostic factor with respect to tolerance and response to therapy is the CD4 lymphocyte count, with patients having low levels of CD4 cells doing poorly.

A major limiting factor to the use of chemotherapy in AIDS-related NHL, either alone or with drugs such as AZT, is hematologic toxicity. This is particularly a problem in patients who have depleted bone marrow reserves as a result of long-term AZT therapy. Bone marrow-stimulating cytokines such as granulocyte-macrophage colony-stimulating factor (GM-CSF) or granulocyte colony-stimulating factor (G-CSF) are currently being incorporated into treatment regimens with

encouraging preliminary results [105, 106]. This may allow for the use of AZT from the initiation of chemotherapy rather than after completion of this treatment. Newer, less myelosuppressive antiretroviral agents like dideoxinosine may also prove useful in this setting [107–109].

A preliminary report of the administration of central nervous system prophylaxis early in the treatment of these lymphomas appears promising [110], and further investigation into the appropriate timing and means of such prophylaxis needs to continue. In addition, the use of aerosolized pentamidine for the prophylaxis of *Pneumocystis carinii* pneumonia may help to reduce the high morbidity and mortality associated with this complication of treatment of AIDS-related NHL.

Besides measures to allow more intensive treatment of these lymphomas with current regimens or their derivatives, newer agents that are more active and less toxic need to be developed. For example, in a trial of suramin, an agent used for years to treat trypanosomiasis in Africa, in patients with AIDS, one patients was found to have a long-lasting complete response of his NHL [111]. Also, as mentioned before, a model of Burkitt's lymphoma was found to be inhibited by an antisense construct directed at the c-*myc* region, and such an approach could conceivably be used in humans in the not-too-distant future. These and other novel approaches need to be explored for their potential role in the therapy of AIDS-related NHL. Also, new combination regimens employing currently known active agents in novel ways in an attempt to decrease toxicities and increase activity are also worth pursuing. Finally, with current regimens unable to induce sustained responses, there may be a role for the administration of chronic, nonmyelosuppressive maintenance therapy to patients achieving complete responses to initial therapy.

Conclusion

It would appear that HIV infection and the associated immunosuppression will have a substantial impact on the incidence of NHL in the near future. Research into the pathogenesis of these tumors may yield clinically useful information leading to the development of newer, more effective therapies, as well as the means to prevent NHL. Improved antiretroviral therapies and strategies to stop the spread of HIV infection are needed to prevent the severe immunosuppression caused by this virus which predisposes patients to develop lymphomas at an increased rate. In addition, work needs to continue both in the public health sector and the research laboratory to find ways to prevent the spread of this devastating illness.

References

1. Gottlieb MS, Schroff R, Schanker HM et al. Pneumocystis carinii pneumonia and mucosal candidiasis in previously

198

healthy homosexual men. N Engl J Med 1981; 305: 1425–31.

2. Hymes KB, Greene FB, Marcus A et al. Kaposi's sarcoma in homosexual men – A report of eight cases. Lancet 1981; 2: 598–600.

3. Masur H, Michelis MA, Greene JB et al. An outbreak of community-acquired Pneumocystis carinii pneumonia: Initial Manifestation of cellular immune dysfunction. N Engl J Med 1981; 305: 1431–8.

4. Siegal FP, Lopez C, Hammer GS et al. Severe acquired immunodeficiency in male homosexuals, manifested by chronic perianal ulcerative herpes simplex lesions. N Engl J Med 1981; 305: 1439–44.

5. Doll DC, List AF. Burkitt's lymphoma in a homosexual. Lancet 1982; 1: 1026–7.

6. Bermudez MA, Grant K, Rodvien R et al. Non-Hodgkin's lymphoma in a population with or at risk for acquired immunodeficiency syndrome: Indications for intensive chemotherapy. Am J Med 1989; 86: 71–6.

7. Kalter SP, Riggs SA, Cabanillas F et al. Aggressive non-Hodgkin's lymphomas in immunocompromised homosexual males. Blood 1985; 66: 655–9.

8. Kaplan LD, Abrams DI, Feigal E et al. AIDS-associated non-Hodgkins lymphoma in San Francisco. JAMA 1989; 261: 719–24.

9. Knowles DM, Chamulak GA, Subar M et al. Lymphoid neoplasia associated with the acquired immunodeficiency syndrome (AIDS): The New York University Medical Center experience with 105 patients (1981–1986). Ann Intern Med 1988; 108: 744–53.

10. Levine AM, Gill PS, Meyer PR et al. Retrovirus and malignant lymphoma in homosexual men. JAMA 1985; 254: 1921–5.

11. Lowenthal DA, Straus DJ, Campbell SW et al. AIDS-related lymphoid neoplasia: The Memorial Hospital experience. Cancer 1988; 61: 2325–37.

12. Ziegler JL, Miner RC, Rosenbaum E et al. Outbreak of Burkitt's-like lymphoma in homosexual men. Lancet 1982; 2: 631–3.

13. Ziegler JL, Becksted JA, Volberding PA et al. Non-Hodgkin's lymphoma in 90 homosexual men: Relation to generalized lymphadenopathy and the acquired immunodeficiency syndrome. N Engl J Med 1984; 311: 565–70.

14. Centers for Disease Control. Revision of the case definition of acquired immunodeficiency syndrome for national reporting – United States. MMWR 1985; 34: 373–373.

15. Biggar RJ, Burnett W, Mikl J et al. Cancer among New York men at risk of acquired immunodeficiency syndrome. Int J Cancer 1989; 43: 979–85.

16. Biggar RJ, Horm J, Goedert JJ et al. Cancer in a group at risk of acquired immunodeficiency syndrome (AIDS) through 1984. Am J Epidemiol 1987; 126: 578–86.

17. Centers for Disease Control. HIV/AIDS Surveillance Report. 1990; January, 1990: 1–22.

18. The Non-Hodgkin's Lymphoma Pathologic Classification Project. National Cancer Institute sponsored study of classifications of non-Hodgkin's lymphomas: Summary and description of a working formulation for clinical usage. Cancer 1982; 49: 2112–35.

19. Gill PS, Levine AM, Krailo M et al. AIDS-related malignant lymphoma: Results of prospective treatment trials. J Clin Oncol 1987; 5: 1322–8.

20. Filipovich AH, Heinitz KJ, Robison LL et al. The immunodeficiency cancer registry: A research resource. Am J Pediatr Hematol Oncol 1987; 9. 183–4.

21. Kersey JH, Spector BD, Good RA. Primary immunodeficiency diseases and cancer: The immunodeficiency-cancer registry. Int J Cancer 1973; 12: 333–47.

22. Perry GSI, Spector BD, Schuman LM et al. The Wiskott-Aldrich syndrome in the United States and Canada (1892–1979). J Pediatr 1980; 97: 72–8.

23. Frizzera G, Rosai J, Dehner LP et al. Lymphoreticular disorders in primary immunodeficiencies: New findings based on an up-to-date histologic classification of 35 cases. Cancer 1980; 46: 692–99.

24. Cotelingam JD, Witebsky FG, Hsu SM et al. Malignant Lymphoma in patients with the Wiskott-Aldrich syndrome. Cancer Invest 1985; 3: 515–22.

25. Penn I. Tumors arising in organ transplant recipients. Adv Cancer Res 1978; 28: 31–61.

26. Penn I. Kaposi's sarcoma in organ transplant recipients. Transplantation 1979; 27: 8–11.

27. Penn I. The occurrence of malignant tumors in immunosuppressed states. Prog Allergy 1986; 37: 259–300.

28. The Surveillance Program Division of Cancer Prevention and Control National Cancer Institute. Table II–1. Summary of 15 year trends: Age adjusted cancer incidence rates. In: Ries LAG, Barrett MJ and Labbe RR (eds). Cancer Statistics Review: 1973–1987. 1990: II–4.

29. Hardell L, Eriksson M, Lenner P et al. Malignant lymphoma and exposure to chemicals, especially organic solvents, chlorophenols and phenoxy acids: A case-control study. Br J Cancer 1981; 43: 169–76.

30. Woods JS, Polissar L, Severson RK et al. Soft tissue sarcoma and non-Hodgkin's lymphoma in relation to phenoxyherbicide and chlorinated phenol exposure in western Washington. JNCI 1987; 78: 899–910.

31. Burmeister LF, Everett GD, Van Lier SF et al. Selected cancer mortality and farm practices in Iowa. Am J Epidemiol 1983; 118: 72–7.

32. Hoar SK, Blair A, Holmes FF et al. Agricultural herbicide use and risk of lymphoma and soft-tissue sarcoma. JAMA 1986; 256: 1141–7.

33. Cantor KP. Farming and mortality from non-Hodgkin's lymphoma: A case-control study. Int J Cancer 1982; 29: 239–47.

34. Wigle DT, Semenciw RM, Wilkins K et al. Mortality study of Canadian male farm operators: Non-Hodgkin's lymphoma mortality and agricultural practices in Saskatchewan. JNCI 1990; 82: 575–82.

35. Persson B, Dahlander A-M, Fredriksson M et al. Malignant lymphomas ans occupational exposures. Br J Ind Med 1989; 46: 516–20.

36. Cartwright RA, McKinney PA, O'Brien C et al. Non-Hodgkin's lymphoma: A case control epidemiologic study in Yorkshire. Leukemia Res 1988; 12: 81–8.

37. Ott MG, Teta MJ, Greenberg HL. Lymphatic and hematopoietic tissue cancer in a chemical manufacturing environment. Am J Ind Med 1989; 16: 631–43.

38. Olsson H, Brandt L. Risk of non-Hodgkin's lymphoma among men occupationally exposed to organic solvents. Scan J Work Environ Health 1988; 14: 246–51.

39. Blakley BR, Schiefer BH. The effect of topically applied n-butylester of 2,4-dichlorophenoxyacetic acid on the immune response in mice. J Appl Toxicol 1986; 6: 291–5.

40. Blakley BR. The effect of oral exposure to the n-butylester of 2,4-dichlorophenoxyacetic acid on the immune response in mice. Int J Immunopharmac 1986; 8: 93–9.

41. Blakley BR, Blakley SM. The effect of prenatal exposure to the n-butylester of 2,4-dichlorophenoxyacetic acid (2,4-D) on the immune response in mice. Teratology 1986; 33: 15–20.

42. Harris MW, Moore JA, Vos JG et al. General biological effects of TCDD in laboratory animals. Environ Health Perspect 1973; 5: 101–9.

43. Vos JG, Moore JA, Zinkl JG. Effect of 2,3,7,8 tetrachlorodibenzo-p-dioxin on the immune system of laboratory animals. Environ Health Perspect 1973; 5: 149–62.

44. Burmeister LF. Cancer mortality in Iowa farmers, 1971–8. JNCI 1981; 66: 461–4.

45. Cantor KP, Fraumeni JF Jr. Distribution of non-Hodgkin's lymphoma in the United States between 1950 and 1975. Cancer Res 1980; 40: 2645–52.

46. Pearce NE, Smith AH, Fisher DO. Malignant lymphoma and

multiple myeloma linked with agricultural occupations in a New Zealand cancer registry-based study. Am J Epidemiol 1985; 121: 225–37.

47. Pearce NE, Sheppard RA, Smith AH et al. Non-Hodgkin's lymphoma and farming: An expanded case-control study. Int J Cancer 1987; 39: 155–61.

48. Johnson ES, Fischman HR, Matanoski GM et al. Cancer mortality among white males in the meat industry. J Occup Med 1986; 28: 23–32.

49. Francis DP, Essex M, Cotter SM et al. Epidemiological association between virusnegative feline leukemia and the horizontally transmitted feline leukemia cirus. Cancer Lett 1981; 12: 37–42.

50. Fraumeni JF Jr. Epidemiological studies of cancer. In: Griffin AC and Shaw CR (eds). Carcinogens: Identification and Mechanisms of Action. New York: Raven Press 1979; 51–63.

51. Lemp GF, Payne SF, Neal D et al. Survival trends for patients with AIDS. JAMA 1990; 263: 402–6.

52. Allegra CJ, Chabner BA, Tuazon CU et al. Trimetrexate for the treatment of Pneumocystis carinii pneumonia in patients with the acquired immunodeficiency syndrome. N Engl J Med 1987; 317: 978–85.

53. Kovacs JA, Ng VL, Masur H et al. Diagnosis of Pneumocystis carinii pneumonia: Improved detection in sputum with use of monoclonal antibodies. N Engl J Med 1988; 318: 589–93.

54. Zaman MK, Wooten OJ, Suprahmanya B et al. Rapid non-invasive diagnosis of Pneumocystis carinii from induced liquefied sputum. Ann Intern Med 1988; 109: 7–10.

55. Girard P-M, Gaudebout C, Lottin P et al. Prevention of Pneumocystis carinii pneumonia relapse by pentamidine aerosol in zidovudine-treated AIDS patients. Lancet 1989; 1: 1348–53.

56. Golden JA, Hollander H, Chernoff D et al. Prevention of Pneumocystis carinii pneumonia by inhaled pentamidine. Lancet 1989; 1: 654–7.

57. Fischl MA, Richman DD, Grieco MH et al. The efficacy of azidothymidine (AZT) in the treatment of patients with AIDS and AIDS-related complex: a double-blind, placebo-controlled trial. N Engl J Med 1987; 317: 185–91.

58. Montgomery AB, Leoung GS, Wardlaw LA et al. Effect of zidovudine on mortality rates and Pneumocystis carinii (PCP) incidence in AIDS and ARC patients on aerosol pentamidine. Am Rev Resp Dis 1989; 139: A250 (abstract).

59. New York State Department of Health. Survival of AIDS cases by risk factors and year of diagnosis. In: AIDS in New York State through 1989. Albany, N.Y.: New York State Department of Health 1990; 92–93.

60. Pluda JM, Yarchoan R, Jaffe ES et al. Development of non-Hodgkin lymphoma in a cohort of patients with severe human immunodeficiency virus (HIV) infection on long-term antiretroviral therapy. Ann Int Med 1990; 113: 276–82.

61. Gill PS, Loureiro C, Bernstein-Singer M et al. Clinical effect of glucocorticoids on Kaposi's sarcoma related to the acquired immunodeficiency syndrome (AIDS). Ann Intern Med 1989; 110: 937–40.

62. Real FX, Krown SE, Koziner B. Steroid-induced development of Kaposi's sarcoma in a homosexual man with Burkitt's lymphoma. Am J Med 1986; 80: 119–22.

63. Burroughs Wellcome Company. Lifetime Bioassay Studies. In: (eds) Comprehensive Information for Investigators, RETROVIR. Research Triangle Park, North Carolina: Burroughs Wellcome Company; 1989: 48.

64. Ayers KM, Preclinical toxicology of zidovudine: An overview. Am J Med 1988; 85: 186–8.

65. Pelicci P-G, Knowles DM II, Arlin ZA et al. Multiple monoclonal B cell expansions and c-myc oncogene rearrangements in acquired immune deficiency syndrome-related lymphoproliferative disorders. J Exp Med 1986; 164: 2049–76.

66. Lippman SM, Volk JR, Spier CM et al. Clonal ambiguity of human immunodeficiency virus-associated lymphomas. Arch Pathol Lab Med 1988; 122: 128–32.

67. Egerter DA, Beckstead JH. Malignant lymphomas in the acquired immunodeficiency syndrome: Additional evidence for a B-cell origin. Arch Pathol Lab Med 1988; 112: 602–6.

68. Pahwa S, Pahwa R, Saxinger C et al. Influence of the human T-lymphotropic virus/lymphadenopathy-associated virus on functions of human lymphocytes: Evidence for immunosuppressive effects and polyclonal B-cell activation by banded viral preparations. Proc Natl Acad Sci USA. 1985; 82: 8198–202.

69. Schnittman SM, Lane HC, Higgins SE et al. Direct polyclonal activation of human B lymphocytes by the acquired immune deficiency syndrome virus. Science 1986; 233: AIDS-lymphoma pathogenesis.

70. Yarchoan R, Redfield RR, Broder S. Mechanisms of B cell activation in patients with acquired immunodeficiency syndrome and related disorders. Contribution of antibodyproducing B cells, of Epstein-Barr virus-infected B cells, and of immunoglobulin production induced by human T cell lymphotropic virus, Type III/lymphadenopathy-associated virus. J Clin Invest 1986; 78: 439–47.

71. Birx DL, Redfield RR, Tosato G. Defective regulation of Epstein-Barr virus infection in patients with acquired immunodeficiency syndrome (AIDS) or AIDS-related disorders. N Engl J Med 1986; 314: 874–9.

72. Ganser A, Carlo-Stella C, Bartram CR et al. Establishment of two Epstein-Barr virus negative Burkitt cell lines from a patient with AIDS and B-cell lymphoma. Blood 1988; 72: 1255–60.

73. Groopman JE, Sullivan JL, Mulder C et al. Pathogenesis of B cell lymphoma in a patient with AIDS. Blood 1986; 67: 612–5.

74. Subar M, Neri A, Inghirami G et al. Frequent c-myc oncogene activation and infrequent presence of Epstein-Barr virus genome in AIDS-associated lymphoma. Blood 1988; 72: 667–71.

75. McGrath MS, Feigal E, Reyes GR et al. Evidence that Epstein-Barr virus (EBV) may infect B lymphoma cells after transformation in the small subgroup of AIDS-associated lymphomas (A-NHL) that are ABV positive. IV International Conference on AIDS, Stochholm, Sweden, June 12–16. 1988; 325.

76. Whang-Peng J, Lee EC, Sieverts H et al. Burkitt's lymphoma in AIDS: Cytogenetic study. Blood 1984; 63: 818–22.

77. Chaganti RSK, Jhanwar SC, Koziner B et al. Specific translocations characterize Burkitt's-like lymphoma of homosexual men with the acquired immunodeficiency syndrome. Blood 1983; 61: 1269–72.

78. Haluska FG, Russo G, Kant J et al. Molecular resemblance of an AIDS-associated lymphoma and endemic Burkitt lymphomas: Implications for their pathogenesis. Proc Natl Acad Sci USA 1989; 86: 8907–11.

79. Rechavi G, Ben-Bassat I, Berkowicz M et al. Molecular analysis of Burkitt's leukemia in two hemophilic brothers with AIDS. Blood 1987; 70: 1713–7.

80. Klein G. Multiple phenotypic consequences of the Ig/Myc translocation in B-cell-derived tumors. Genes Chrom Cancer 1989; 1: 3–8.

81. Friedman-Kien AE, Salzman BR, Cao Y et al. Kaposi's sarcoma in HIV-negative homosexual men. Lancet 1990; 335: 168–9.

82. Beral V. Peterman TA, Berkelman RL et al. Kaposi's sarcoma among persons with AIDS: a sexually transmitted infection. Lancet 1990; 335: 123–8.

83. McManaway ME, Neckers LM, Loke SL et al. Tumor-specific inhibition of lymphoma growth by ab antisense oligodeoxynucleotide. Lancet 1990; 335: 808–11.

84. Saxon A, Stevens RH, Golde DW. T-lymphocyte variant of hairy-cell leukemia. Ann Intern Med 1978; 88: 323–6.

85. Kalyanaraman VS, Sarngadharan MG, Robert-Guroff M et al. A new subtype of human T-cell leukemia virus (HTLV-II) as-

sociated with a T-cell variant of hairy cell leukemia. Science 1982; 218: 571–3.

86. Rosenblatt JD, Golde DW, Wachsman W et al. A second isolate of HTLV-II associated with atypical hairy-cell leukemia. N Engl J Med 1986; 315: 372–7.

87. Uchiyama T, Yodoi J, Sagawa K et al. Adult T-cell leukemia: Clinical and hematologic features of 16 cases. Blood 1977; 50: 481–92.

88. Poiesz BF, Ruscetti FW, Gazdar AF et al. Detection and isolation of type C retrovirus particles from fresh and cultured lymphocytes of a patient with cutaneous T-cell lymphoma. Proc Natl Acad Sci USA 1980; 77: 7415–9.

89. Bunn PA, Schlechter GP, Jaffe E et al. Clinical course of retrovirus-associated adult t-cell lymphoma in the United States. N Engl J Med 1983; 309: 257–64.

90. Broder S, Bunn PA, Jaffe ES et al. T-cell lymphoproliferative syndrome associated with human T-cell leukemia/lymphoma virus. Ann Int Med 1984; 100: 543–57.

91. Tanaka A, Takahashi C, Yamaoka S et al. Oncogenic transformation by the tax gene of human T-cell leukemia virus type I in vitro. Proc Natl Acad Sci USA 1990; 87: 1071–5.

92. Waldmann TA, Junghans RP. Interleukin-2 receptor directed therapy: a model for immune intervention. AIDS Res Hum Retroviruses 1990; 6–96.

93. Mann DL, DeSantis P, Mark G et al. HTLV-I-associated B-cell CLL: Indirect role for retrovirus in leukemogenesis. Science 1987; 236: 1103–6.

94. Bartholomew C, Saxinger C, Clark JW et al. Transmission of HTLV-I and HIV among homosexual men in Trinidad. JAMA 1987; 257: 2604–8.

95. Robert-Guroff M, Weiss SH, Giron JA et al. Prevalence of antibodies to HTLV-I, -II, and -III in intravenous drug abusers from an AIDS endemic region. JAMA 1986; 255: 3133–7.

96. Hahn RA, Onorato IM, Jones S et al. Prevalence of HIV infection among intravenous drug users in the United States. JAMA 1989; 261: 2677–84.

97. Zack JA, Cann AJ, Lugo JP et al. HIV-1 production from infected peripheral blood T cells after HTLV-I induced mitogenic stimulation. Science 1988; 240: 1026–9.

98. Rimsky L, Hauber J, Dukovich M et al. Functional replacement of the HIV-I rev protein by the HTLV-1 rex protein. Nature 1988; 335: 738–40.

99. Harper ME, Kaplan MH, Marselle LM et al. Concomitant infection with HTLV-I and HTLV-III in a patient with T8 lymphoproliferative disease. N Engl J Med 1988; 315: 1073–8.

100. Volberding PA, Lagakos SW, Koch MA et al. Zidovudine in asymptomatic human immunodeficiency virus infection: A controlled trial in persons with fewer than 500 CD4-positive cells per cubic millimeter. N Engl J Med 1990; 322: 941–9.

101. Fischl MA, Richman DT, Hansen N et al. The safety and efficacy of zidovudine (AZT) in the treatment of subjects with mildly symptomatic human immunodeficiency virus type 1 (HIV) infection: A double-blind, placebo-controlled trial. Ann Int Med 1990; 112: 727–37.

102. Neudorf SML, Filipovich AH, Kersey JH. Immunoreconstitution by bone marrow transplantation decreases lymphoproliferative malignancies in Wiskott-Aldrich and severe combined immune deficiency syndromes. In: Purtilo DT (eds). Immune Deficiency and Cancer: Epstein-Barr Virus and Lymphoproliferative Malignancies. New York: Plenum Medical Book Company 1984; 471–80.

103. Till MA, Ghetie V, Gregory T et al. HIV-infected cells are killed by rCD4-ricin A chain. Science 1988; 242: 1166–8.

104. Berger EA, Clouse KA, Chaudhary VK et al. CD4-Pseudomonas exotoxin hybrid blocks the spread of human immunodeficiency virus infection in vitro and is active against cells expressing the envelope glycoproteins from diverse primate immunodeficiency retroviruses. Proc Natl Acad Sci USA 1989; 86: 9539–43.

105. Kaplan LD, Kahn JO, Grossberg H et al. Chemotherapy with and without granulocytemacrophage colony stimulating factor (rGM-CSF) in patients with AIDS-associated non-Hodgkin's lymphoma (NHL). V International Conference on AIDS: The Scientific and Social Challenge, Montreal, Canada, June 4–9. 1989 (abstract): 334.

106. Walsh C, Wernz J, Laubenstein L et al. Phase I study of m-BACOD and GM-CSF in AIDS-associated non-Hodgkin's lymphoma (NHL): Preliminary results. Blood 1989 (abstract); 74 (Suppl 1): 126a.

107. Yarchoan R, Mitsuya H, Thomas RV et al. In vivo activity against HIV and favorable toxicity profile of 2′,3′-dideoxyinosine. Science 1989; 245: 412–5.

108. Lambert JS, Seidlin M, Reichman RC et al. 2′,3′-dideoxyinosine (ddl) in patients with the acquired immunodeficiency syndrome or the AIDS-related complex: A phase I trial. N Engl J Med 1990; 322: 1333–40.

109. Cooley TP, Kunches LM, Saunders CA et al. Once-daily administration of 2′,3′-dideoxyinosine (ddl) in patients with the acquired immunodeficiency syndrome or AIDS-related complex. N Engl J Med 1990; 322: 1340–5.

110. Levine AM, Wernz JC, Kaplan L et al. Low dose chemotherapy with CNS prophylaxis and zidovudine (AZT) maintenance for AIDS-related lymphoma: Preliminary results of a multi-institutional study. Proc Am Soc Clin Oncol 1989 (abstract); 8:5.

111. Cheson BD, Levine AM, Mildvan D et al. Suramin therapy in AIDS and related disorders: Report of the US suramin working group. JAMA 1987; 258: 1347–51.

Correspondence to:
James M. Pluda, M.D.
National Cancer Institute
National Institutes of Health
9000 Rockville Pike
Building 10, Room 13N248
Bethesda, MD, USA 20892

Annals of Oncology, Supplement 2 to Volume 2: 201–205, 1991.
© 1991 *Kluwer Academic Publishers.*

Original article ⎯⎯⎯⎯⎯⎯⎯⎯⎯⎯⎯⎯⎯⎯⎯⎯⎯⎯⎯⎯⎯⎯⎯⎯⎯⎯⎯

Hodgkin's disease in 63 intravenous drug users infected with human immunodeficiency virus*

S. Monfardini, U. Tirelli, E. Vaccher, R. Foà & F. Gavosto
for the Gruppo Italiano Cooperativo AIDS & Tumori (GICAT)*
(See the Appendix for participating members and institutions)

Summary. Sixty-three cases of Hodgkin's disease in intravenous drug users (IVDUs) have been collected by the Italian Cooperative Group on AIDS-Related Tumors (GICAT). In most patients (74%) the histological pattern was that of mixed cellularity and lymphocyte depletion. In 39% of patients the initial symptom was a persistent lymph node enlargement due to persistent generalized lymphadenopathy (PGL). Unusual presentations included Waldeyer's ring, skin, meninges, colon, and pleura. After MOPP alternated or followed by ABVD, MOPP alone, or ABVD alone, 15 of 32 patients (47%) had a complete remission (CR) and 15 of 32 (47%) had a partial remission (PR). The median duration of CR was 14 months, while the median survival of patients with CR has not been reached; the median survival of patients treated with chemotherapy who had CD4 levels at presentation $\geqslant 400/mm^3$ was significantly superior to that of those who had CD4 $< 400/mm^3$. The overall median survival was only 14 months. Forty-four percent of patients receiving chemotherapy, with or without radiotherapy, developed opportunistic as well as nonopportunistic infections. Lethal hepatic toxicity was observed in one patient. Among IVDUs, unusual presentations of Hodgkin's disease occurred at a lower rate than was previously reported for homosexuals. Complete remissions could be achieved in almost half the patients, but non opportunistic infections, in addition to parenchymal function impairment due to drug abuse, may limit treatment administration in IVDUs.

Introduction

In Italy, as in other countries of southern Europe where the AIDS epidemic affects predominantly intravenous drug users (IVDUs) [1], Hodgkin's disease has been described mainly in IVDUs rather than in homosexual men as it has been documented in the United States [2–6]. At the present time, it is not clear whether the natural history of the HIV infection may differ between IVDUs and homosexual men, although infectious complications may partially vary between the two groups [7, 8]. Furthermore, intravenous drug abuse may seriously affect pharmacokinetics and scheduling of drugs, as well as evaluation of response and overall follow-up. Drug abuse and dependency have been defined as a psychiatric disorder [9], and one of the established rules of clinical research protocols concerns the exclusion of patients with this mental problem. Therefore, by definition, these patients have been excluded from therapeutic trials. The purpose of this article is to describe the diagnostic and therapeutic aspects of one of the largest case series of Hodgkin's disease in IVDUs, which was collected through the Italian Cooperative Group on AIDS-Related Tumors (GICAT),

with particular emphasis on the differences in homosexual men suffering from the same disease. In view of the very low number of Italian patients in the homosexual risk group (5 cases), the comparison has been carried out with series from other countries.

Patients and methods

Participating investigators of the GICAT were asked to identify all known patients at risk for AIDS (homosexual men, IVDUs, hemophiliacs, and polytransfused persons) in whom a malignant lymphoma had developed between January 1980 and December 1989. A second integrated form was then sent to investigators who had previously reported to the Secretarial Office of the Cooperative Group cases of malignant lymphomas, to better collect data regarding the initial localizations, histological subtypes, clinical stages, treatment response, toxicities, causes of death, and duration of survival from time of antineoplastic treatment to death or to March 1990. This evaluation was carried out on the basis of the data collected through the initial and then integrated questionnaire and

* Supported by a grant of the Istituto Superiore di Sanità, Rome, Italy.

through case-by-case discussion with the medical staff responsible in each center for each patient, but without pathological review of the material.

The criteria used to diagnose persistent generalized lymphadenopathy (PGL) and AIDS were those established by the Centers for Disease Control (CDC) [10, 11]. Serology was performed by enzyme-linked immunosorbent assay and confirmed by Western blot (immunoblot). Survival distributions were estimated according to the product-limit method of Kaplan and Meier [12] and distribution comparisons were made with the method of Mantel [13]. Significance tests for proportions were computed by chi-square test [14].

Results

Owing to the peculiar features of this population of patients, complete clinical information could not be obtained from all cases. Therefore not all patients were evaluable for all parameters.

Three IVDUs with Hodgkin's disease were observed in 1984, 10 in 1985, 15 in 1986, 18 in 1987, 8 in 1988, and 9 in 1989. By December 1989, 74 cases of Hodgkin's disease had been reported in Italy. Sixty-three (85%) were IVDUs, and 11 fell into other risk groups (3 IVDUs and homosexuals, 5 homosexuals, and 3 heterosexuals).

Table 1 shows the presently available information on the clinical and pathological features of IVDU patients with HIV infection and Hodgkin's disease in Italy. Ninety-four per cent were males; the median age was 27 years; 44% of patients had persistent generalized lymphadenopathy (PGL); 31% were HIV-positive but met no other criteria for a diagnosis of AIDS, PGL, or AIDS-related complex (ARC); 17% of patients had ARC; and 7% had AIDS. Among the histological sub-types, most patients (74%) presented mixed cellularity and lymphocyte depletion. Lymphocyte predominance was not represented. Fifty-two per cent of the patients had stage IV disease. Unusual initial extranodal presentations included Waldeyer's ring (1 case), skin (1 case), meninges (1 case), colon (1 case), and pleura (1 case). However, a complete pathological staging with bone marrow biopsy, laparoscopy (7 of 44 cases), or laparotomy (2 of 10 cases) was performed in only 20% of patients. A clinical staging with bone marrow biopsy was performed in 50% and a simple clinical staging in 28% of patients. The reasons for the incomplete staging procedures were: postmortem diagnosis (3 patients), opportunistic infections or rapid progression of Hodgkin's disease (13 patients), and refusal (6 cases). In 8 patients the cause of the incomplete staging was not reported.

PGL was associated with lymphoma in 33 of 51 cases (65%) and preceeded the lymphoma in 20 of 27 evaluable cases (74%). The median latency between PGL and Hodgkin's disease was 8 months (range 1–37.5). The initial clinical presentation was an increase in size of preexistent adenopathies (i.e., of PGL) in 14 of 36 (39%) evaluable patients; 8 of the 36 had B symptoms whereas 6 of 36 did not, and the appearance of systemic symptoms in patients without PGL in 6% (2 patients); 44% (16/36) presented a 'de novo' lymph node enlargement with or without B symptoms, while an incidental diagnosis occurred in 4 patients, 3 at autopsy and 1 following a biopsy to document histologically a PGL.

Nineteen percent of patients presented with opportunistic infections at onset (C-1 and C-2 according to the CDC definition). The median number of CD4 lymphocytes/mm^3 in 38 evaluable patients was low (254, range 27–1316). Seventeen of 38 (45%) had CD4 values lower than 200/mm^3.

Table 1. Clinicopathological features of Hodgkin's disease in 63 intravenous drug users (IVDUs).

Total number	63		
Male	59/63 (94%)	Female	4/63 (6%)
Median age (yr)	27 (range 20–44)		
HIV-Seropositivity	63/63 (100%)		

Diagnosis of			
PGL*	ARC**	AIDS	Only HIV +
24/54 (44%)	9/54 (17%)	4/54 (7%)	17/54 (31%)

Grade					
Lymphocyte predominance	Nodular sclerosis	Mixed cellularity	Mixed cellularity + nodular sclerosis	Lymphocyte depletion	Lymphocyte depletion + mixed cellularity
0/62 (−)	14/62 (23%)	30/62 (48%)	2/62 (3%)	14/62 (23%)	2/62 (3%)

Stage			
I	II	III	IV
3/62 (5%)	8/62 (13%)	19/62 (31%)	32/62 (52%)

Abbreviations:
PGL* = persistent generalized lymphadenopathy.
ARC** = Aids-related complex.

Only 46 of 63 patients were treated. Of the 17 remaining patients, 5 could not receive any treatment because of rapid disease progression complicated by opportunistic infections. In 3 cases only postmortem diagnosis was obtained, and in 4 patients the reason for lack of treatment was not reported. In 5 cases no information on therapy was available. Owing to a lack of data on treatment response, 11 patients were not evaluable. Thirty-five patients evaluable for response were treated with MOPP/ABVD alternating regimens +/− radiotherapy (8 patients), MOPP followed by ABVD +/− radiotherapy (4 patients), MOPP alone +/− radiotherapy (10 patients), ABVD alone (3 patients), EBV (Epiadriamycin-Bleomycin-Vinblastine) + radiotherapy (4 patients), other combinations (3 patients). Three patients were treated with radiotherapy alone. Six or more cycles of combination chemotherapy could be administered in only 17 patients. Fourteen patients received three or more cycles of chemotherapy, but failed to complete treatment. In 1 of the 32 patients evaluable for response to chemotherapy, information on the number of cycles could not be obtained. Among 14 patients who did not complete treatment (six cycles), 1 died because of hepatic toxicity, 2 died because of opportunistic infections and/or rapid disease progression, 2 were lost to follow-up, and 1 refused therapy. In 3 patients therapy was still ongoing at the time of this evaluation, and in 5 patients the causes of incomplete treatment could not be determined. Severe hepatic toxicity was also observed in 1 patient not evaluable for response but still alive at the time of this evaluation.

After combination chemotherapy, a complete remission (CR) was observed in 15 of 32 patients (47%), while of the other 17 cases, 15 patients (47%) achieved a partial remission (PR). Two CRs were observed in the group of 3 patients treated with radiotherapy alone. The median duration of CR was 14 months (range 5–47). Among 16 evaluable patients with CR, only 2

(13%) had initial opportunistic infections (C-2 according to CDC) and only 3 (18%) had CD4 lymphocytes <400/mm³. Six presented with PGL, 1 with ARC, and 8 were asymptomatic (only HIV-positive); but none had AIDS.

Forty-four percent of patients receiving chemotherapy with or without radiotherapy developed infections during the follow-up. Opportunistic infections were diagnosed in 12 of 36 patients (33%) (C-1 nine cases, C-2 three cases) and non-opportunistic infections (pneumonia, enteric bacterial infections and bacteremia) in 4 of 36 (11%). Among patients who did not undergo therapy, 6 of 9 presented with opportunistic infections (C-1), and 2 of 9 with non opportunistic infections during the follow-up. However, in 2 patients opportunistic infections were already present at the onset of Hodgkin's disease.

The majority of patients died of tumor progression or opportunistic infections alone or associated with disease progression (Table 2). The overall median survival was only 14 months (Fig. 1). Opportunistic infections were the most important cause of death among treated patients, while tumor progression and opportunistic infections were the leading cause of death for untreated patients.

Median survival for patients achieving PR was 17 months, whereas median survival for patients with CR was not reached at the time of this analysis (Fig. 1). Patients receiving therapy survived a median of 17 months, whereas patients who could not receive any therapy survived less than 1 month. Patients receiving treatment and with CD4 lymphocytes <400/mm³ at onset had a median survival of 13.5 months, while the median survival for those with CD4 lymphocytes ≥400/mm³ was not reached.

Discussion

Sixty-six percent of Italian AIDS cases occur in IVDUs, and only 18% in homosexual men (Italian Ministry of Health, personal communication). Therefore it is not surprising that this large series of patients with HIV infection and Hodgkin's disease consists pre-

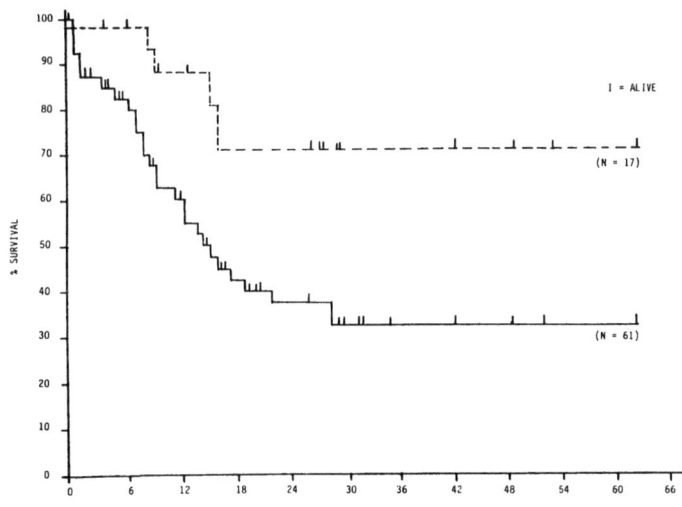

Fig. 1. Overall actuarial survival (————) and actuarial survival by complete response to therapy (− − − −) of IVDUs with HIV-related Hodgkin's disease.

Table 2. Mortality and causes of death in 57 evaluable IVDUs with Hodgkin's disease.

Mortality	32/57	(56%)
Cause of death:		
– Tumor progression	7/32	(22%)
– OI[a]	7/32	(22%)
– Non OI[b]	3/32	(9%)
– Tumor progression + OI	8/32	(25%)
– Other[c]	2/32	(6%)
– Unknown	5/32	(16%)

[a] Opportunistic infections.
[b] Bacterial pneumonia.
[c] Anaphylaxis 1, Hepatic toxicity 1.

dominantly of IVDUs. Histological subtype and stage distribution are similar to those described in other series in the United States (2–6) and other European countries where homosexual men are the main group affected by Hodgkin's disease in the HIV setting [15–18]. Atypical presentations (CNS, skin, endobronchial site, or lung involvement with lack of mediastinal adenopathy), which have been almost regularly observed in North American homosexual men [2–6], were not common in this IVDU series.

The majority of patients had persistent generalized lymphadenopathy, and in 39% of cases the diagnosis of malignant lymphoma was obtained in lymph nodes already known to be affected by PGL. Hodgkin's disease may be confused with PGL, therefore any increase in size of a preexistent adenopathy in patients with PGL should be evaluated with a biopsy. The initial diagnostic work-up may also require, in particular cases, lymph node biopsies at multiple sites. To avoid over- or understaging in patients with PGL, particular attention should be paid to the peculiar aspects of lymphangiography which may be confused with those of malignant lymphomas [19].

Almost half of our patients died of opportunistic infections alone or associated with tumor progression, while more than 20% died of tumor progression alone. Did chemotherapy produce a positive effect on survival, or possibly play a negative role by increasing immunodeficiency in our case series? The achievement of a CR in 47% of our patients was reflected in an increased survival in comparison to the remaining 47% of patients who obtained a PR. It should be noted that none of the patients achieving CR had AIDS at onset, the majority had PGL or were only HIV-positive. Patients who could not receive treatment survived less than one month. Survival was significantly increased after chemotherapy in patients with CD4 $\geqslant 400/mm^3$ at onset. Based on these considerations, it can be suggested that chemotherapy had a positive effect in patients at an early stage of the HIV infection who had no opportunistic infections, who had a good initial level of CD4 lymphocytes, and who were able to receive adequate therapy.

Myelodysplasia due to HIV infection, and the presence of opportunistic infections, are probably the main limiting factors to antineoplastic chemotherapy administration in homosexual men and IVDUs with malignant lymphoma. Hodgkin's disease in IVDUs should be approached, however, by taking into consideration that some peculiar complications may be due to the underlying drug abuse. It has been shown among IVDUs in the New York area that hepatic insufficiency due to previous hepatitis, bacterial pneumonia, and endocarditis are leading to an excess of non-AIDS-related deaths in comparison with homosexual men [7]. The same increases in bacterial pneumonia and endocarditis have been shown among IVDUs in Milan [20]. In our series of IVDUs, serious hepatic toxicity, observed in 2 cases, was the major limiting factor in the administration of chemotherapy; also, a negative role was played by the development of non opportunistic infections. Based on these considerations, the use of antitumor drugs with potential lung and cardiac toxicity should be carefully evaluated in IVDUs with Hodgkin's disease.

Appendix

The following persons and institutions participated in the Cooperative Study Group on AIDS-Related Tumors (GICAT):

S. Monfardini, U. Tirelli, E. Vaccher, D. Errante, A. Carbone, R. Talamini, Centro di Riferimento Oncologico, Via Pedemontana Occ., 33081 Aviano (PN) – F. Albericci, Ospedale Civile di Piacenza, Divisione Malattie Infettive, 29100 Piacenza – T. Barbui, Ospedale Civile di Bergamo, Divisione di Ematologia, 24100 Bergamo – C. Bernasconi, Policlinico S. Matteo, Divisione di Ematologia, Via Mentana 4, 27100 Pavia – A. Cajozzo, Istituto di Clinica Medica III, Divisione di Malattie Cardiovascolari, Via del Vespro 127, Palermo – A. Cargnel, A. Lazzarin, N. Moroni, G. Rizzardini, Ospedale L. Sacco, Divisione Malattie Infettive, Via G. B. Grassi 74, 20157 Milano – M. Clerici, Ospedale S. Carlo Borromeo, Divisione Oncologia Medica, Via Pio III n. 3, Milano – F. De Lalla, Ospedale Generale Provinciale S. Anna, Divisione Malattie Infettive, Via Napoleone 60, Como – P. Dessalvi, Ospedale A. Businico, Divisione di Ematologia, Via Jenner, Cagliari – F. Fiaccadori, Università degli Studi di Parma, Cattedra di Malattie Infettive, Via Gramsci 14, Parma – P. L. Garavelli, Ospedale Civile di Alessandria USL 70, Divisione di Malattie Infettive, Via Comunale 33, Valmadonna (AL) – M. Giudici, Arcispedale S. Maria Nuova, Divisione Malattie Infettive, Via Risorgimento, Reggio Emilia – F. Gherlinzoni, Policlinico S. Orsola, Istituto di Ematologia, Via G. Massarenti 9, Bologna – G. Lambertenghi-Deliliers, Ospedale Maggiore Milano, Istituto di Scienze Mediche, Via F. Sforza 35, Milano – G. Luzi, Cattedra di Allergologia ed Immunologia, Università La Sapienza, Pol. Umberto, Viale Università 37, Roma – R. Luzzati, Ospedale B. Trento, Divisione Malattie Infettive, Verona – A. Malfitano, Istituto IRCCS, Divisione Malattie Infettive, Piazzale Golgi, 27100 Pavia – F. Mandelli, Cattedra di Ematologia, Dipartimento di Biopatologia Umana, Via Benevento 6, 00161 Roma – S. Marigo, Ospedale S. Andrea, Via Veneto 197, Divisione Malattie Infettive, Via Veneto 197, 19100 La Spezia – V. Montesarchio, Cattedra di Oncologia Medica, Università degli Studi di Napoli, Via Sergio Pansini 5, 80131 Napoli – F. Puppo, Istituto Scientifico di Medicina Interna, Università degli Studi di Genova, Viale Benedetto XV 6, 16132 Genova – E. Raise, Ospedale Maggiore di Bologna, Divisione Malattie Infettive ed Immunopatologia. Via L. B. Nigrisoli 2, 40133 Bologna – G. Rezza, Ministero della Sanità, Istituto Superiore di Sanità, Piazzale dell'Industria, 00185 Roma – M. Rizzi, Ospedali Riuniti, Divisione Malattie Infettive, Largo Barozzi 11, 24100 Bergamo – E. Rossi, Ospedali Civili di Brescia, III Medicina Sezione Ematologia, 25125 Brescia – G. Saliva, Ospedale S. Andrea, Divisione Malattie Infettive, C.so M. Abbiate 31, 13100 Vercelli – A. Scanni, Ospedale Fatebenefratelli e Oftalmico, Corso di Porta Nuova 23, 20121 Milano – A. Sinicco, Università di Tornino-Ospedale Amedeo di Savoia, Divisione Malattie Infettive, Corso Svizzera 164, 10149 Torino – A. Vaglia, Ospedale Civile di Vicenza, Viale F. Rodolfi, 36100 Vicenza – R. Foà, F. Gavosto, Università di Torino, Dipartimento di Scienze Biomediche, Clinica Medica A, Via Genova 3, 10126 Torino.

References

1. World Health Organization – Geneva. Acquired immunodeficiency Syndrome (AIDS) surveillance update to 31 December

1988 in the WHO European Region. Weekly Epidemiological Record 1988; 64: 109–16.

2. Robert NJ, Schneiderman H. Hodgkin's disease and the Acquired Immunodeficiency Syndrome. Annals of Internal Medicine 1984; 101 (1): 142–3.

3. Lowenthal DA, Straus DJ, Campbell SW et al. AIDS-related neoplasia. The Memorial Hospital Experience. Cancer 1988; 61: 2325–7.

4. Kaplan LD, Abrams DI, Volberding PA et al. Clinical course and epidemiology of Hodgkin's disease (HD) in homosexual men in San Francisco. In Third International Conference on AIDS 1987; abstract n.9. Washington.

5. Schoeppel SL, Hoppe R, Abrams D et al. Hodgkin's disease (HD) in homosexual men: the San Francisco Bay area experience. In: Proceedings of the American Association of Clinical Oncology (ASCO) 1986; Abstract. Vol. 5 (3). Los Angeles.

6. Knowles DM, Chamulak GA, Suber M et al. Lymphoid neoplasia associated with the AIDS. The New York Medical Center experience with 105 patients. Annals of Internal Medicine 1988; 108: 744–53.

7. Stoneburner RL, Des Jarlais DC, Benetsra D et al. A larger spectrum of severe HIV-one-related disease intravenous drug users in New York City. Science 1988; 242: 916–9.

8. Selwin PA, Hartel D, Wasserman W, Drucker E. Impact of the AIDS epidemic on morbidity and mortality among Intravenous drug users in a New York City methadone maintenance program. American Journal of Public Health 1989; 79: 1358–62.

9. Mendelson SH, Mello NK. Commonly abused drug. In: Harrison's principles of internal medicine. 11th edition, Edited by Bramwald E, Isselbacher KJ, Petersdorg RG, Wilson JD, Martini JB, Fanci AS, pp 2115–8. St. Louis New York, San Francisco, Auckland, Bogota, Hamburg, Joliannesburg, London, Madrid, Moscow, Milan, Montreal, New Delphi, Panama, Paris, Sao Paulo, Singapore, Tokyo, Toronto: Mc Grace-Hill Book Company, 1987.

10. Centers for Disease Control. Classification system for human T-Lymphotropic virus type III/Lymphadenopathy-associated virus infections. Annals of Internal Medicine 1986; 105: 234–7.

11. Centers for Disease Control. Revision of the CDC surveillance case definition for Acquired Immunodeficiency Syndrome. Morbidity & Mortality Weekly Reports 1987; 36: 19–155.

12. Kaplan EL, Meier P. Comparametric estimation from incomplete observations. Journal of the American Statistics Association 1958; 53: 457–81.

13. Mantel N. Evaluation of survival data and two new rank order statistics arising in its consideration. Cancer Chemotherapy Reports 1966; 50: 163–120.

14. Armitage P, Barry G. 2×2 – and x^2 tests. In Statistical methods in medical research. 2nd Edition, pp 125–32. Blackwell Scientific Publications, 1987.

15. Raphael M, Tulliez M, Bellefqih S et al. Las Lymphomas et la Sida. Annales de Pathologie 1986; 6: 278–81.

16. Andrieu JM, Tourani JM, Raphael M et al. HIV associated Hodgkin's disease. In: Proceedings of ESMO 1988; Abstracts C6, 24P.

17. Schurman D, Dienemann D, Ruf B et al. Malignant lymphomas in HIV infected patients: clinical and pathological features. V° International Conference on AIDS (Montreal) 1989; Abstract 206, WBO 20.

18. Alfonso GP, Saundo FE, Galinso CR et al. Hodgkin's disease in HIV infected patients. In: Proceedings ECCO-4 (Madrid) 1987; Abstract 1051.

19. Tirelli U, Vaccher E, Carbone A et al. Lymphangiography computerised tomography in persistent generalized lymphadenopathy. AIDS Research 1986; 2 (2), 149–53.

20. Galli M, Carito M, Cruccu V et al. Causes of death in IV drug abusers (IVDAs) a retrospective survey on 4883 subjects. IV° International Conference on AIDS (Stockholm) 1988; Abstract 194: 4520.

Correspondence to:
Dr. Silvio Monfardini, Chief
Division of Medical Oncology
Centro di Riferimento Oncologico
Via Pedemontana Occidentale, 33081 Aviano (PN), Italy

Annals of Oncology, Supplement 2 to Volume 2: 207–211, 1991.
© 1991 *Kluwer Academic Publishers.*

Original article

Workshop on growth factors

Derek Crowther,[1] Michael B. Sporn,[2] Anita B. Roberts[2] & Brian G. M. Durie[3]

[1] *Christie Hospital, Manchester, UK;* [2] *National Cancer Institute, Bethesda, Md., USA;* [3] *Charing Cross and Westminster Medical School, London, UK*

Summary. The 'Workshop on Growth Factors' which took place at the Lugano Lymphoma Conference on June 8, 1990, included a presentation by Michael Sporn on the concept that loss of inhibitory control mechanisms may be important in the development and growth of human cancer. Examples illustrating this were taken from current experimental biology research into transforming growth factor β (TGF-β) interactions. Brian Durie presented recent data on the biology of interleukin-6 (IL-6) and its putative role in plasma cell diseases. These studies have culminated in the first clinical study of the role of an antibody to a growth factor as therapy for a human cancer (anti-IL-6 antibody as therapy for patients with myeloma). Derek Crowther presented data concerning the current clinical role of the haematopoietic growth factors in patients undergoing chemotherapy for cancer. Recent clinical research has established the role of granulocyte colony-stimulating factor (G-CSF) and granulocyte-macrophage colony-stimulating factor (GM-CSF) in improving the safety of high-dose or accelerated chemotherapy, and their use is associated with enhanced neutrophil recovery following ablative therapy and bone marrow rescue. This session was followed by the presentation of three papers concerning the use of G-CSF and GM-CSF in association with chemotherapy for patients with malignant lymphoma.

Transforming growth factor-β (TGF-β) and negative growth control, with special relevance to leukaemia and lymphoma

Michael B. Sporn & Anita B. Roberts

TGF-β1 was first purified to homogeneity from human platelets, human placenta, and bovine kidney, using its ability to induce normal rat kidney fibroblasts to grow and form colonies in soft agar in the presence of epidermal growth factor (EGF) as the assay system to monitor the purification. Subsequently, two other isoforms of TGF-β, known as TGF-β2 and TGF-β3, have been isolated, characterised, and cloned from various mammalian cells. All three isoforms have very similar biological activities in most assay systems, and all can now be produced in bulk amounts using recombinant DNA expression systems. Following the original characterisation of TGF-β, it was found to be a multifunctional agent, with many different actions on many different cell types. Although it can stimulate proliferation in some cells, especially in connective tissue, it is a potent inhibitor of proliferation in many others, especially epithelial cells, as well as both T lymphocytes and B lymphocytes.

TGF-β is the most potent known endogenous suppressor of lymphocyte proliferation and function; it is 10 000 to 100 000 times more potent on a molar basis than cyclosporine. It is an endogenous product of both T and B cells, serving as a negative autocrine signal to inhibit the action of the various interleukins and other cytokines that stimulate lymphocyte proliferation and function. Thus, TGF-β can inhibit DNA synthesis in T cells stimulated with either IL-1 or IL-2, inhibit antibody production in B cells stimulated by a variety of activating factors, and inhibit the generation of cytotoxic T cells. It is a particularly potent inhibitor of the action of tumour necrosis factor in many assay systems.

It is now well established in many situations that as cells become malignant, they may lose their responsiveness to negative regulatory signals such as TGF-β and become autonomous in their growth properties. The mechanisms whereby this loss of regulation occurs are not well understood, but may involve processes as diverse as the inability to synthesise TGF-β, the loss of its receptor, or loss of steps in the intracellular signalling pathways controlled by TGF-β.

Recent work in the laboratory of Dr. Francis Ruscetti and colleagues (National Cancer Institute, USA) has begun to shed some light on the failure of this negative autocrine pathway in human leukaemia and lymphoma cells. In both HL-60 human promyelocytic leukaemia cells and a variety of human B-lymphoma cell lines, they have found that there may be a failure to express the cell surface receptor for TGF-β, although the gene for the receptor is still present in these cells. Thus, these cells do not respond to TGF-β with an appropriate growth inhibitory response. However, if these malignant cells are treated with differentiating agents such as retinoic acid or phorbol ester, they then are induced to express the TGF-β receptor, as determined in cross-linking experiments using iodinated TGF-β. After treatment with retinoic acid or phorbol ester, these leukaemia or lymphoma cells become responsive to TGF-β, which then inhibits DNA synthesis. Ruscetti and colleagues have also shown that retinoic acid or phorbol ester can induce synthesis of mRNA or TGF-β, as well as of the peptide itself, in these cells. Thus, there is a failure of a negative autocrine loop in the malignant leukaemia or lymphoma cells, and one of the actions of differentiating agents appears to be the restoration of the function of such a loop. These pioneering studies shed new light on potential mechanisms that conceivably can be exploited for chemoprevention of epithelial cancer, as well as for treatment of leukaemia and lymphoma.

The biology of interleukin 6: The role in plasma cell diseases

Brian G. M. Durie

Introduction

Interleukin-6 (IL-6) is a pleotropic cytokine. It has a molecular weight of 26 kd and consists of 184 amino acids with 2 glycosylation sites and 4 cysteine residues. Of interest, there is amino acid sequence homology with G-CSF. Before IL-6 was cloned and the amino acid sequence completely known, activities similar to IL-6 were ascribed to a number of molecules including B-cell stimulatory factor 2, interferon beta 2, myeloma/plasmacytoma growth factor, hepatocyte-stimulating factor, macrophage/granulocyte-inducing factor 2, and cytotoxic T-cell differentiation factor. It is now known that IL-6 has all these diverse actions. Specific effects of IL-6 within the immune system include the induction of immunoglobulin production by plasma cells as well as the induction of both proliferation and differentiation of plasma cells. In the T-cell system there is stimulation of IL-2 production by T cells. In the bone marrow, haematopoietic stem cells are stimulated towards multilineage haematopoietic growth. Pronounced effects on the liver include both the stimulation of C-reactive protein production as well as inhibition of albumin synthesis.

Production of IL-6

A variety of cells have the capacity to synthesize IL-6, including lymphoid cells (both B and T cells), monocytes, fibroblasts, bone marrow cells, endothelial cells, keratinocytes, astrocytes, and kidney mesangial cells.

Several tumour cell lines have been found to produce significant amounts of IL-6, including T-cell lines (HTLV-1 transformed), plus the MG 63 osteosarcoma, T24 bladder carcinoma, A549 lung carcinoma, SK-MGk4 glioblastoma and U373 astrocytoma lines. In addition, several types of direct tumour cell specimens have been found to produce IL-6, including cardiac myxoma cells, myeloma cells, and hypernephroma tumour cells.

IL-6 plasma cell disorders

A controversial area of IL-6 biology is its role in the pathogenesis of myeloma and related plasma cell disorders. Several studies have indicated the potential for an autocrine loop, i.e., that myeloma cells both produce and are sensitive to IL-6 and that an enhancement of this loop (mechanism?) is an integral part of the disease process. This argument is supported by experiments involving the insertion of c-DNA for IL-6 into IL-6-dependent murine B cells. A disease process, very similar to mouse plasmacytomata or myeloma, develops. Although this process is possible, the question remains as to whether or not it is the primary mechanism in human myeloma.

Most direct human myeloma specimens as well as myeloma cell lines spontaneously synthesize very little or no IL-6 or mRNA for IL-6. It is very difficult even to induce IL-6 mRNA or IL-6 synthesis by human myeloma cells. Conversely, several groups have now demonstrated that the accessory cells in human bone marrow produce very large amounts of IL-6, specifically macrophages and fibroblasts as well as endothelial cells. In separation studies the accessory cells are the major source of IL-6 in human myeloma bone marrow. These accessory cells are also the predominant source of elevated serum IL-6 levels which have been noted in the plasma cell diseases and correspond to disease activity. For example, very high serum IL-6 levels occur in patients with plasma cell leukaemia.

As shown in Figure 1 (see discussion in [6]), paracrine loops have been proposed indicating positive feedback with the release of IL-6 from accessory cells and an associated production of IL-1 beta or possibly other cytokines with feedback stimulation of the accessory cells, as well as bone cells (direct stimulation of osteoblasts with secondary stimulation of osteoclasts via a coupling factor [as yet unidentified]). Stimulation of the bone cells represents an important trigger for bone destruction, a crucial identifying feature of human myeloma. The current consensus is that this type of paracrine loop mechanism is most likely an important part of the pathogenesis of myeloma. There is therefore interest in the therapeutic manipulation of this loop using inhibitors of cytokines and/or cytokine receptors.

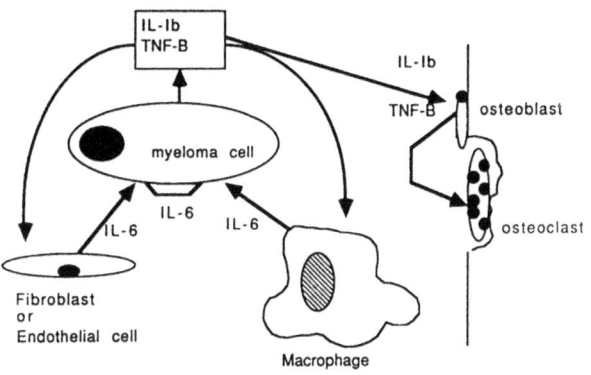

PARACRINE LOOPS IN MYELOMA

Fig. 1. Paracrine loops in myeloma.

Initial studies using antibody to IL-6 have proved promising in the inhibition of disease activity in two patients with plasma cell leukaemia.

Molecular biology of IL-6 dysregulation

The dysregulation of IL-6 occurs not just in myelomas and related plasma cell disorders, but also in other diseases, including Castleman's disease, rheumatoid arthritis, and mesangial proliferative glomerulonephritis. The exact basis for the dysregulation in myeloma and these other diseases remains to be determined. Crucial to the understanding of these entities is the function of the IL-6 receptor which has a very unusual function-to-structure relationship. The ligand-binding component is a single polypeptide with a molecular mass of 80 kd. It has extracellular, transmembrane, and intracellular components (Fig. 2 [diagram based upon data published in [11]).

When IL-6 binds to IL-6 regulatory (IL-6R), a process of signal transduction occurs between IL-6R and the extracellular portion of an adjacent membrane glycoprotein called GP-130 which is non ligand binding and has a molecular mass of 130 kd. The intracellular portion of this membrane glycoprotein is responsible

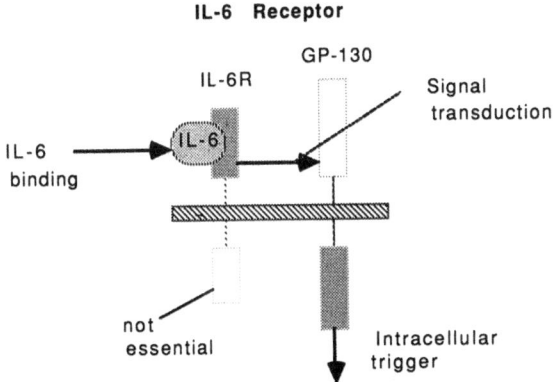

IL-6 Receptor

Fig. 2. IL-6 Receptor.

Table 1. Potential IL-6 defects in myeloma.

1. Mutation
   - IL-6 structural gene
   - IL-6 regulatory segments
   - IL-6 receptor (IL-6R or GP130 component)

2. Abnormal trigger for
   paracrine IL-6 production
   (eg, IL-1b, TNFb, BCGF2 [IL-5])

3. Dysfunction of IL-6
   dependent cofactors
   (eg, GM-CSF)

for the intracellular trigger mechanism for the IL-6 receptor. The exact sequence of events following IL-6 receptor activation remains to be clarified. However, the effects include the incorporation of TdR into activated cells. Obviously a dysregulation of this system could include specific mutations involving either one or both components of the IL-6 receptor as well as the IL-6 molecule itself. In addition (Table 1), in myeloma for example, there could be a specific defect involving the paracrine loop mechanism incorporating such molecules as IL-1 beta, as well as cofactors, such as G-CSF or GM-CSF.

It is very important to investigate these details in terms of extracellular cytokine levels and function (including binding and activation of IL-6R) as well as the detailed molecular biology of intracellular structure/ function relationships. It will be important, for example, to evaluate interrelationships with other known molecular abnormalities including RAS mutations and aberrant P-glycoprotein and other membrane antigen expression. The very promising results in initial studies treating plasma cell leukaemia with antibody to IL-6 suggests that further understanding of this IL-6 system could prove therapeutically useful.

The clinical role of the haemopoietic growth factors

Derek Crowther

Since the first publication in 1987 showing that G-CSF given by continuous intravenous infusion ameliorates the neutropenia and reduces the incidence of infection following intermittent combined chemotherapy for cancer [12], there have been a number of reports indicating beneficial effects in this context using both G and GM-CSF [13]. In our first study the period of neutropenia was significantly shortened (by a median of 80%) and the neutrophil count levels were above normal again by 14 days following chemotherapy. In view of these results a further study was undertaken to examine the possibility of using intensive chemotherapy every two weeks under cover of G-CSF. Treatment with doxorubicin at doses of 75, 100, 125, and 150 mg/m^2 was followed by infusion of G-CSF for 11 days. Again the neutrophil counts returned to normal within 12–14 days, allowing the delivery of up to three cycles of high-dose chemotherapy at 14-day intervals. These studies demonstrated that intensive chemotherapy with dose-limiting myelosuppression can be given with increased frequency under cover of G-CSF. Our studies using GM-CSF have also shown that administration can reduce the period of life-threatening neutropenia following high-dose melphalan (120 mg/m^2) without resort to autologous bone marrow transplantation (ABMT). In this study the period of granulocytopenia ($<500 \times 10^9$ granulocytes per litre) following melphalan was less than 15 days. This compares favourably with other series using high-dose melphalan followed by ABMT without CSF where the duration of severe neutropenia was prolonged beyond three weeks. Current studies from a number of centres have shown an improved neutrophil recovery using both G-CSF and GM-CSF following ablative therapy (high-dose chemotherapy with or without total body irradiation) and bone marrow rescue. This has been associated with a reduced risk of infection and fewer days in hospital requiring antibiotic therapy. Enhanced neutrophil recovery has been demonstrated following conventional and high-dose chemotherapy allowing the use of accelerated chemotherapy of higher dose intensity than would have been possible without the use of a myelopoietic growth factor.

Improvement in the neutrophil count using G-CSF and GM-CSF has been observed in patients with marrow graft failure, bone marrow failure from a variety of causes, myelodysplastic syndrome, AIDS undergoing therapy with AZT, cyclic neutropenia, or Kostman's syndrome and in patients undergoing chemotherapy for acute myelogenous leukaemia. To date, most of these studies have involved relatively few patients, but major large randomised studies are under way to confirm these findings. Crawford recently published preliminary results from a large, multicentre, randomised, double-blind, placebo-controlled trial of G-CSF in patients with small-cell lung cancer undergoing chemotherapy. Episodes of febrile neutropenia, days in hospital, and days of antibiotic use were all significantly reduced in patients receiving G-CSF following chemotherapy.[14]

Although enhanced platelet recovery has been observed following the use of GM-CSF, effects on platelets have been relatively modest. Nevertheless, early trials with IL-3 and the combined use of growth factors are showing more beneficial effects on platelet counts in patients with some forms of bone marrow failure [15]. The administration of haematopoietic growth factors has increased the yield of peripheral blood stem cells, allowing the use of these cells as rescue following ablative chemotherapy; and it would appear that the combined use of growth factors including IL-3 is likely to further increase the yield [16]. Data showed marked enhancement of peripheral blood progenitors following G-CSF in patients with non-Hodgkin's lymphoma who had received combined chemotherapy given using a weekly schedule over a period of three months. These progenitors had the capacity to survive in long-term culture, and sufficient numbers of progenitors for rescue from ablative therapy were present in as little as 350 ml of blood taken at the appropriate time. However, there was considerable variation in the number of progenitors available, depending on the amount of previous chemotherapy and the timing of harvest. Although a great deal has been accomplished in the three to four years that some of the haemopoietic growth factors have been available for clinical use, a great deal more needs to be done before their optimal role in therapy can be established. Proteins (such as macrophage inhibitory protein-1α and TGF-β) and several small peptides have been identified which are capable of inhibiting haemopoiesis, and their future use in reducing bone marrow toxicity associated with chemotherapy is an exciting prospect. Studies of the possible use of GM-CSF and M-CSF in enhancing host antitumour activity are currently under way. Although continuous intravenous infusion has been accompanied by more pronounced effects than bolus intravenous or subcutaneous administration, optimal routes and schedules of administration have not been established for the various therapeutic indications. The use of combinations of growth factors is only just beginning, and more work is required to optimise the way these are delivered.

References

1. Kishimoto T. The Biology of Interleukin-6. Blood 1989; 74: 1, 1–10.
2. Kawano M, Hirano T, Matsuda T, Taga T, Horil Y, Iwato K, Asoku H, Tang B, Tanabe O, Tanaka H, Kuramoto A, Kishimoto T. Autocrine generation and essential requirement of BSF-2/IL-6 for human multiple myelomas. Nature 1988; 332: 83.
3. Heinrich PC, Castell JV, Andus T. Interleukin-6 and the acute phase response. Biochemical J 1990; 265: 621.
4. Lichtenstein A, Berenson J, Norman D, Chang MP, Carlile A. Production of Cytokines by Bone Marrow Cells Obtained from Patients with Multiple Myeloma. Blood 1989; 74: 1266–73.
5. Zhang XG, Klein B, Bataille R. Interleukin-6 is a Potent Myeloma-Cell Growth Factor in Patients with Aggressive Multiple Myeloma. Blood 1989; 74: 11–3.
6. Durie BGM, Vela EE, Frutiger Y. Macrophages as an Important Source of Paracrine IL-6 in Myeloma Bone Marrow. In: Proceedings of Mechanisms in B Cell Neoplasia 1990. (In press)
7. Bataille R, Jourdan M, Zhang XG, Klein B. Serum Levels of Interleukin-6, A Potent Myeloma Cell Growth Factor, As A Reflect of Disease Severity in Plasma Cell Dyscrasias. J Clin Invest (In Press).
8. Freeman GJ, Freedman AS, Rabinowe SN, Segil JM, Horowitz J, Rosen K, Whitman JF, Nadler LM. Interleukin-6 Gene Expression in Normal and Neoplastic B cells. J Clin Invest 1989; 83: 1512–8.

9. Jourdan M, Bataille R, Sequin J, Zhang XG, Chaptal PA, Klein B. Constitutive Production of Interleukin and Immunologic Features in Cardiac Myxomas. Arthritis & Rheumatism 1990; 33: 1–5.

10. Tohyama N, Karasuyama H, Tada T. Growth Autonomy and Tumorigenicity of Interleukin 6-Dependent B Cells Transfected with Interleukin 6 cDNA. J Exp Med 1990; 171: 389–400.

11. Taga T, Hibi M, Hirata Y, Yamasaki K, Yasukawa K, Matsuda T, Hirano T, Kishimoto T. Interleukin-6 Triggers the Association of Its Receptor with a Possible Signal Transducer, gp130. Cell 1989 58: 573–81.

12. Bronchud MH, Scarffe JH, Thatcher N, Crowther D, Souza M, Alton NK, Testa NG, Dexter TM. Phase I/II study of recombinant human granulocyte colony-stimulating factor in patients receiving intensive chemotherapy for small cell lung cancer. Br J Cancer 1987; 56: 809–13.

13. Gurney H, Crowther D. Hemopoietic growth factors: their clinical role (Ed: J. R. Prous). Drugs of the Future 1990; 15: No. 6, 581–595.

14. Crawford J, Ozer H, Johnson. The G-CSF study group. Granulocyte colony stimulating factor: prevention of chemotherapy induced neutropneia in patients with small cell lung cancer. A randomised bould eblind placebo controlled trial. Proc Amer Soc Clin Oncol 1990; 9: 229.

15. Ganser A, Lindemann A, Seipelt G, Ottmann OG, Herrmann F, Schulz G, Mertelsman R, Hoelzer D. Effect of recombinant human interleukin-3 (rhIL-3) in patients with bone marrow failure – A phase I/II trial. Blood 1989; 74 (7), Suppl. 1, 50a.

16. Gianni AM, Siena S, Bregni M, Tarella C, Stern AC, Allessandro P, Bonadonna G. Granulocyte-macrophage colony stimulating factor to harvest circulating haemopoietic stem cells for autotransplantation. Lancet 1989; 2: 580.

13. Gurney H, Crowther D. Hemopoietic growth factors: their clinical role. Drugs of the Future 1990; 15: No. 6, (In press).

Correspondence to:
Professor Derek Crowther
Christie Hospital and Holt Radium Institute
Wilmslow Road
Manchester M20 9BX
England

Annals of Oncology, Supplement 2 to Volume 2: 213–217, 1991.
© 1991 Kluwer Academic Publishers.

Original article

Report of the first workshop on prognostic factors in large-cell lymphomas

B. Coiffier,[1] M. A. Shipp,[2] F. Cabanillas,[3] D. Crowther,[4] J. O. Armitage[5] & G. P. Canellos[2]

[1]Hematology Service, Centre Hospitalier Lyon-Sud, Pierre-Bénite, France; [2]Division of Clinical Oncology, Dana-Farber Cancer Institute and Harvard Medical School, Boston, Massachusetts, USA; [3]Lymphoma Department, M. D. Anderson Hospital Center and Tumor Institute, Houston, Texas, USA; [4]CRC Department of Medical Oncology, Christie Hospital and Holt Radium Institute, Manchester, England; [5]Department of Internal Medicine, University of Nebraska Medical Center, Omaha, Nebraska, USA

Malignant lymphomas are a group of extremely heterogeneous diseases. This heterogeneity is seen in histological subtype as well as in clinical presentation, response to treatment, and prognosis. The natural diversity of histologic subtypes of malignant lymphomas was complicated by the number of classifications used around the world, including the Rappaport [1], Lukes-Collins [2], and Kiel [3]. However, the development of the Working Formulation [4] allowed pathologists and physicians to speak the same language. The most frequent subtype of non-Hodgkin's lymphoma is called 'diffuse large-cell' lymphoma. It includes diffuse large cell and immunoblastic (groups G and H) from the Working Formulation, and is also known as diffuse histiocytic lymphoma (Rappaport), or immunoblastic and centroblastic (Kiel). In this subtype, clinical presentation can vary from localized adenopathy or localized visceral infiltration in some patients to extensive adenopathy and visceral involvement in others. Non-Hodgkin's lymphomas are usually classified by the Ann Arbor staging system, which was primarily devised for Hodgkin's disease [5].

The demonstration that a fraction of patients with large-cell lymphoma could be cured by chemotherapy [6] was followed by a proliferation of trials attempting to improve on these results [7, 8, 9, 10, 11, 12]. Active regimens were based on the combination of doxorubicin, vincristine and cyclophosphamide, or their analogues, and encompassed two major ideas: the importance of dose intensity and the need for giving drugs in sequence [13]. With these intensive regimens, response to treatment and survival vary according to prognostic factors [14]. These new regimens sometimes produce a higher incidence of morbidity and mortality than was seen with the classic CHOP regimen. As would be expected, toxicity has occurred primarily in patients with more advanced disease and impaired performance status. Therapeutic results are a subtle interaction of tumor mass and site as well as intensity of chemotherapy, tolerance, and performance status. Interpretation of results of these new regimens must be gauged to the clinical characteristics of the patient population [13].

For these reasons, studies of prognostic factors have been performed and several institutions have each proposed a prognostic scheme. The importance of some factors is relatively difficult to assess because they are studied in too few patients or in retrospective studies where a number of therapeutic regimens have been used.

Regardless of the lymphoma subtype and type of treatment, numerous prognostic parameters are related to the mass of lymphoma and its effects on the host (Table 1) [15–25]. The earliest prognostic factor amongst the non-Hodgkin's lymphomas is histological type [4, 26]. But, among the large cell lymphomas, no significant differences have been observed according to whether they are immunoblastic, cleaved or noncleaved large cells, with the exception of follicular large cell lymphoma which has a more favorable prognosis. Peripheral T cell lymphomas are associated with a worse prognosis in most studies independent of the other prognostic factors [27–29]. Most of the prognostic factors described in Table 1 are related to response to treatment and overall survival, reflecting the close relationship between the two determinants in aggressive lymphomas [30]. Some of these parameters are also related to disease-free survival but the relation is generally weaker than for survival. M. A. Shipp, B. Coiffier and F. Cabanillas presented results of studies effected in Boston [23, 31], Lyon [14, 16], and Houston [15, 21, 24]. Their conclusions were (a) that patients with aggressive lymphoma can be partitioned into subgroups of different outcome, (b) that such a partitioning is useful for interpreting and comparing results, and (c) that prognostic factors that permit this partition are related to tumor burden and not very different from one study to another.

Other features have been described as potentially important for survival in large cell lymphomas (Table 2). It is difficult to know the impact of these parameters compared to those described in Table 1 because the studies have rarely been reproduced or analyzed with multiparametric methods. The study of chromosomal rearrangements is a recent addition [32–34] and this may be a major factor when the specific

214

Table 1. Parameters associated with response to treatment, disease-free survival and overall survival in large cell lymphomas according to major regimens.

Initial parameters	Response to treatment	Disease-free survival	Overall survival
Age	MSKCC, CHHRI, SWOG, GELA		MDAH, MSKCC, CHHRI, SWOG, UNMC, GELA
Increased alkaline phosphatase level	CHHRI, JLSG		CHHRI, JLSG
B symptoms	DFCI, MSKCC, CHHRI, SWOG, JLSG, GELA, NCI	MDAH	DFCI, MDAH, CHHRI, NCI, SWOG, GELA
Increased β2-microglobulin level	MDAH	MDAH	MDAH
Bone marrow involvement	CHHRI, DFCI, JLSG, GELA, NCI	CHHRI, GELA	CHHRI, JLSG, NCI, DFCI, GELA
Low hemoglobin level	CHHRI, NCI		CHHRI, NCI, JLSG
Increased LDH level	MSKCC, CHHRI, JLSG, GELA, NCI	MDAH, GELA	MDAH, NCI, JLSG, GELA, MSKCC, CHHRI
Liver involvement	NCI, GELA		NCI, GELA
Impaired performance status	SWOG, GELA, DFCI, CHHRI	GELA	SWOG, GELA, DFCI, CHHRI
Pleural effusion	DFCI, GELA		DFCI, GELA
Low serum albumin level	CHHRI, GELA		CHHRI, GELA
Splenic involvement	DFCI		GELA
Disseminated stage	CHHRI, SWOG, DFCI, JLSG, NCI, GELA	CHHRI, MDAH, GELA	DFCI, CHHRI, NCI, JLSG, GELA
Bulky abdominal mass	NCI		MSKCC, NCI
Bulky tumor mass	DFCI, MSKCC, CHHRI, GELA	MDAH, GELA	DFCI, MDAH, MSKCC, GELA
Weight loss ≥10%	GELA		GELA
≥2 extranodal sites	CHHRI, GELA, DFCI	CHHRI, MDAH, GELA	CCHRI, GELA, DFCI

CHHRI: Christie Hospital and Holt Radium Institute, Manchester, England [17].
DFCI: Dana-Farber Cancer Institute, Boston, MA [23, 31].
GELA: Groupe d'Etude des Lymphomes Agressifs, Lyon, France [16].
JLSG: Japanese Lymphoma Study Group, Tokyo, Japan [22].
MDAH: M.D. Anderson Hospital and Tumor Institute, Houston, TX [15, 21, 24].
MSKCC: Memorial Sloan-Kettering Cancer Center, New York, NY [8].
NCI: National Cancer Institute, Bethesda, MD [20].
SWOG: Southwest Oncology Group, USA [19].
UNMC: University of Nebraska Medical Center, Omaha, NE [25].

Table 2. Potentially important prognostic parameters associated with poorer survival in large cell lymphomas.

Chromosomal abnormalities:
Chromosome 5 [34]
Chromosome 6 [34]
Chromosome 7 [32]
Chromosome 17 [32, 33, 34]
Chromosome 18 [34]

Proliferative index:
^{3}H-thymidine labelling index [35]
DNA-malignancy grade [36]
Ki-67 antigen positive-cells [38, 43]
Mitotic index [36]
% of cells in S-phase [38, 39]

karyotypic abnormalities are known. J. O. Armitage summarized studies done on this subject. Some chromosomal abnormalities are correlated with disease characteristics. At present, the number of patients with any specific chromosomal abnormality is too small to allow the definitive assessment of the individual specific abnormalities' independent prognostic significance [34]. Clearly, further studies on specific chromosomal abnormalities, gene alterations, and protooncogene modifications should be carried out before such parameters could be included in the initial staging of lymphoma patients.

Studies of proliferative activity of lymphoma cells are highly correlated with survival [35–40] (Table 2). A higher percentage of cells in S phase or S + G_2M phase has been associated with a poorer outcome [36, 37] but was not found statistically associated with survival in large trials analyzed with multiparametric methods. DNA aneuploidy and low proliferative activity predict a favorable outcome [41]. D. Crowther presented results of flow cytometric estimation of DNA content to correlate outcome and DNA ploidy or cell proliferative activity [42]. If proliferative activity correlates with histological subtype and response to therapy, it is not a clearly independent predictor of outcome. Ki-67 monoclonal antibody detects a nuclear antigen associated with cell proliferation. High proliferative activity, defined as nuclear Ki-67 expression in the majority of lymphoma cells was found to be a strong independent predictor of poor survival [43].

The significance of most of the factors described in Table 1 disappears when multiparametric statistics are applied. Features associated with poor response to treatment and poor survival are age older than 60 or 65 year, impaired performance status (2 or greater), stage III and IV, presence of multiple extranodal sites, tumor mass greater than or equal to 10 cm, particularly if abdominal, low serum albumin level, and elevated LDH level. One recent series also defined β2-microglobulin levels as reflective of tumor mass and prognosis, especially when combined with LDH [24].

Prognostic index in large cell lymphomas

Several interested institutions have analyzed their data with multiparametric methods and have described a prognostic index. A prognostic index takes parameters remaining significant in the multiparametric study and described the relative risk of death for each association. Using this technique, the whole group of patients can be partitioned into smaller subgroups, each with a different risk of relapse or death. Consistently, then, three groups with increasing risk of death are identified. In large cell lymphomas, five such analyses have been published from four institutions.

The Dana-Farber Cancer Institute first presented an analysis on 121 patients in 1986, then an extended analysis on 215 patients in 1990 [23, 31]. All patients were treated with the m/M-BACOD regimen. Risk groups were defined as: low risk, patients with good performance status with no more than one extranodal site of disease and the largest mass size less than 10 cm; moderate risk, patients with good performance status with either a small mass and two or more extranodal sites of disease or massive (≥10 cm) bulky disease and less than two extranodal involvement; high risk, patients with good performance status but massive bulky disease and two or more extranodal sites of disease, or with poor performance status regardless of other factors. In the expanded study, disseminated stage (Ann Arbor stage III or IV), that is more easily measurable than performance status, assumed more importance for

survival than in the initial analysis with smaller numbers.

The Memorial Sloan-Kettering Cancer Center study, presented in 1986 [18], described four subgroups of patients with decreasing survival: group I, patients with normal LDH level; group II, patients with medium LDH level with peripheral lymph nodes and/or extranodal sites; group III, patients with either high LDH level and peripheral lymph nodes and/or extranodal sites, or with medium LDH level and mediastinal or retroperitoneal lymph nodes; group IV, patients with high LDH level and mediastinal or retroperitoneal lymph nodes.

The M. D. Anderson Hospital and Tumor Institute has presented two indexes, the first in 1986 based on LDH level and tumor burden [21] which was recently modified [44], and the second in 1989 based on LDH and serum β2-microglobulin levels [24]. In the first prognostic index, low risk patients (stage A) have a normal LDH level and a low tumor burden; stage B (intermediate risk) patients have either low tumor burden and high LDH level or intermediate tumor burden and low LDH level; stage C (intermediate risk) patients have either intermediate tumor burden and high LDH level or high tumor burden and low LDH level; high risk (stage D) patients have high tumor burden and high LDH level. The clinical estimate of tumor burden is based on the number of bulky areas and extranodal sites of disease. For the second prognostic index, β2-microglobulin level was found to be highly correlated with tumor burden and stage and thus incorporated in the index. Low risk patients have normal LDH level and β2-microglobulin level less than 3 mg/L; medium risk patients have either increased LDH or β2-microglobulin levels; high risk patients have elevated LDH and β2-microglobulin levels.

The 'Groupe d'Etude des Lymphomes Agressifs' has presented an index described after analysis of the 737 patients included in the LNH-84 regimen [16]. There are three risk groups: low risk, patients with localized disease, Ann Arbor stage I or II, with tumor mass less than 10 cm, with less than 2 extranodal sites of disease, and with normal LDH level; medium risk, patients with either elevated LDH level and localized disease and no bulky tumor and less than 2 extranodal sites of disease, or normal LDH level and one or two of the following adverse parameters, advanced Ann Arbor stage, 2 or more extranodal sites of disease, or tumor ≥10 cm; high risk, patients with either normal LDH level and advanced stage and 2 or more extranodal sites of disease and tumor mass ≥10 cm, or elevated LDH level and advances Ann Arbor stage or 2 or more sites of extranodal involvement or tumor mass greater than or equal to 10 cm. This index applies to overall survival and disease-free survival.

The prognostic indexes described by these institutions do not differ greatly. They are all based on the same clinical parameters: tumor mass and tumor dissemination and biological factors reflecting the tumor mass or growth characteristics of the tumor such as LDH or β2-microglobulin levels. Due to the discrepancies associated with the measurement of proliferative activity by DNA content or percentage of cells in S phase, it seems too early to incorporate such a parameter in a prognostic schema. Data obtained to date from cytogenetic analysis suggest that this prognostic information is independent of that provided by clinical and histologic features but these data are too fragmentary to be used for a prognostic system in 1990. However, all participants to the Workshop agreed that a useful and powerful prognostic factor classification should be described and that such a prognostic index should be clinically and biologically sound, easy to remember, broadly applicable, and reproducible. Ideally, it should apply to all patients with lymphoma and be able to identify patients with high risk of early relapse and death.

In conclusion, participants to the Workshop agreed that a common prognostic scheme should be used by physicians reporting treatment of lymphoma patients. This common prognostic system would permit identification of risk categories for patients. The Workshop proposed a new Lugano Prognostic Index as an initial attempt to establish an easy, widely-applicable prognostic classification for large-cell lymphomas. The next step will be to analyze patients treated by major institutions around the world in order to validate this proposed prognostic index.

References

1. Rappaport H. Tumors of the hematopoietic system. In Atlas of Tumor Pathology. Section III, Fasc. 8. Washington DC: Armed Forced Institute of Pathology, 1966.
2. Lukes RJ, Collins RD. Immunologic characterization of human malignant lymphomas. Cancer 1974; 34: 1488–1503.
3. Lennert K. Histopathology of non-Hodgkin's lymphomas (based on the Kiel classification). Springer-Verlag, Berlin 1981.
4. The non-Hodgkin's lymphoma pathologic classification project. National Cancer Institute sponsored study of classifications of non-Hodgkin's lymphomas. Summary and description of a Working Formulation for clinical usage. Cancer 1982; 49: 2112–35.
5. Carbone PP, Kaplan HS, Musshoff K et al. Report of the committee on Hodgkin's disease staging classification. Cancer Res 1971; 31: 1860–1.
6. DeVita VT, Chabner B, Hubbard SP et al. Advanced diffuse histiocytic lymphoma, a potentially curable disease. Results with combination chemotherapy. Lancet 1975; 1: 248–50.
7. Skarin AT, Canellos GP, Rosenthal DS et al. Improved prognosis of diffuse histiocytic and undifferentiated lymphoma by use of high dose methotrexate alternating with standard agents (M-BACOD). J Clin Oncol 1983; 1: 91–8.
8. Klimo P, Connors JM. MACOP-B chemotherapy for the treatment of diffuse large-cell lymphoma. Ann Int Med 1985; 102: 596–602.
9. Coleman M, Gerstein G, Topilow A et al. Advances in chemotherapy for large cell lymphoma. Sem Hematol 1987; 24, S1: 8–20.
10. Jagannath S, Velasquez WS, Tucker SL et al. Stage IV diffuse large cell lymphoma: a long term analysis. J Clin Oncol 1985; 3: 39–47.
11. Coiffier B, Bryon PA, Berger F et al. Intensive and sequential combination chemotherapy for aggressive malignant lymphomas (Protocol LNH-80). J Clin Oncol 1986; 4: 47–153.
12. Fisher RI, DeVita VT, Hubbard SM et al. Diffuse aggressive lymphomas: increased survival after alternating flexible sequences of ProMACE and MOPP chemotherapy. Ann Int Med 1983; 98: 304–9.
13. Armitage JO, Cheson BD. Interpretation of clinical trials in diffuse large-cell lymphoma. J Clin Oncol 1988; 6: 1335–47.
14. Coiffier B, Lepage E. Prognosis of aggressive lymphomas: a study of five prognostic models with patients included in the LNH-84 regimen. Blood 1989; 74: 558–64.
15. Cabanillas F, Burke JS, Smith TL et al. Factors predicting for response and survival in adults with advanced non-Hodgkin's lymphoma. Arch Int Med 1978; 138: 413–8.
16. Coiffier B, Gisselbrecht C, Vose JM et al. Prognostic factors in aggressive malignant lymphomas: description and validation of a prognostic index that could identify patients requiring a more intensive therapy. J Clin Oncol 1990 (to be published).
17. Cowan RA, Jones M, Harris M et al. Prognostic factors in high and intermediate grade non-Hodgkin's lymphoma. Brit J Cancer 1989; 59: 276–82.
18. Danieu L, Wong G, Koziner B et al. Predictive model for prognosis in advanced diffuse histiocytic lymphoma. Cancer Res 1986; 46: 5372–9.
19. Dixon DO, Neilan B, Jones SE et al. Effect of age on therapeutic outcome in advanced diffuse histiocytic lymphoma: the Southwest Oncology Group experience. J Clin Oncol 1986; 4: 295–305.
20. Fisher RI, Hubbard SM, DeVita VT et al. Factors predicting long-term survival in diffuse mixed, histiocytic, or undifferentiated lymphoma. Blood 1981; 58: 45–51.
21. Jagannath S, Velasquez WS, Tucker SL et al. Tumor burden assessment and its implication for a prognostic model in advanced diffuse large-cell lymphoma. J Clin Oncol 1986; 4: 859–65.
22. Shimoyama M, Ota K, Kikuchi M et al. Chemotherapeutic results and prognostic factors of patients with advanced non-Hodgkin's lymphoma treated with VEPA or VEPA-M. J Clin Oncol 1988; 5: 128–41.
23. Shipp MA, Harrington DP, Klatt MM et al. Identification of major prognostic subgroups of patients with large-cell lymphoma treated with m-BACOD or M-BACOD. Ann Inter Med 1986; 104: 757–65.
24. Swan F, Velasquez WS, Tucker S et al. A new serologic staging system for large-cell lymphomas based on initial β2-microglobulin and lactate dehydrogenase levels. J Clin Oncol 1989; 7: 1518–27.
25. Vose JM, Armitage JO, Weisenburger DD et al. The importance of age in survival of patients treated with chemotherapy for aggressive non-Hodgkin's lymphoma. J Clin Oncol 1988; 6: 1838–44.
26. Simon R, Durrleman S, Hoppe RT et al. The non-Hodgkin lymphoma pathologic classification project. Long-term follow-up of 1153 patients with non-Hodgkin's lymphomas. Ann Int Med 1988; 109: 939–45.
27. Coiffier B, Brousse N, Peuchmaur M et al. Peripheral T-cell lymphomas have a worse prognosis than B-cell lymphomas: a prospective study of 361 immunophenotyped patients treated with the LNH-84 regimen. Ann Oncol 1990; 1: 45–50.
28. Lippman SM, Miller TP, Spier CM et al. The prognostic significance of the immunotype in diffuse large-cell lymphoma: a comparative study of the T-cell and B-cell phenotype. Blood 1988; 72: 436–441.
29. Shimizu K, Hamajima N, Ohnishi K et al. T-cell phenotype is associated with decreased survival in non-Hodgkin's lymphoma. Jap J Cancer Res 1989; 80: 720–6.
30. Armitage JO, Weisenburger DD, Hutchins M et al. Chemotherapy for diffuse large-cell lymphoma. Rapidly responding patients have more durable remissions. J Clin Oncol 1986; 4: 160–4.

31. Shipp MA, Yeap BY, Harrington DP et al. The M-BACOD combination chemotherapy regimen in large-cell lymphoma: analysis of the completed trial and comparison with the M-BACOD regimen. J Clin Oncol 1990; 8: 84–93.

32. Cabanillas F, Pathak S, Grant G et al. Refractoriness to chemotherapy and poor survival related to abnormalities of chromosomes 17 and 7 in lymphoma. Amer J Med 1989; 87: 167–72.

33. Levine EG, Arthur DC, Frizzera G et al. Cytogenetic abnormalities predict clinical outcome in non-Hodgkin lymphoma. Ann Inter Med 1988; 108: 14–20.

34. Schouten HC, Sanger WG, Weisenburger DD et al. Chromosomal abnormalities in untreated patients with non-Hodgkin's lymphoma: associations with histology, clinical characteristics, and treatment outcome. Blood 1990; 75: 1841–7.

35. Silvestrini R, Costa A, Giardini R et al. Prognostic implications of cell kinetics, histopathology and pathologic stage in non-Hodgkin's lymphomas. Hematol Oncol 1989; 7: 411–22.

36. Akerman M, Brandt L, Johnson A et al. Mitotic activity in non-Hodgkin's lymphoma. Relation to the Kiel classification and to prognosis. Brit J Cancer 1987; 55: 219–23.

37. Bocking A, Chatelain R, Auffermann W et al. DNA-grading of malignant lymphomas. I. Prognostic significance, reproducibility and comparison with other classifications. Anticancer Res 1986; 6: 1205–16.

38. Christensson B, Lindemalm C, Johansson B et al. Flow cytometric DNA analysis: a prognostic tool in non-Hodgkin's lymphoma. Leukemia Res 1989; 13: 307–14.

39. Jalkanen S, Joensuu H, Klemi P. Prognostic value of lymphocyte homing receptor and S-phase fraction in non-Hodgkin's lymphoma. Blood 1990; 75: 1549–56.

40. Weiss LM, Strickler JG, Madeiros LJ et al. Proliferative rates of non-Hodgkin's lymphomas as assessed by Ki-67 antibody. Hum Pathol 1987; 18: 1155–9.

41. Wooldridge TN, Grierson HL, Weisenburger DD et al. Association of DNA content and proliferative activity with clinical outcome in patients with diffuse mixed cell and large cell non-Hodgkin's lymphoma. Cancer Res 1988; 48: 6608–13.

42. Cowan RA, Harris M, Jones M, Crowther D. DNA content in high and intermediate grade non-Hodgkin's lymphoma. Prognostic significance and clinicopathological correlations. Brit J Cancer 1989; 60: 904–10.

43. Grogan TM, Lippman SM, Spier C et al. Independent prognostic significance of a nuclear proliferation antigen in diffuse large cell lymphomas as determined by the monoclonal antibody Ki-67. Blood 1988; 71: 1157–60.

44. Velasquez WS, Jagannath S, Tucker SL et al. Risk classification as the basis for clinical staging of diffuse large-cell lymphoma derived from 10-year survival data. Blood 1989; 74: 551–7.

Correspondence to:
Professeur B. Coiffier
Hematology Service
Centre Hospitalier Lyon-Sud
69310 Pierre-Bénite, France

Annals of Oncology, Supplement 2 to Volume 2: 219–223, 1991.
© 1991 Kluwer Academic Publishers.

Original article —————————————————————————————————

Workshop on pediatric lymphomas: Current results and prospects

Sharon B. Murphy[1] & Ian T. Magrath[2]

[1] Chief, Division of Hematology/Oncology, Children's Memorial Hospital and Professor of Pediatrics, Northwestern University School of Medicine; [2] Head, Lymphoma Biology Section, Pediatric Oncology Branch, Division of Cancer Treatment, National Cancer Institute

Introduction and scope

In the last 15 years we have witnessed a remarkable improvement in the survival rates of children and adolescents with Hodgkin's disease (HD) and non-Hodgkin's lymphoma (NHL) – an improvement that continues today. Just 20 years ago, only some 30–40% of children with localized NHL could be expected to achieve long-term survival, and vanishingly few with extensive disease survived. Currently 80–90% of all lymphomas, HD and NHL, are curable. This progress has been the result of many factors, not the least of these being the conduct of controlled clinical trials. The well-organized and disciplined trials conducted during the last decade by the German group for pediatric HD (see Table 1) are a model in this regard [1].

In the present Lugano conference, the major focus in the field of pediatric NHL was on the excellent results that have been recently obtained in patients with small noncleaved (B) cell neoplasia involving the bone marrow and (or) central nervous system – the worst prognostic category. Three different groups of investigators, the Pediatric Oncology Group (POG), the French Pediatric Oncology Society (SFOP), and the Berlin-Frankfurt-Munster (BFM) Group described chemotherapy regimens [2, 3, 4] that result in survival rates of 70–80% among stage III and IV patients with childhood B-cell NHL, bringing the overall survival of all childhood NHL cases to approximately 80–90%. This is a remarkable accomplishment, particularly in view of the fact that, until now, patients with stage IV disease have had an expected survival of only 10–40% (lower figures obtaining in patients with CNS disease) in most reported studies. None of the three protocols described include systemic irradiation, and there can no longer be any doubt that the application of the latter modality would serve only to increase toxicity without any therapeutic gain, and could result in therapeutic loss. One of these protocols (the BFM protocol) and another primary protocol described in this meeting incorporated ifosfamide into the regimen, and phase II protocols that included this drug were also discussed. Finally, the immunophenotype, clinical features, and response to treatment of Ki-1-positive anaplastic large-cell lymphomas, a quite recently described group of diseases, were discussed.

Table 1. Outline of 4 German therapy studies for Hodgkin's disease.

	HD-78	HD-82		HD-85	HD-87
Lymphography	–	–		–	–
Ultrasonography	–	most patients		all patients	all patients
Laparotomy	all patients	all patients		selectively	selectively
Splenectomy	all patients	selectively		selectively	selectively
Chemotherapy	OPPA / COPP	OPPA / COP		OPA / COMP	
I / IIA	2 cycles	2		2	2 OPA
IIB / IIIA	6 cycles	4		4	2 OPA + 2 COPP
IIIB / IV	6 cycles	6		6	2 OPPA + 4 COPP
Radiotherapy					
field	extended	involved		involved	involved
dose	IF 36–40 Gy	I / IIA	35 Gy	35 Gy	30 Gy
	AF 36–40 Gy versus	IIB / IIIA	30 Gy	30 Gy	25 Gy
	AF 18–20 Gy	IIIB / IV	25 Gy	25 Gy	20 Gy

220

Hodgkin's disease

The continuing challenge of management of HD remains the refinement and development of risk-adapted therapies designed to maintain high rates of curability (85–90% overall) while simultaneously reducing the acute and long-term adverse consequences of therapy, particularly sterility and second malignant neoplasms. It was therefore disheartening to learn the results of the recent German trial (DAL-HD-85) which demonstrated that the elimination of procarbazine from the combination chemotherapy regimens resulted in an unacceptable frequency of relapse.

Schellong et al. [5] reported that the aim of their trial, DAL-HD-85, was to reduce chemotherapy in comparison to trial HD-82, primarily to avoid the gonadotoxic effects in males. In their experience, at least 40–60% of surviving young men treated on HD-82 had elevated follicle-stimulating hormone (FSH) levels. Consequently, in HD-85, procarbazine was eliminated from OPPA (resulting in OPA) and replaced by methotrexate in COPP, resulting in COMP. Other aspects of staging and management are outlined in Table 1.

It is worth noting that the German algorithm to limit invasive staging only to those with the highest probability of intraabdominal involvement allowed for selective performance of laparotomy (in 60%) and splenectomy (in 32%) in DAL-HD-85. Unfortunately, the strategy to omit procarbazine resulted in relapse in 24 of the 98 patients who attained a CR, i.e., event-free survival (EFS) of only 45–55% for stages IIB-IV at four years, compared to 90–96% in HD-82, a clearly unacceptable result which led to study closure and the need to salvage the relapsing patients.

Concerning salvage, Bessa et al. [6] presented their experience with 22 children and adolescents with relapsed or refractory HD who were treated with high-dose combination chemotherapy regimens (mainly BCNU, cyclophosphamide, and VP-16) followed by autologous bone marrow transplant (ABMT). This French experience with ABMT for HD is the largest yet reported in childhood (median age 13, range 5–17). Results confirm the experience in adults, i.e., about half of the patients survived (58% EFS at 24 months), and the status of the patient prior to the high-dose chemotherapy is predictive of outcome (i.e., 6 of 6 treated in complete remission are alive).

Improved results in stage IV B cell lymphomas and B cell ALL

In discussing the reported results, a word must first be said about nomenclature. Firstly, the term *B-cell disease* (implying the presence of surface immunoglobulin) is used even though not all tumors are immunophenotyped, so that a small number of patients may not, in fact, have B-cell disease. The group of childhood

Table 2. Results reported in childhood B cell ALL / stage IV B cell lymphoma.

Group	No. Pts.	B ALL	St IV NHL	BM + CNS	BM − CNS
POG	51	51%	78%		
SFOP	34[a]			72%	82%
BFM	53	74%	77%		

[a] 23 had CNS involvement.

B-cell lymphomas is generally taken to include the large-cell and small, noncleaved lymphomas, sometimes jointly referred to as the 'nonlymphoblastic lymphomas,' which many pediatric oncologists treat according to the same protocols. A small proportion of lymphoblastic lymphomas do, however, express B-cell markers, but not surface immunoglobulin, i.e., they are of pre-B phenotype. Secondly, the arbitrary division between leukemia and lymphoma – based upon greater than or less than 25% blast cells in the bone marrow, respectively – appears to serve no useful purpose. None of the three groups reported a significant difference in outcome between patient groups divided according to this criterion, although the POG group showed a trend that favored stage IV NHL. Yet this highly questionable distinction, (the diagnosis could depend upon the adequacy of bone marrow sampling or simply on temporal factors) has led to the current use of the cumbersome rubric of 'stage IV B-cell lymphoma and B-cell leukemia.' Biologically, these diseases are identical in terms of immunophenotype and karyotype although more detailed molecular characterization (of chromosomal breakpoint locations) would be of interest. Nonetheless, from the clinical perspective, it would seem that a good case could be made for allaying confusion by using the same nomenclature for both. Why not simply abandon the term B-cell leukemia, and abolish the <25% bone marrow blasts as a requirement for a patient to qualify as B-cell lymphoma (purists might prefer the term *B-cell neoplasm*)? This would force investigators to focus upon the most important issue, which is not the percentage of blast cells in the bone marrow, but rather the overall tumor burden. Serum lactate dehydrogenase (LDH) and soluble IL-2 receptor levels have been shown to be useful correlates of tumor burden, and it would be of interest to determine whether the three series were comparable with each other (as well as with other reported series) in this respect, as well as with respect to the presence of extensive disease outside the bone marrow; and whether such factors remain of prognostic significance in spite of the very good results achieved.

Whilst we could, perhaps, rest on the laurels of the outstanding achievements reported at the Lugano meeting (Table 1) and treat all future patients with one or other of these protocols [2, 3, 4], it might be more appropriate to turn our attention to such questions as, If we can cure 80% of patients, can we cure 100%? and

Could equally good results be achieved with less toxic and perhaps simpler, or even shorter-duration, therapy? The POG protocol, for example, resulted in a 20% incidence of grade 3–4 neurotoxicity, which was also seen in some of the French patients, and six to eight months of therapy may be more than is necessary. In order to answer these questions, it is necessary to attempt to determine the reasons for the improved results, so that future modifications to the chemotherapeutic regimens maintain those elements or principles that are essential, and remove noncontributory components.

How, then, do these protocols compare with their predecessors and with other, apparently less successful, protocols? Are drug doses higher? Are new drugs added? Is the duration of therapy different? And how is successful CNS prophylaxis or treatment accomplished? The authors have implied that changes made in their protocols, particularly the inclusion of higher doses of S-phase-specific agents as intravenous infusions, are responsible for their improved results. The BFM protocol includes a substantially higher dose of methotrexate ($5 g/m^2$), while the POG protocol has been modified to include a higher dose of cytarabine (Ara-C) from the outset (it already included $1 g/m^2$ methotrexate), and the French protocol includes both high-dose methotrexate ($8 g/m^2$) and high-dose Ara-C. Attainment of cytotoxic levels of these agents within the central nervous system by high-dose systemic intravenous therapy is also intended – and, no doubt, contributes to the success of these efforts – to control to disease in this sanctuary site. It would seem probable that these high-dose infusions of S-phase-specific agents are important. But are they particularly important in the context of bone marrow disease and/or of CNS disease? And are both drugs needed? At present, there are no answers to these questions, since controlled studies have not been done (and, indeed, would be very difficult in view of the small number of such cases accrued, even to cooperative group studies). An alternative possibility that should be considered is whether at least some component of the improved results has not simply resulted from increased experience, i.e., a confidence born of familiarity with the side effects of these or similar protocols and their successful management, with resultant improved adherence to planned dosage. A precedent for this exists is testicular cancer. In his recent Karnofsky Memorial Lecture at the 1990 meeting of the American Society of Clinical Oncology, Einhorn pointed out that disease-free survival rates have improved in disseminated testicular cancer from 57% in 1976 to 80% today without any change in the chemotherapy regimen. Similarly, in the Children's Cancer Group trial designed to investigate the role of an anthracycline in nonlymphoblastic lymphomas, treatment in the control arm (which was identical to that used more than 10 years ago and reported upon in 1983) has resulted in EFS rates about 20% higher than those originally published. Have pediatric oncologists in the United States and Europe simply improved their skills over the years?

One possible explanation as to how experience may translate into improved survival, when improved outcome is not simply a consequence of a reduction in toxic deaths, is that the achieved dose intensity – i.e., the dose per square meter per week of protocol drugs – has been increased. In a recent analysis of a National Cancer Institute (NCI) protocol (77–04), one of us (I.M.) found that dose intensity during the first two cycles was significantly associated with EFS in patients with small noncleaved-cell lymphomas. Improvements in survival rates of more than 20% were observed in patients with dose intensities of cyclophosphamide and methotrexate above 70% of the planned dose compared to patients in whom dose intensity was less than this. It would be of interest to submit the three protocols reported here to similar analysis. Indeed, a comparison of dose intensity achieved in these protocols and in less successful ones, with account being taken of the additional delay in bone marrow recovery incurred by patients with bone marrow involvement, would be of considerable interest. If dose intensity significantly affects outcome, it would be important to build this into the protocol design, and to plan dosage in terms of the optimal dose (i.e., that dose and schedule which results in the highest dose intensity) of the most effective agents. Such protocols could prove to be less toxic insofar as superfluous therapy would be avoided. In addition, dose intensity could be monitored during therapy and steps taken to ensure that the highest possible dose intensity is achieved. Perhaps this would result in both streamlining the protocols and even further improving the results.

An additional change made in the BFM '86 protocol was the introduction or ifosfamide. Two other presentations in this session discussed the use of this drug in patients with NHL [7, 8]. The NCI phase I and Phase II data clearly demonstrated that ifosfamide is an active drug in small noncleaved-cell lymphoma, even in a group of very high-risk patients with progressive, recurrent disease. Many of the patients had previously been treated with very high-dose cyclophosphamide-containing regimens such as BACT, raising the possibility that ifosfamide may be non-cross-resistant with cyclophosphamide, and perhaps even a better drug in this disease. The data from Egyptian trials, in which alternating cyclophosphamide and ifosfamide cycles are used, are also of interest in this regard. In the Egyptian series, most of the deaths occurred during induction – a number of the patients were in extremely poor condition at presentation, and resources for supportive care are not as advanced in Egypt. Nonetheless, all patients who achieved complete response (82%) attained prolonged survival, attesting to the efficacy of this protocol. These data raise the question as to how important it is to include ifosfamide in the treatment regimen – possibly even to the exclusion of cyclophosphamide. Only randomized comparisons will provide an answer to this question, and we must decide whether it is important enough to ask.

As pediatric oncologists, influenced by the successful results of the long-duration therapy use as standard treatment for acute lymphoblastic leukemia, we have taken many years to realize that the B-cell lymphomas can be effectively treated with much shorter durations of therapy (although the earliest regimens for Burkitt's lymphoma, which cured a number of patients, were often only two to three cycles. But what is the minimum of cycles that, from the perspective of outcome can safely be given? In the NCI experience, an association with dose intensity could only be demonstrated for cycles 1 and 2 in protocol 77-04 (the commencement of cycle 3 determined the dose intensity of cycle 2). This could be interpreted as indicating that any treatment given after cycle 3 may take no contribution to outcome – a conclusion that is consistent with the empirical experience of the BFM group's use of short-duration therapy, the earlier experience in Africa, the NCI results with only two or three cycles of therapy, and the data reported from Egypt, which showed that an eight-cycle protocol was as effective, if not more effective, than a protocol including three years of maintenance therapy. If so few cycles are necessary, then providing that the best drugs at the highest dose intensity are used, the introduction of different agents after two or more cycles of therapy (as is done in the French protocol) may accomplish little. Or, if the introduction of new agents changes outcomes, perhaps the induction regimen itself is suboptimal.

It would seem that a major task that we must now undertake is to determine which drugs or which components of each protocol are the most important, and which are superfluous. Such fine tuning is likely to further improve survival rates, but with a simultaneous lessening of toxicity, since the use of less active agents could well result in a lessening of the dose intensity of more active agents, and so detract from the efficacy of the protocol.

One seemingly remarkable finding in the French study, is the excellent survival of patients with central nervous system (CNS) disease. As recently as 1987, Philip and colleagues suggested that patients with CNS disease at presentation constituted one of two groups of patients in whom further intensification of therapy is indicated [9]. He has also presented results suggesting that high-dose therapy with autologous bone marrow support may improve the outcome of such patients. These results, coupled with the SFOP results reported in this meeting, support a contention that was made several years ago, namely that CNS disease is not per se an obstacle to cure (intrathecal therapy combined with methotrexate or Ara-C infusions must clearly be highly effective). On the contrary, it may be that CNS disease occurs most often in patients with the highest tumor burden, and that the latter is the cause of the poor prognosis. In the NCI series, although admittedly with an inferior outcome, we have not been able to discern a difference between patients with and without CNS disease when both groups have similarly high tumor burdens. This is also consistent with data from Africa, where patients with CNS disease, unlike their Western counterparts, often have rather small tumor burdens and, in this circumstance, a correspondingly better outcome. But regardless of whether high-dose systemic administration of these agents is necessary to eliminate CNS disease, a possibility that is supported by the French results presented at this meeting, high-dose infusions of S-phase specific agents are likely to be effective against both systemic and CNS disease. Therefore, high-dose infusions of these agents probably represent an important component of therapy, and one of the reasons for the improved overall results reported. We simply need to decide whether to use one or both drugs, and to identify the dose and schedule that will produce the best result with the least toxicity. In this regard, the fact that activation of Ara-C to Ara-CTP by kinases – particularly the first step, which is catalyzed by deoxycytidine kinase – is saturable needs to be taken into account. Too high an infusion rate will have no advantage in terms of survival, but a distinct disadvantage with respect to toxicity.

It is questionable whether CNS irradiation played a role in the results of the French group, the only investigators who used this therapeutic modality. The BFM group has been unimpressed by its efficacy, and has excluded it from its most recent protocol; but since systemic therapy was also less effective in former trials, and the present BFM trial has too few patients with CNS disease to draw any conclusions, this issue remains unresolved. Based on the general experience with radiation in the B-cell lymphomas, however, it would seem likely that this modality makes little or no contribution to the outcome of therapy. It is an important issue, because when radiation is combined with high-dose systemic infusions of methotrexate and Ara-C, it is to be expected that there will be a significant price to pay in terms of CNS toxicity.

Large-cell anaplastic lymphomas bearing the Ki-1 antigen (CD30)

For a long time it has been apparent that the large-cell lymphomas are a heterogenous mixture of tumors. A subset of these tumors, identified by a rather typical morphology, express an antigen (Ki-1, CD30) originally identified by a monoclonal antibody that reacts with Reed-Sternberg and Hodgkin cells raised against a Hodgkin's disease-derived cell line. The antigen is now considered to be a lymphoid activation antigen and provides an objective marker which considerably aids the diagnosis of the anaplastic large-cell lymphomas. These lymphomas have in the past often been confused with nonlymphoid tumors, including atypical malignant histiocytosis and even amelanotic melanomas and carcinomas. Kadin et al. [10] originally described this entity and recently reported 19 cases of Ki-1 + lymphomas in detail, (including six previously reported) and speculated that a retrovirus of the human T-cell lymphoma virus family could play a role in the pathogenesis of this tumor of activated T cells.

Two groups – a combined Austrian/German consortium and the University of Bologna – reported their findings in children and adolescents with Ki-1+ anaplastic large-cell lymphomas (ALC) in this meeting [11, 12]. Eleven of the Austrian/German patients were originally diagnosed as having malignant histiocytosis; 28 were included in the BFM B-cell lymphoma protocols, and 8 were identified per primum. The 13 patients studied in Bologna were identified among 78 NHL patients. Both groups made the point that while some (but apparently not all) ALC lymphomas expressed the Ki-1 antigen, there were three immunophenotypes: T (the majority), B (the minority), and null, possibly histiocytic (rare patients). This reported immunophenotypic heterogeneity differs from the original series reported by Kadin and certainly blurs the distinctiveness of this new syndrome. Indeed, until further reports demonstrate the reproducibility in recognition of this morphologic subtype of large-cell lymphomas, the limits of this syndrome remain indistinct.

References

1. Schellong G, Brämswig H, Schwarze EW, Wannemacher M. An approach to reduce treatment and invasive staging in childhood Hodgkin's disease: the sequence of the German DAL Multicenter Studies. Bull Cancer 1988; 75: 41–52.
2. Bowman WP, Shuster J, Cook B, Behm F, Berard C, Murphy SB. Results of treatment for advanced stage (IV) diffuse small non-cleaved cell non-Hodgkins (NHL) lymphomas and B(SIg+) cell acute lymphoblastic leukemia (ALL): The Pediatric Oncology Group (POG) Experience, 1986–89. Abstract –40. Fourth International Conference on Malignant Lymphoma, Lugano, June, 1990.
3. Patte C, Perel Y, Leverger G, Rubie H, Otten J, Plantaz D, Munzer M, Boutard P, Benz-Lemoine E, Pautard B, Kalifa C. High survival rate of B-cell non Hodgkin's lymphomas (B-NHL) with CNS involvement (CNS+) and B-ALL. Results of the LBM 86 protocol of the French Pediatric Oncology Society (SFOP). Abstract –39. Fourth International Conference on Malignant Lymphoma, Lugano, June 1990.
4. Reiter A, Sauter S, Müller-Weihrich S, Kühl J, Gadner H, Riehm H. BFM therapy strategy and results in advanced childhood B-cell neoplasias (stage-IV B-NHL; B-ALL). Abstract –38. Fourth International Conference on Malignant Lymphoma, Lugano, June 1990.
5. Schellong G, Hörnig-Franz I, Brämswig J, Wannenmacher M. Hodgkin's disease in children: treatment reduction by elimination of procarbazine from OPPA/COPP chemotherapy. Results of the German Cooperative Study DAL-HD-85. Abstract –32. Fourth International Conference on Malignant Lymphoma, Lugano, June 1990.
6. Bessa E, Oberlin O, Hartman O, Michon J, Bordigoni J, Hervé P, Demeocq, Plantaz D, Philip T, Michel G, Baruchel A, Leverger G. High-dose combination chemotherapy for childhood Hodgkin's disease: The French Pediatric Oncology Society Experience. Abstract –33. Fourth International Conference on Malignant Lymphoma, Lugano, June 1990.
7. Magrath IT, Adde M, Sandlund J, Jain V. Ifosfamide (IF) in the treatment of high-grade, recurrent B cell lymphomas: experience of the Pediatric Branch, National Cancer Institute. Abstract –37. Fourth International Conference on Malignant Lymphoma, Lugano, June 1990.
8. Gad-El-Mawla N, Hamza MR, Abdel-Hadi S, Hussein MH, El-Tannir O, Magrath I. Prolonged disease free survival in pediatric non-Hodgkin's lymphoma using ifosfamide containing combination chemotherapy. Abstract –36. Fourth International Conference on Malignant Lymphoma, Lugano, June 1990.
9. Philip T, Pinkerton R, Hartmann O, Patte C, Philip I, Biron P, Favrot M. The role of massive therapy with autologous bone marrow transplantation in Burkitt's lymphoma. Clinics in Haematology 1986; 15: (1) 205–17.
10. Agnarsson BA, Kadin ME. Ki-1 positive large cell lymphoma: a morphologic and immunologic study of 19 cases. Am J Surg Pathol 1988; 12(4): 264–74.
11. Bucsky P, Feller AC, Reiter A, Heitger A, Gadner H, Riehm H. Malignant histiocytosis and large cell anaplastic (Ki-1) lymphoma in children and adolescents – preliminary experiences of the BFM Study Group. Abstract –34. Fourth International Conference on Malignant Lymphoma, Lugano, June 1990.
12. Vecchi V, Pileri S, Burnelli R, Rosito P, Pession A, Rondelli R, Borghetti A, Paolucci G. Anaplastic large-cell lymphoma (Ki-1+/CD30+) in childhood. Abstract –35. Fourth International Conference on Malignant Lymphoma, Lugano, June 1990.

Correspondence to:
Sharon B. Murphy
2300 Children's Plaza
Chicago, IL 60614, USA

Annals of Oncology, Supplement 2 to Volume 2: 225–228, 1991.
© 1991 *Kluwer Academic Publishers*.

Conference program ⎯⎯⎯⎯⎯⎯⎯⎯⎯⎯⎯⎯

Wednesday, June 6, 1990

Bone marrow transplantation
J. O. Armitage, Omaha, USA
Peripheral T-cell lymphomas
R. Zittoun, Paris, France
CNS-lymphoma
B. P. O'Neill, Rochester, USA
Follicular lymphomas
T. A. Lister, London, United Kingdom
Special situations in HD and NHL
J. E. Ultmann, Chicago, USA
Modern radiology in the staging of lymphomas
R. Musumeci, Milan, Italy

Poster Session I/Biological studies

Opening ceremony/Welcome and introductory remarks
F. Cavalli, Bellinzona, Switzerland

Henry Kaplan Memorial Lecture/The influence of information on drug resistance on protocol design
V. T. DeVita, New York, USA

Session 1 — Biology of lymphomas I
Chairmen: C. W. Berard and B. Coiffier

Nature of Sternberg-Reed cells and other biological problems
H. Stein, Berlin, Germany
Low serum interleukin-2 receptor levels correlate with a good prognosis in patients with Hodgkin's disease
M. Pfreundschuh, Cologne, Germany
An epidemiologic view of the new cytogenetic findings in Hodgkin's disease
N. E. Mueller, Boston, USA
Non Hodgkin's lymphoma arising in patients treated for Hodgkin's disease in the BNLI – A 20 year experience
M. H. Bennett et al, London, United Kingdom
Hodgkin's disease and its relation to non Hodgkin's lymphoma
M. L. Hansmann, Kiel, Germany
Peripheral T-cell lymphomas
H. Stein, Berlin, Germany
Current epidemiologic and therapeutic situation in AIDS
S. Broder, Bethesda, USA
Quantitative magnetic resonance studies of lumbar vertebral marrow in patients with refractory or relapsed Hodgkin's disease
S. R. Smith et al, Liverpool, United Kingdom
Key note lecture/Molecular genetics of human B cell neoplasia
C. M. Croce, Philadelphia, USA

Session 2 — General session on HD
Chairman: T. J. McElwain

The continuing challenge of Hodgkin's disease
S. A. Rosenberg, Stanford, USA
Alternating versus hybrid MOPP-ABVD in Hodgkin's disease: The Milan experience
G. Bonadonna, Milan, Italy
Long term toxicity of Hodgkin's disease treatment
J. M. Cosset, Villejuif, France

Session 3 — Proffered papers on HD
Chairmen: S. A. Rosenberg and D. Crowther

A randomised study of adjuvant MVPP chemotherapy after Mantle radiotherapy in PS IA–IIB Hodgkin's disease: 10 year follow up
H. Anderson et al, Manchester, United Kingdom
Evaluation of the toxicity of three courses of ABVD and mediastinal irradiation in favorable Hodgkin's disease
P. Brice et al, Paris, France
Combination chemotherapy with chlorambucil, vinblastine, prednisolone and procarbazine in Hodgkin's disease: 14 year follow up on 284 patients
T. J. McElwain et al, Sutton, United Kingdom
MOPP versus ABVD versus MOPP alternating with ABVD as treatment for advanced Hodgkin's disease: Results at a median follow-up of 4 years
J. R. Anderson et al, Omaha, USA
Management of relapse and survival in advance stages Hodgkin's disease: The EORTC experience
J. M. V. Burgers et al, Amsterdam, The Netherlands
Salvage radiotherapy in recurrent Hodgkin's disease
M. Brada et al, Sutton, United Kingdom
Autologous bone marrow transplantation for refractory or relapsed Hodgkin's disease. The Memorial Sloan-Kettering Cancer Center experience using high dose chemotherapy with and without hypefractionated accelerated total lymphoid irradiation
J. Yahalom et al, New York, USA
100 cases of relapsed Hodgkin's disease treated with

beam chemotherapy and ABMT in a single centre
A. *McMillan et al*, London, United Kingdom
Treatment outcome in Hodgkin's disease in patients above the age of 60: A population-based study
G. *Enblad et al*, Uppsala, Sweden
HIV-related Hodgkin's disease in 50 intravenous users
S. *Monfardini et al*, Aviano, Italy

Poster Session II/Hodgkin's disease

Session 4 — Workshop on 'new diagnostic tools in lymphoma'
Chairmen: C. W. Berard and J. Costa

Some animal models suggesting new links between immunosuppression and lymphoma development
P. *Ebbesen*, Aarhus, Denmark
The impact of molecular biology on the diagnosis, prediction of prognosis, and clinical management of the lymphoma patient
C. L. *Willman*, Albuquerque, Mexico
Phenotypic and functional markers relevant to the diagnosis and prognosis of non Hodgkin's lymphomas
D. *Delia*, Milan, Italy
High frequency of Epstein-Barr virus genome in lymph nodes involved by Hodgkin's disease in HIV+ patients
S. *Uccini et al*, Rome, Italy
Expression of the BCL-2 oncogene product in follicular lymphoma
D. Y. *Mason et al*, Oxford, United Kingdom
Direct sequence analysis of 14Q+ and 18Q- chromosome junctions at the MBR and MCR revealing clustering within the MBR in follicular lymphoma
F. E. *Cotter et al*, London, United Kingdom
Heterogeneity of aggressive lymphomas by ploidy and proliferative activity. Morphologic and prognostic implications
P. *Felman et al*, Lyon, France
α, β and γ, δ T-cell receptors in peripheral T-cell lymphoma
Ph. *Gaulard et al*, Creteil, France
KI67 and 4F2 antigen expression as well as DNA synthesis predict survival at relapse/tumour progression in low-grade B-cell lymphoma
H. *Holte et al*, Oslo, Norway

Session 5 — Lymphoma in childhood
Chairmen: S. B. Murphy and G. Schellong

Hodgkin's disease in children: Treatment reduction by elimination of procarbazine from OPPA/COPP chemotherapy. Results of the German Cooperative Study DAL-HD-85.
G. *Schellong et al*, Münster, Germany
High-dose combination chemotherapy for childhood Hodgkin's disease: The French Pediatric Oncology Society experience

O. *Oberlin et al*, Villejuif, France
Malignant histiocytosis and large cell anaplastic (KI-1) lymphoma in children and adolescents – Preliminary experiences of the BFM study group
P. *Bucsky et al*, Hannover, Germany
Anaplastic large-cell lymphoma (KI-1+/CD30+) in childhood
V. *Vecchi et al*, Bologna, Italy
Prolonged disease free survival in pediatric non-Hodgkin's lymphoma using ifosfamide containing combination chemotherapy
N. *Gad-El-Mawla et al*, Cairo, Egypt
Ifosfamide in the treatment of high-grade, recurrent B-cell lymphomas: Experience of the pediatric branch, National Cancer Institute
I. T. *Magrath et al*, Bethesda, USA
BFM therapy strategy and results in advanced childhood B-cell neoplasias (stage-IV, B-NHL, B-ALL)
A. *Reiter et al*, Hannover, Germany
High survival rate of B-cell non Hodgkin's lymphomas with CNS involvement and B-ALL
C. *Patte et al*, Villejuif, France
Results of treatment for advanced stage diffuse small-non-cleaved cell non-Hodgkin's lymphomas and B-cell acute lymphoblastic leukemia: The Pediatric Oncology Group experience, 1986–89
S. B. *Murphy*, Chicago, USA
Panel discussion: Treatment of stage IV (B) NHL and B-ALL
A. *Reiter, C. Patte and S. B. Murphy*
Rapporteur: *I. Magrath*

Friday, June 8, 1990

Poster Session III/Studies in NHL

Session 6 — Biology of lymphomas II
Chairmen: M. Pfreundschuh and R. Zittoun

Epidemiological, pathological, serological and clinical studies of malignant lymphomas in China
Y. *Sun*, Beijing, China
T-cell lymphoma in Japan
M. *Shimoyama*, Tokyo, Japan
New insights in the biology of lymphomas
L. M. *Nadler*, Boston, USA
The significance of B-clonal excess in peripheral blood in patients with non-Hodgkin's lymphoma in clinical complete remission
A. *Johnson et al*, Lund, Sweden

Intermission

Idiotype expression, sharing and remodeling in follicular lymphoma
R. *Levy*, Stanford, USA
Analysis of T (14; 18) chromosomal breakpoints by

polymerase chain reaction and direct DNA sequencing in B-cell lymphoma
M. Kneba et al, Göttingen, Germany
Expression of growth-related genes and drug-resistance genes in HTLV-1-positive and HTLV-1-negative post-thymic T-cell malignancies
I. J. Su, Taipei, Taiwan
Prognostic significance of proliferative activity in non-Hodgkin's lymphoma
J. Armitage et al, Omaha, USA
Clinical relevance of myelomonocytic antigen CD13 (aminopeptidase N) expression in B-cell chronic lymphocytic leukemia
A. Pinto et al, Aviano, Italy
Key note lecture/The role of growth factors in haemopoiesis: Biological and clinical implications
T. M. Dexter, Manchester, United Kingdom

Session 7 — General session on NHL
Chairman: J. E. Ultmann

Management of follicular lymphoma
T. A. Lister, London, United Kingdom
The present status of therapy for patients with aggressive non Hodgkin's lymphoma
J. O. Armitage, Omaha, USA

Session 8 — Proffered papers on NHL
Chairmen: S. Horning and R. Somers

Morphologic prognostic factors in follicular lymphomas. A retrospective study of 127 patients
B. Coiffier et al, Pierre Benite, France
Stage I–II low-grade lymphomas: A prospective trial of combination chemotherapy and radiotherapy
P. McLaughlin et al, Houston, USA
Interferon-α_{2B}. As initial therapy in combination with chlorambucil and as maintenance therapy in follicular lymphoma
G. Price, London, United Kingdom
Report about workshop on prognostic factors in aggressive NHL
G. P. Canellos, Boston, USA
Superiority of second versus first generation chemotherapy in a randomized trial for stage III–IV aggressive non Hodgkin's lymphoma: The 1980–1985 EORTC trial
P. Carde et al, Villejuif, France
Prospective multicenter trial for the response-adapted treatment of high-grade malignant non-Hodgkin lymphomas: Updated results of the COP-BLAM/IMVP-16 protocol with randomized adjuvant radiotherapy
M. Engelhard et al, Essen, Germany
Treatment of intermediate and high grade non-Hodgkin's lymphomas with third generation chemotherapy regimens: Analysis of southwest oncology group, phase II studies

R. I. Fisher et al, Maywood, USA
Chemotherapy for elderly patients with advanced stage large cell lymphoma – A little goes a long way
S. O'Reilly et al, Vancouver
Non Hodgkin's lymphomas associated with human immunodeficiency virus: Treatment by LNH 84 regimen
C. Gisselbrecht et al, Paris, France
Treatment of relapses in the SFOP LMB 0384 protocol. Role of bone marrow transplantation as salvage therapy
T. Philip et al, Lyon, France
Autologous bone marrow transplantation for adult lymphoblastic lymphoma in first complete remission. A pilot study of the non-Hodgkin's lymphoma co-operative study group
G. Santini et al, Genua, Italy
Autologous bone marrow transplantation for incurable advanced stage B-cell non-Hodgkin's lymphoma in first remission
A. Freedman et al, Boston, USA

Session 9 — Workshop on growth factors
Chairman: D. Crowther

Regulation of normal and malignant lymphocyte differentiation and function by transforming growth factor-β.
M. B. Sporn, Bethesda, USA
The biology of interleukin 6: The role in plasma cell diseases
B. G. M. Durie, London, United Kingdom
Haemopoietic growth factors: Clinical role
D. Crowther, Manchester, United Kingdom
Role of GM-CSF in treatment of malignant lymphomas
D. Hovgaard et al, Copenhagen, Denmark
Recombinant human GM-CSF and mitoxantrone/high-dose ARA-C in the treatment of refractory non-Hodgkin lymphoma
A. D. Ho et al, Heidelberg, Germany
A prospective randomized trial comparing recombinant granulocyte colony stimulating factor vs placebo for neutropenia induced by chemotherapy in patients with non-Hodgkin lymphoma
M. Ogawa et al, Tokyo, Japan

Session 10 — Clinical-pathological correlation
Chairmen: H. Rappaport and K. Lennert

Association of lymphocyte HOMIMG receptor expression and staining intensity with S-phase fraction, stage, and prognosis in non-Hodgkin's lymphoma
H. Joensuu et al, Turku, Finland
Secondary B-cell lymphomas developing in two patients with adult T-cell leukemia
K. Tobinai et al, Tokyo, Japan

Large cell anaplastic KI-1 positive lymphoma. A study of 5 cases
C. C. De Bruyn et al, Natal, South Africa
Mediastinal large cell lymphomas. A histopathological and immunohistochemical study
M. F. D'Agay et al, Paris, France
Primary gastric non-Hodgkin lymphomas. Does the concept of 'mucosa-associated lymphoma' have any clinical relevance?
A. Johnsson et al, Lund, Sweden
Primary gastric lymphoma: Clinical and prognostic features of 145 cases
S. B. Cogliatti et al, Kiel, Germany
The prognostic significance of histological pattern in primary gastric lymphoma: An analysis of 80 patients
K. A. MacLennan et al, London, United Kingdom
Malignant lymphoma of gastrointestinal tract: Analysis of clinicopathological features and treatment results
M. Ben-Shahar et al, Jerusalem, Israel
Non-Hodgkin lymphoma of Waldeyer's ring lymphoid tissue: Presentation and prognosis
J. Raemaekers et al, Nijmegen, The Netherlands
Primary cerebral malignant non-Hodgkin's lymphomas. Histological and immunomorphological findings on stereotactic brain biopsies
K. Schwechheimer et al, Freiburg, Germany
Chromosomal abnormalities in untreated patients with non-Hodgkin's lymphoma have an independent prognostic value for treatment outcome
H. C. Schouten et al, Maastricht, The Netherlands
Longterm follow-up of 1520 NHL patients classified according to the Kiel classification – Experiences of a single institution
R. Heinz, Vienna, Austria

Saturday, June 9, 1990

Session 11 — Future prospects
Chairmen: F. Cavalli and J. E. Ultmann

Treatment of aggressive lymphomas in patients older than 69 years. First interim report of a randomized study from the G.E.L.A.
B. Coiffier et al, Pierre Benite, France
Summary of workshop on new diagnostic tools
C. W. Berard, Memphis, USA
Ablative therapy with autologous bone marrow transplantation as consolidation therapy for follicular lymphoma
A. Z. S. Rohatiner, London, United Kingdom
Therapy with immunotoxins
L. M. Nadler, Boston, USA
Radio-immunotherapy of non-Hodgkin's lymphoma with single high dose I-131 radiolabeled antibodies
J. F. Eary, Seattle, USA
Autologous lymphocytes as vectors to target therapeutic radiation in patients with diffuse lymphoma lymphocytic
R. A. Cowan et al, Manchester, United Kingdom
Summary of the conference
J. E. Ultmann, Chicago, USA

Subject index

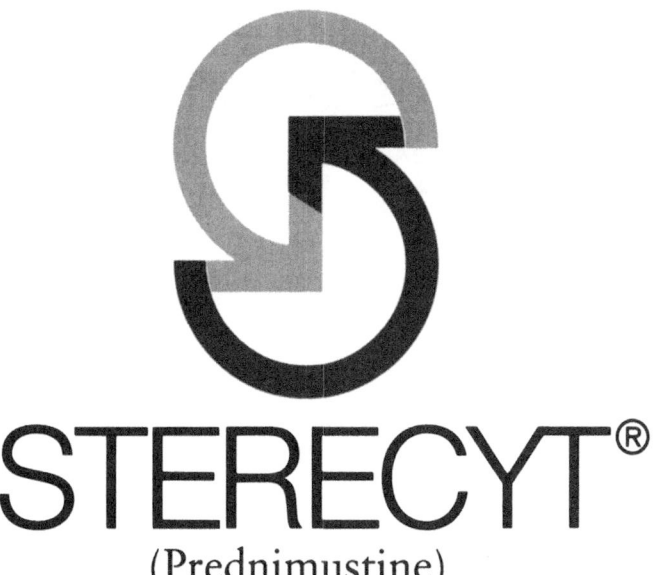

STERECYT®

(Prednimustine)

FOR YOUR LOW GRADE NON-HODGKIN´S PATIENT

Sterecyt versus CVP

1:ST LINE THERAPY
OVERALL RESPONSE

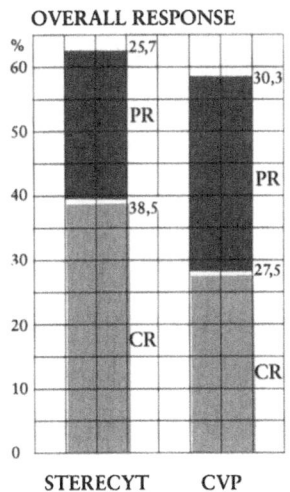

2:LINE THERAPY AFTER CROSSOVER
OVERALL RESPONSE

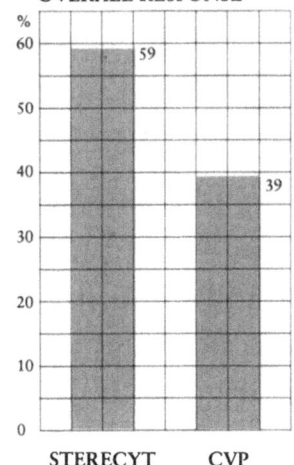

In each group 109 patients similar regarding age, sex, histological subtype, presence of B-symptoms and clinical stage were available for response.

After treatment failure, crossover to the other treatment arm was advocated.

Nilsson B. Clinical experiences with Sterecyt in the treatment of malignant lymphomas - a review. In: Sterecyt Proc. Sat. Symp. Hamburg, September 1987.

Tablets à 20 mg and 100 mg.

For more information:

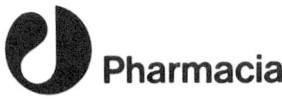 **Pharmacia**

Pharmacia LEO Therapeutics AB
Box 491, 251 09 Helsingborg, Sweden.

CANCER GROWTH AND PROGRESSION

(Series Editor: Hans E. Kaiser)

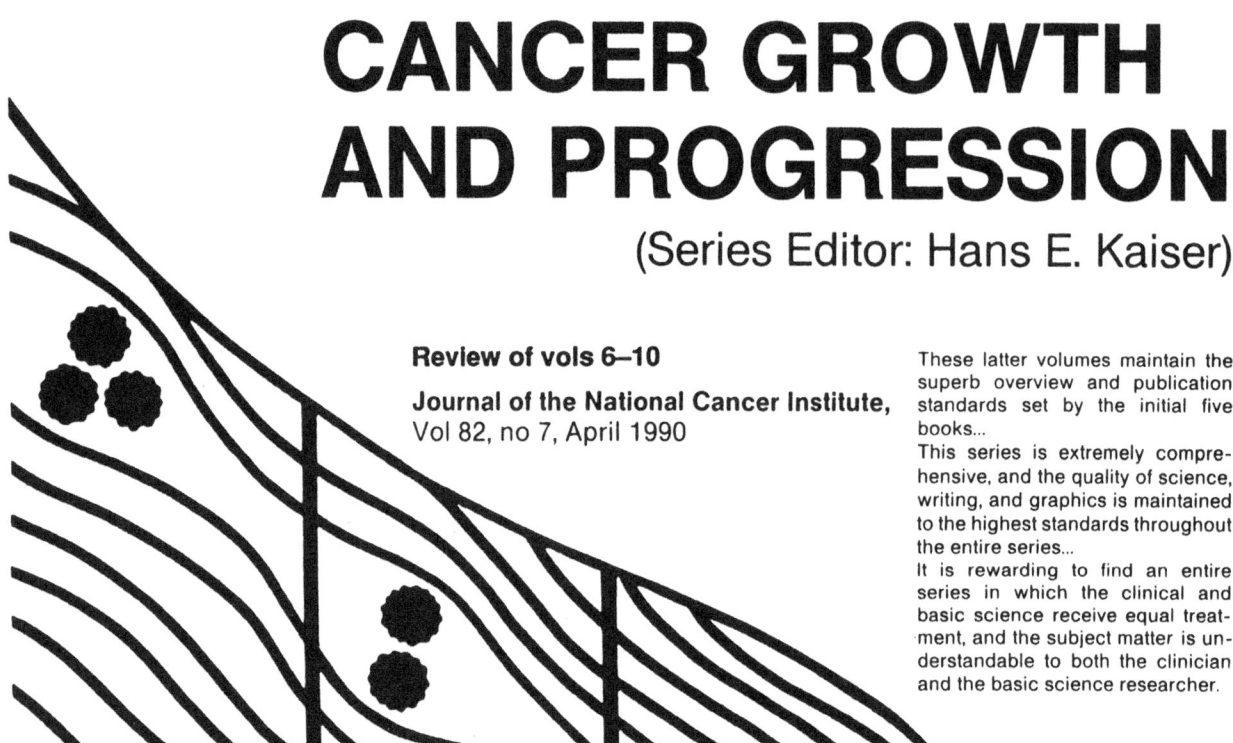

Review of vols 6–10

Journal of the National Cancer Institute,
Vol 82, no 7, April 1990

These latter volumes maintain the superb overview and publication standards set by the initial five books...
This series is extremely comprehensive, and the quality of science, writing, and graphics is maintained to the highest standards throughout the entire series...
It is rewarding to find an entire series in which the clinical and basic science receive equal treatment, and the subject matter is understandable to both the clinician and the basic science researcher.

Fundamental Aspects of Cancer

Edited by
Ronald H. Goldfarb, *Pittsburgh Cancer Institute, PA, USA*

CANCER GROWTH AND PROGRESSION 1

This volume introduces the reader to the themes that will be emphasized in subsequent volumes of this series; tumor biology in various species; tumor progression and metastatic spread, immune intervention, comparative tumor development, animal models of malignant disease and the clinical relevance of cancer growth and progression to the diagnosis and treatment of human malignancies.

1989, 214 pp. ISBN 0–89838–990–9
Hardbound Dfl. 199.00/£67.25

Mechanisms of Carcinogenesis

Edited by
Elisabeth K. Weisburger, *National Cancer Institute, National Institutes of Health, Bethesda, MD, USA*

CANCER GROWTH AND PROGRESSION 2

The topics of this volume encompass premalignant non-invasive lesions, species-specific aspects of carcinogenesis, oncogenes, and selected environmental carcinogens.

1989, 204 pp. ISBN 0–89838–991–7
Hardbound Dfl. 200.00/£67.50

Influence of Tumor Development on the Host

Edited by
Lance A. Liotta, *Dept. of Pathology, National Cancer Institute, National Institutes of Health, Bethesda, MD, USA*

CANCER GROWTH AND PROGRESSION 3

This volume reviews the current knowledge on the biochemistry and molecular biology of tumor invasion and metastatic spread.

1989, 236 pp. ISBN 0–89838–992–5
Hardbound Dfl. 199.00/£67.25

Influence of the Host on Tumor Development

Edited by
Ronald B. Herberman, *Pittsburgh Cancer Institute, PA, USA*

CANCER GROWTH AND PROGRESSION 4

This volume deals with the host properties that influence tumor development, including tumor dormancy, tumor regression, and tumor recurrence.

1989, 186 pp. ISBN 0–89838–993–3
Hardbound Dfl. 199.00/£67.25

Comparative Aspects of Tumor Development

Edited by **Hans E. Kaiser**, Dept. of Pathology, University of Maryland, Baltimore, USA

CANCER GROWTH AND PROGRESSION 5

This volume reviews comparative aspects of tumor development in cancer growth and progression. Particular emphasis is placed on both taxonomic aspects as well as on environmental oncology or species-specific aspects of environmental chain reactions.

1989, 258 pp.   ISBN 0-89838-994-1
Hardbound Dfl. 199.00/£67.25

Etiology of Cancer in Man

Edited by
Arthur S. Levine, National Institute of Child Health & Human Development, National Institutes of Health, Bethesda, MD, USA

CANCER GROWTH AND PROGRESSION 6

This volume reviews our current knowledge concerning cancer growth and progression as it relates to the etiology of human cancer.

1989, 236 pp.   ISBN 0-89838-995-X
Hardbound Dfl. 195.00/£59.95

Local Invasion and Spread of Cancer

Edited by
Kenneth W. Brunson, Dept. of Immunology and Infectious Diseases, Pfizer Central Research, Groton, CN, USA

CANCER GROWTH AND PROGRESSION 7

This volume reviews, in detail, the characteristics of local, direct tumor spreading in various organ systems: head and neck, the coelomic surface, and neuroendocrine tumors; spreading of neoplasm by implantation on epithelial surfaces; the spread of occult primary malignancies, and rare types of neoplastic progression.

1989, 240 pp.   ISBN 0-89838-996-9
Hardbound Dfl. 195.00/£59.95

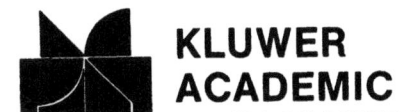

KLUWER
ACADEMIC
PUBLISHERS

Metastasis/Dissemination

Edited by
Elizier Gorelik, Pittsburgh Cancer Institute, PA, USA

CANCER GROWTH AND PROGRESSION 8

This volume emphasizes metastasis/dissemination as important processes in cancer growth and progression. Following a review of general patterns of metastatic spread in man, metastasis to or progression of neoplasms in several organ systems are highlighted including: the central nervous system, esophageal cancer, the lung, the large intestine, the liver, bone, epithelial neoplasms, endocrine cells, pigmented tissues, supporting tissues, connective tissues, muscle, neuronal sources and teratomas.

1989, 304 pp.   ISBN 0-89838-997-6
Hardbound Dfl. 195.00/£59.95

Cancer Management in Man
Detection, diagnosis, surgery, radiology, chronobiology, endocrine therapy

Edited by
Alfred L. Goldson, Dept. of Radiotherapy, Howard University, College of Medicine and Howard University Hospital, Washington DC, USA

CANCER GROWTH AND PROGRESSION 9

Cancer Management in Man consists of two parts (volumes 9 and 10 of the series *Cancer Growth and Progression*). This part critically reviews approaches at the levels of detection, diagnosis, surgery, radiology, chronobiology and endocrine treatment

1989, 292 pp.   ISBN 0-89838-998-4
Hardbound Dfl. 195.00/£59.95

Cancer Management in Man
Biological response modifiers, chemotherapy, antibiotics, hyperthermia supporting measures

Edited by
Paul V. Woolley, Division of Oncology, Vincent T. Lombardi Cancer Research Center, Georgetown University School of Medicine, Washington, DC, USA

CANCER GROWTH AND PROGRESSION 10

Volume 10 deals with the subjects of biological response modifiers, chemotherapy, antibiotics, hyperthermia, and supporting measures.

1989, 234 pp.   ISBN 0-89838-999-2
Hardbound Dfl. 195.00/£59.95

Set of 10 volumes   ISBN 0-89838-989-5
Dfl. 1950.00/£599.50

P.O. Box 322, 3300 AH Dordrecht, The Netherlands
P.O. Box 358, Accord Station, Hingham, MA 02018-0358, U.S.A.

In addition to surgery,
radiation and chemotherapy

a new dimension
in cancer treatment

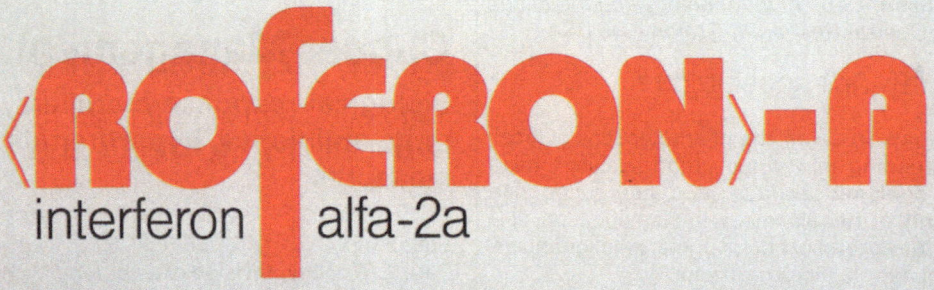

Full details on composition, indications,
contraindications, side effects, dosage and precautions
are available on request.

‹Roferon› is a Trade Mark

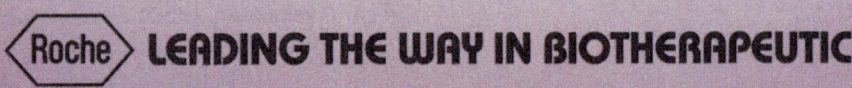

F. Hoffmann-La Roche Limited Company,
Basle, Switzerland

GPSR Compliance

The European Union's (EU) General Product Safety Regulation (GPSR)
is a set of rules that requires consumer products to be safe and our
obligations to ensure this.

If you have any concerns about our products, you can contact us on
ProductSafety@springernature.com

In case Publisher is established outside the EU, the EU authorized
representative is:

Springer Nature Customer Service Center GmbH
Europaplatz 3
69115 Heidelberg, Germany

Batch number: 09635764

Printed by Printforce, the Netherlands